Nurse Notes

Psychiatric-Mental Health

Core Content At-A-Glance

Nurse Notes

Psychiatric-Mental Health
Core Content At-A-Glance

Sally Lambert Lagerquist, RN, MS
Former Instructor of Undergraduate, Graduate, and
Continuing Education in Nursing, University of California,
San Francisco, School of Nursing; President, Review for
Nurses, Inc., and RN Tapes Company, San Francisco

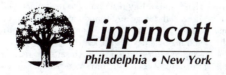

Lippincott
Philadelphia • New York

Acquisitions Editor: Susan Glover
Assistant Editor: Bridget Blatteau
Project Editor: Tom Gibbons
Production Manager: Helen Ewan
Production Coordinator: Nannette Winski
Design Coordinator: Doug Smock
Indexer: Nancy Newman

Library of Congress Cataloging in Publications Data
  Lagerquist, Sally L.
  Nurse Notes: psychiatric-mental health / Sally Lambert Lagerquist.
      p.   cm.
  Includes bibliographical references and index.
  ISBN 0-781-71127-4
  1. Psychiatric nursing—Outlines, syllabi, etc. 2. Psychiatric nursing—Examinations, questions, etc. I. Title.
  [DNLM: 1. Psychiatric Nursing—examination questions. 2. Psychiatric Nursing—outlines. 3. Mental Disorders—nursing—examination questions. 4. Mental Disorders—nursing—outlines. WY 18.2 L174L 1996]
  RC440.L34   1996
  610.73'68'076—dc20
  DNLM/DLC
  for Library of Congress   96-9116
                                                                                      CIP

Care has been taken to confirm the accuracy of the information presented and to describe generally accepted practices. However, the authors, editors, and publisher are not responsible for errors or omissions or for any consequences from application of the information in this book and make no warranty, express or implied, with respect to the contents of the publication.

The authors, editors and publisher have exerted every effort to ensure that drug selection and dosage set forth in this text are in accordance with current recommendations and practice at the time of publication. However, in view of ongoing research, changes in government regulations, and the constant flow of information relating to drug therapy and drug reactions, the reader is urged to check the package insert for each drug for any change in indications and dosage and for added warnings and precautions. This is particularly important when the recommended agent is a new or infrequently employed drug.

Some drugs and medical devices presented in this publication have Food and Drug Administration (FDA) clearance for limited use in restricted research settings. It is the responsibility of the health care provider to ascertain the FDA status of each drug or device planned for use in their clinical practice.

9 8 7 6 5 4 3 2 1

This book is dedicated to . . .

Tom, my husband, my soul mate.

In honor of 30 years of devoted friendship and unconditional love.

The time is here . . . we can now smell our roses and wisteria; do the hora, Cajun, and Svenska dancing; and hum a few bars from Kalinka. L'chaim!

Elana, our first born, our very talented daughter.

You are a significant part in the success of my books. Without your diligent, dependable, side-by-side help during the early and final stages of manuscript production, my six new nursing review books wouldn't have gotten off our dining room table and into print! You were my proofreading eyes. You nurtured my books—and their author—with skill, sensitivity, perspective, humor, and caring.

Thank you for sharing with us your own successes in academia and theater productions. We are full of pride, joy, and love for you.

Kalen, our special son. In honor of your significant first year as a university graduate.

You have the enthusiasm, the sense of humor, and the aptitude to give of yourself, to succeed in making a difference in social conditions and in the life of others.

May you follow the spirit of *carpe diem* (in taking actions that bring results) as well as a *laissez les bon temps rouler* spirit.

With gratitude for being a special caring son when we needed it the most this year (and many other times before!).

Lourdes Perez, our friend and colleague.

Ever supportive, ever committed to us, and to the success of our nursing review company.

With untold gratitude for being very flexible and filling so many vital roles in skillfully managing our business on a daily basis, especially when I was flailing away at meeting manuscript deadlines.

Sally

This book is a special tribute to victims of all crimes and to the advocates who relentlessly *speak out* for victims' rights and everyone's right not to become a crime victim.

Tom and I want to especially recognize the following individuals for their sensitivity to victims' despair, for hearing us, and giving *voice* to the serious concerns of all victims of crime:

Jim Nielsen (Former California State Senator), Chairman of the California Board of Prison Terms; *John Monday*, Chief Deputy Commissioner of the California Board of Prison Terms; *Curt Soderland*, Deputy Executive Officer of California State Board of Control; *Sandi Menefee*, Coordinator of Victims of Crime Services in the California Department of Corrections, Special Projects Branch of the Victims Services Program; *Solange Brooks*, Assistant Agency Secretary, Program Oversight of California Youth and Adult Correctional Agency; and California State Senators *John Burton* and *Quentin Kopp*. You all made a significant difference! *You do not follow where the path may lead. You go instead where there is no path and leave a trail.*

A special tribute to Harriet and Mike Salarno who have become my symbols of perseverance and dedication. They are two advocates who insist on justice for *victims* of all crimes. I honor them for the courage of their convictions to make changes. They have been our inspiration for the work that Tom and I must continue to do to help victims of all crimes.

Sally Lagerquist

This book was written with the intention of helping my colleagues and nursing students to be successful. I offer the following reflections; do go beyond traditional health care. You will be rewarded beyond measure.

What is Success?
To laugh often and to love much;
To win the respect of intelligent people and affection of children;
To earn the appreciation of honest critics and endure the betrayal of false friends;
To appreciate beauty;
To find the best in others;
To give of one's self;
To leave the world a bit better, whether by a healthy child, a garden patch or a
    redeemed social condition;
To have played and laughed with enthusiasm and sung with exaltation;
To know even one life has breathed easier because you have lived.
This is to have succeeded.

modified from *Ralph Waldo Emerson*

Foreword

Nursing practice has become a fast-moving, rapidly-changing, essential service for individuals, families, and communities. Nurses are moving into the community as home-care, ambulatory-care, and advance-practice nurses. As managed care becomes more of a norm than a fad, the practice will continue to change.

Being a nursing student today means there is a great deal to know and to apply to patient care in these many environments. As a clinician there is much to keep up with. If one were to use the textbooks prepared for each aspect of nursing care, it would mean searching through several very large books. However, there is an easier way to do both.

Sally Lagerquist has prepared four small nursing review books (*Nurse Notes: Maternal-Newborn; Nurse Notes: Medical-Surgical; Nurse Notes: Pediatric;* and *Nurse Notes: Psychiatric-Mental Health*). These books are quick references for almost any nursing situation. Each book focuses on a different aspect of nursing; each one also contains many features that make success possible for both students and clinicians alike. Test-taking tips, summaries of important points, activities for memory aids, and outlines that help with note taking are just a few of the features in these books. A very popular supplement to each of the four books in this series is the accompanying disk that allows for review with questions and answers. Because these books have a variety of uses, they should be in the library of every nurse and every nursing student.

These reference books can help you in a variety of ways. You can get prepared for and succeed on nursing exams (as well as on the NCLEX or a certifying exam) and keep current on nursing practice whether you are a student or a practicing nurse. As a resource for keeping current, preparing for an exam, note taking during a class, or learning new and useful ways to remember, this book surpasses any other book.

Sally Lagerquist has been preparing study guides for nursing students for over 22 years and thus has the experience necessary for the preparation of a quality product. She knows what students need and she knows how to prepare materials that are consistent with current theory and practice. She has kept abreast of the changes in the NCLEX and the certifying exams offered by ANA and other specialty associations; thus these books are excellent resources for the preparation for either kind of exam.

There are no other books like these review books. There is no product that covers so much in such a small space and there is no text that offers so many tips for success. I frankly cannot imagine being a student or a nurse without these quick referral texts. And best of all, you can easily carry one with you so you will never be without a resource. Home health care nurses, community health nurses, hospital nurses, and those nurses in skilled nursing facilities and nursing homes will find these books very useful. Nurses everywhere will find that this very new book is a "must have" item.

Fay L. Bower, PhD, FAAN
President, Clarkson College
Past President, Sigma Theta Tau International

Preface

Is your required course textbook overwhelming? Do you have time to use it as a study guide?

This book reduces the overwhelming task of having to ferret your way through voluminous pages in a reference book by providing a useful study tool with "just enough" information about each subject and topic area. We have limited the information presented here to **"above all—this is what you need to know."** The best thing about this book is that it quickly gives you the big picture, with concise descriptions.

How to Use This Book

Depending on *your* purpose, there is more than one way to use this book. If your primary concern is passing nursing exams, this book will give you a quick review of the content with which you should be familiar before taking an exam.

To make the task of taking the exam easier, quicker, and more effective—while efficiently using your time—we have included *many charts* and *figures, study and memory aids* (e.g., acronyms and mnemonic tools), *summaries of key points*, and *test-taking tips* that go with the practice questions and answers at the end of each chapter. Even the *glossary* in each chapter serves as a review tool.

If you want a handy guide to use when you are in a *clinical* setting, this book gives you a comprehensive review of each topic in *outline* format (with succinct and thorough coverage), utilizing many *charts* to cover a great deal of information in the shortest possible time.

This book is meant for use in *both* academic and clinical settings. For example:

1. Undergraduate and graduate nursing students can use this book as a succinct *textbook in theory classes*. It contains many short chapters, which make it easy to correlate with your classroom lectures in nursing school.
2. Nursing students, as well as practicing nurses, can use this book as a *quick reference* in the *clinical setting*. By using the index, or the outlines at the beginning of each chapter, the nursing student or practicing nurse can quickly locate information about a specific topic.
3. Practicing nurses can use this book to *update* their knowledge, as well as to prepare for *certification* exams.

This book can *stand alone* in its coverage of the major topics related to mental health nursing (psychiatric nursing). It can also be used *in conjunction* with the standard, larger textbooks. Most existing required texts seem to be more than 1000 pages long, with much information unrelated to what you need to know "here and now." This book's goal is to make learning relevant as well as easier and enjoyable.

How This Book is Organized

For each topic listed, we include a brief description or definition, main concepts and principles, assessment, nursing diagnosis, nursing care plan/implementation (long and short-term goals), and evaluation/outcome criteria. Health teaching is also included. To serve as a short *course review*, this book includes "thumbnail" discussions of the most significant information, with lots of practice questions (500 in the book and on the practice disk), which is something completely different from the large reference texts.

The best features of this book:

1. Lots of concise, short chapters followed immediately by practice questions, *right after* you have studied a topic (e.g., schizophrenia, depression, substance abuse, etc.).
2. An excellent framework for making your own condensed notes, to facilitate quick review.
3. Complete outline of each topic at the beginning of each chapter.
4. A portable size that makes it a take-along book that you can skim through between classes.
5. Use of unique symbols and boldface and italic type will help you to quickly identify each of the five steps of the nursing process, hands-on nursing care, medications, lab and diagnostic tests.

The unique visual features offered in this book will assist you to more readily understand the material covered in this subject area. Each chapter is short and easy to digest. The content of each chapter focuses on essential information. Each chapter includes a *glossary* that in itself is useful as a review of key points and provides information in *addition* to what is included in the chapter.

A set of self-test questions is also included at the end of each chapter, along with step-by-step (option-by-option) explanations of how to eliminate the three incorrect answer options and select the best answer. As an added learning feature—*in addition* to what is in the text of each chapter and in the glossaries—supplementary content is covered by *questions* with detailed rationale. A free disk with additional questions is included for further practice and self-assessment. By sharpening your problem-solving skills as you go along, you can avoid last-minute, frantic memorization and reviewing.

We welcome any test-taking tips and memory aids that *you* many want to see included in later editions of this book, if you have used them in your own learning-reviewing process and found them helpful. Your contributions will be acknowledged in future editions.

Here's to making your learning easier and more enjoyable!

Sally Lambert Lagerquist, RN, MS

Acknowledgments

This book happened, in large part, because I was fortunate to be working with two of the best and talented professionals: Bonnie Bergstrom and Katie Mascaro.

Bonnie, you have been an incredibly dependable and supportive friend and colleague, and a part-time saint since the conception of this book! You were invaluable in compiling and pulling together what I had to say and in shepherding this book through the complexities of the manuscript production process. You gave generously of your time and contributed insightful comments all along the way. The successful finished product reflects your expertise and nurturing.

Katie, my production editor . . . You are an incredible woman, with unfolding talents and skills and interests—from manuscript production to marketing; from detailed editing to exuberant energy in selling what we created together. You stand out in all that you do! Thank you for your patience, for deciphering my handwriting, for making many allowances and adjustments, for your commitment to our six projects. I feel that these are truly *our* books!

A separate and special paragraph is devoted to you, Tom Gibbons—my Lippincott-Raven editor—for your uncommon editorial expertise and sensitivity, incredible flexibility, and personal commitment to helping this book come into being. I was not only the lucky beneficiary of your attention to detail, but also your *kindness* and listening ear: we talked; you heard; you cared; we did it all—again!

About the Author

Sally Lambert Lagerquist, RN, MS

Sally is the author and editor of *Practice Questions and Answers for NCLEX-RN*, published by Review for Nurses Tapes Co.; *How to Pass Nursing Exams*, published by Review Press; *Little, Brown's NCLEX-RN Examination Review* and *Little, Brown's Nursing Q&A: Critical-Thinking Exercises*. She has coordinated RN licensure exam review courses on campuses nationwide since 1976. She is presently a lecturer on test-taking techniques at workshops held nationwide for graduating senior nursing students. She has produced and developed The *NCLEX-RN Board Game* and audio and video tapes on *Nursing Review* and *Successful Test-Taking Techniques for Nurses*. She originated, developed, and has presented national satellite telecourses for NCLEX-RN review since June 1989. She is also a marriage, family, and child counselor and a member of Sigma Theta Tau. She has been a faculty member at the University of California at San Francisco School of Nursing for over ten years, where she also received her BS and MS degrees.

Contributing Author

Marcia Ann Miller, RN, BSN, MA, MSN

Associate Professor, Nursing Section, Purdue University North Central, Westville, IN

During her career, Professor Miller has served as a nursing administrator, clinical nurse specialist, and nursing educator. She has taught at Purdue University since 1980. She has also published articles about hospital architectural design, selecting and hiring faculty, and chemically impaired students, and has coauthored computerized review questions for psychosocial nursing. Professor Miller has been lecturing nationally for Review for Nurses, Inc. since 1982.

Contents

List of Illustrations

List of Tables

Models of Psychosocial Nursing Care

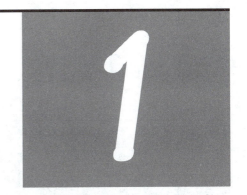

Chapter Outline

Medical/Biologic Model (Kraepelin)

I. **Assumptions:** disturbances seen as diagnosable diseases with classifiable symptoms (or syndromes) that have a characteristic course, prognosis, and treatment.

II. **Focus on diagnostic categories,** such as:
   A. Anxiety, dissociative disorders, phobias.
   B. Psychosis (schizophrenia, affective).
   C. Psychophysiologic conditions.
   D. Personality disorders.

III. **Caused by organic conditions,** such as:
   A. Arrested mental development (Down syndrome).
   B. Infectious (meningitis, tertiary syphilis).
   C. Metabolic (hepatic and renal failure, chronic obstructive pulmonary disease [COPD]).
   D. Drug-induced (alcoholism, lysergic acid diethylamide [LSD]).
   E. Neoplasm (cancer of the brain).
   F. Traumatic (blow on the head).
   G. Endocrine (thyroid disease).

Psychodynamic Model (Freud)

I. **Assumptions and key ideas**
   A. No human behavior is accidental; each psychic event is determined by preceding ones.
   B. Unconscious mental processes occur with great frequency and significance.
   C. Psychoanalysis is used to uncover childhood trauma, which may involve conflict and repressed feelings.
   D. Psychoanalytic methods are used: therapeutic alliance, transference, regression, dream association, catharsis.

II. **Freud**—shifted from classification of behavior to understanding and explaining in psychological terms and changing behavior under structured conditions.
   A. Structure of the mind: id, ego, superego; unconscious, preconscious, conscious.
   B. Stages of psychosexual development (Tables 1.1 and 1.4).
   C. Coping mechanisms. See Patterns of Adjustment (Coping Mechanisms) and Glossary in this chapter.

Stage	Age	Behaviors
Oral	Birth–1 yr	Dependency and oral gratification
Anal	1–3 yr	Creativity, stinginess, cruelty, cleanliness, self-control, punctuality
Phallic or Oedipal	3–6 yr	Sexual, aggressive feelings; guilt
Latency	6–12 yr	Reactivation of pregenital impulses; intellectual and social growth
Genital	12–18 yr	Displacement of pregenital impulses; learns responsibility for self; establishes identity

TABLE 1.1   FREUD'S STAGES OF PSYCHOSEXUAL DEVELOPMENT

Anxiety Model and Coping Mechanisms

Anxiety is a subjective warning of danger in which the specific nature of the danger is usually not known. It occurs when a person faces a new, unknown, or untried situation. Anxiety is also felt when a person perceives threat in terms of past experiences. It is a general concept underlying most disease states. In its milder form, anxiety can contribute to learning and is necessary for problem solving. In its severe form, anxiety can impede a client's treatment and recovery. The general feelings elicited on all levels of anxiety are nervousness, tension, and apprehension.

It is essential that nurses recognize their own sources of anxiety and their behavior in response to anxiety as well as help clients recognize the manifestations of anxiety in themselves.

Anxiety

I. Assessment
  A. Physiologic manifestations:
   1. Increased heart rate and palpitations.
   2. Increased rate and depth of respiration.
   3. Increased urinary frequency and diarrhea.
   4. Dry mouth.
   5. Decreased appetite.
   6. Cold sweat and pale appearance.
   7. Increased menstrual flow.
   8. Increased or decreased body temperature.
   9. Increased or decreased blood pressure.
   10. Dilated pupils.
  B. Behavioral manifestations—stages of anxiety:
   1. *Mild anxiety:*
    a. Increased perception (visual and auditory).
    b. Increased awareness of meanings and relationships.
    c. Increased alertness (notice more).
    d. Ability to utilize problem-solving process.
   2. *Moderate anxiety:*
    a. Selective inattention (e.g., may not hear someone talking).
    b. Decreased perceptual field.
    c. Concentration on relevant data; "tunnel vision."
    d. Muscular tension, perspiration, GI discomfort.
   3. *Severe anxiety:*
    a. Focus on many fragmented details.
    b. Physical and emotional discomfort (headache, nausea, dizziness, dread, horror, trembling).
    c. Not aware of total environment.
    d. Automatic behavior aimed at getting immediate relief instead of problem solving.
    e. Poor recall.
    f. Inability to see connections between details.
    g. Drastically reduced awareness.
   4. *Panic state of anxiety:*
    a. Increased speed of scatter; does not notice what goes on.
    b. Increased distortion and exaggeration of details.
    c. Feeling of terror.
    d. Dissociation (hallucinations, loss of reality, and little memory).
    e. Inability to cope with any problems; no self-control.
  C. Reactions in response to anxiety:
   1. *Fight:*
    a. Aggression.
    b. Hostility, derogation, belittling.
    c. Anger.
   2. *Flight:*
    a. Withdrawal.
    b. Depression.
   3. *Somatization* (psychosomatic disorder).
   4. *Impaired cognition:* blocking, forgetfulness, poor concentration, errors in judgment.
   5. *Learning* about or searching for causes of anxiety, and identifying behavior.

II. Analysis/nursing diagnosis: *Anxiety* related to:
  A. Physical causes: Threats to biologic well-being (e.g., sleep disturbances, interference with sexual functioning, food, drink, pain, fever).
  B. Psychological causes: *Disturbance in self-esteem* related to:
   1. Unmet wishes or expectations.
   2. Unmet needs for prestige and status.
   3. *Impaired adjustment:* inability to cope with environment.

4. *Altered role performance:* not utilizing own full potential.
5. *Altered meaningfulness:* alienation.
6. *Conflict with social order:* value conflicts.
7. Anticipated disapproval from a significant other.
8. *Altered feeling states:* guilt.

III. Nursing care plan/implementation
  A. Moderate to severe anxiety
  1. Provide *motor outlet* for tension energy, such as working at a simple, concrete task, walking, crying, or talking.
  2. Help clients *recognize* their anxieties by talking about how they are behaving and by exploring their underlying feelings.
  3. Help clients *gain insight* into their anxieties by helping them to understand how their behavior has been an expression of anxiety and to recognize the threat that lies behind this anxiety.
  4. Help clients *cope* with the threat behind their anxieties by reevaluating the threats and learning new ways to deal with them.
  5. *Health teaching:*
    a. Explain and offer hope that emotional pain will decrease with time.
    b. Explain that some tension is normal.
    c. Explain how to channel emotional energy into activity.
    d. Explain need to recognize highly stressful situations and to recognize tension within oneself.
  B. Panic state
  1. Give simple, clear, *concise* directions.
  2. *Avoid* decision making by client. Do not try to reason with client, for he or she is irrational and cannot cooperate.
  3. *Stay* with client.
    a. Do not isolate.
    b. *Avoid* touching.
  4. Allow client to seek *motor* outlets (walking, pacing).
  5. *Health teaching:* advise activity that requires no thought.

IV. Evaluation/outcome criteria:
  A. Uses more positive thinking and problem-solving activities and is less preoccupied with worrying.
  B. Uses values-clarification to resolve conflicts and establish realistic goals.
  C. Demonstrates regained perspective, self-esteem, and morale; expresses feeling more in control, more hopeful.
  D. Fewer or absent physical symptoms of anxiety.

Patterns of Adjustment (Coping Mechanisms)

Coping mechanisms (ego defense mechanisms or mental mechanisms) consist of all the *coping* means used by individuals to seek relief from emotional conflict and to ward off excessive anxiety.

I. Definitions of various coping mechanisms°
  blocking A disturbance in the rate of speech when a person's thoughts and speech are proceeding at an average rate but are suddenly and completely interrupted, perhaps even in the middle of a sentence. The gap may last from several seconds up to a minute. Blocking is often a part of the thought disorder found in schizophrenic disorders.
  compensation Making up for real or imagined handicap, limitation, or lack of gratification in one area of personality by overemphasis in another area to counter the effects of failure, frustration, and limitation; e.g., the blind compensate by increased sensitivity in hearing; the unpopular student compensates by becoming an outstanding scholar; a small man compensates for short stature by demanding a great deal of attention and respect; a nurse who does not have manual dexterity chooses to go into psychiatric nursing.
  confabulating Filling in gaps of memory by inventing what appear to be suitable memories as replacements. This symptom may occur in various organic psychoses but is most often seen in Korsakoff's syndrome (deterioration due to alcohol) and in dementia and amnestic disorders.
  conversion Psychological difficulties are translated into physical symptoms *without conscious* will or knowledge; e.g., pain and immobility on moving your writing arm the day of an exam.
  denial An intolerable thought, wish, need, or reality factor is disowned automatically; e.g., a student, when told of a failing grade, acts as if he never heard of such a possibility.
  displacement Transferring the emotional component from one idea, object, or situation to another, more acceptable one. Displacement occurs because these are painful or dangerous feelings that cannot be expressed toward the original object; e.g., kicking the dog after a bad day at school or work; anger with clinical instructor gets transferred to classmate who was late to meet you for lunch.
  dissociation Splitting off or separation of differing elements of the mind from each other. There can be separation of ideas, concepts, emotions, or experiences from the rest of the mind. Dissociated material is deeply repressed and becomes encapsulated and inaccessible to the rest of the mind. This usually occurs as a result of some painful experience, e.g., split of affect from idea in anxiety disorders and schizophrenia.
  fixation A state in which personality development is arrested in one or more aspects at a level short of maturity; e.g., "She is anally fixated" (controlling, stingy, holding on to things and memories).
  idealization Overestimation of some admired aspect or attribute of another person; e.g., "He was a perfect human being."
  ideas of reference Fixed, false ideas and interpretations of external events as though they had direct ref-

°From Kalkman M. *Psychiatric Nursing* (3rd ed). New York: McGraw-Hill, 1967. Pp 83–93. By permission of Mosby-Year Book, Inc.

erence to self; e.g., client thinks that TV news announcer is reporting a story about client.

identification   The wish to be like another person; situation in which qualities of another are unconsciously transferred to oneself; e.g., a boy identifies with his father and learns to become a man; a woman fears she will die in childbirth because her mother did; a student adopts attitudes and behavior of her favorite teacher.

introjection   Incorporation into the personality, without assimilation, of emotionally charged impulses or objects; a quality or an attribute of another person is taken into and made part of self; e.g., a girl in love introjects the personality of her lover into herself—his ideas become hers, his tastes and wishes are hers; this is also seen in severe depression following death of someone close; patient may assume many of deceased's characteristics; similarly, working in a psychiatric unit with a suicidal person brings out depression in a nurse.

isolation   Temporary or long-term splitting off of certain feelings or ideas from others; separating emotional and intellectual content; e.g., talking emotionlessly about a traumatic accident.

projection   Attributes and transfers own feelings, attitudes, impulses, wishes, or thoughts to another person or object in the environment, especially when ideas or impulses are too painful to be acknowledged as belonging to oneself; e.g., in hallucinations and delusions by alcoholics; or, "I flunked the course because the teacher doesn't know how to teach"; "I hate him" reversed into "He hates me"; or a student impatiently accusing an instructor of being intolerant.

rationalization   Justification of behavior by formulating a logical, socially approved reason for past, present, or proposed behavior. Commonly used, conscious or unconscious, with false or real reason; e.g., upon losing a class election, a student states she really did not want all the extra work and is glad she lost.

reaction formation   Going to the opposite extreme from what one wishes to do or is afraid one might do; e.g., being overly concerned with cleanliness when one wishes to be messy, being an overly protective mother through fear of own hostility to child, or showing great concern for a person whom you dislike, going out of your way to do special favors.

regression   When individuals fail to solve a problem with the usual methods at their command they may resort to modes of behavior that they have outgrown but that proved successful at an earlier stage of development; retracing developmental steps; going back to earlier interests or modes of gratification; e.g., a senior nursing student about to graduate becomes dependent on a clinical instructor for directions.

repression   Involuntary exclusion of painful and unacceptable thoughts and impulses from awareness. *Forgetting* these things solves the situation by not solving it; e.g., by not remembering what was on the difficult exam after it was over.

sublimation   Channeling a destructive or instinctual impulse that cannot be realized into a *socially acceptable,* practical, and less dangerous outlet, with some relation to the original impulse for emotional satisfaction to be obtained; e.g., sublimation of sexual energy into other creative activities (art, music, literature) or hostility and aggression into sports or business competition; or an infertile person putting all energies into pediatric nursing.

substitution   When individuals cannot have what they wish and accept something else in its place for symbolic satisfaction; e.g., pin-up pictures in absence of sexual object, or a person who failed an RN exam signs up for an LVN (LPN) exam.

suppression   A deliberate process of blocking from the conscious mind thoughts, feelings, acts, or impulses that are undesirable; e.g., "I don't want to talk about it," "Don't mention his name to me," or "I'll think about it some other time"; or willfully refusing to think about or discuss disappointments with exam results.

symbolism   Sign language that stands for related ideas and feelings, conscious and unconscious. Used extensively by children, primitive peoples, and psychotic patients. There is meaning attached to this sign language that makes it important to the individual; e.g., a student wears dark, somber clothing to the exam site.

undoing   A coping mechanism against anxiety, usually unconscious, designed to negate or neutralize a previous act; e.g., Lady Macbeth's attempt to wash her hands (of guilt) after the murder. A repetitious, symbolic acting out, in reverse of an unacceptable act already completed. Responsible for compulsions and magical thinking.

II. **Characteristics** of coping mechanisms
   A. Coping mechanisms are utilized to some degree by everyone occasionally; they are normal processes by which the ego reestablishes equilibrium—unless they are used to an extreme degree, in which case they interfere with maintenance of self-integrity.
   B. Much overlapping:
      1. Same behavior can be explained by more than one mechanism.
      2. May be used in combination—e.g., isolation and repression, denial and projection.
   C. Common defense mechanisms compatible with mental well-being:
      1. Compensation.
      2. Compromise.
      3. Identification.
      4. Rationalization.
      5. Sublimation.
      6. Substitution.
   D. Typical coping mechanisms in:
      1. *Paranoid disorders*—denial, projection.
      2. *Dissociative disorders*—denial, repression, dissociation.
      3. *Obsessive-compulsive behaviors*—displacement, reaction formation, isolation, denial, repression, undoing.

4. *Phobic disorders*—displacement, rationalization, repression.
5. *Conversion disorders*—symbolization, dissociation, repression, isolation, denial.
6. *Major depression*—displacement.
7. *Bipolar disorder, manic episode*—reaction formation, denial, projection, introjection.
8. *Schizophrenic disorders*—symbolization, repression, dissociation, denial, fantasy, regression, projection.
9. *Organic mental disorders*—regression.

III. **Concepts and principles related to coping mechanisms**
   A. *Unconscious* process—coping mechanisms are used as a substitute for more effective problem-solving behavior.
   B. *Main functions*—increase *self-esteem; decrease,* inhibit, minimize, alleviate, avoid, or eliminate *anxiety;* maintain feelings of personal worth and adequacy and soften failures; *protect the ego; increase security.*
   C. *Drawbacks*—involve high degree of self-deception and reality distortion; may be maladaptive because they superficially eliminate or disguise conflicts, leaving conflicts unresolved but still influencing behavior.

IV. **Nursing care plan/implementation**
   A. Accept coping mechanisms as normal, but not when overused.
   B. Look beyond the behavior to the need that is expressed by the use of the coping mechanism.
   C. Discuss alternative coping mechanisms that may be more compatible with mental health.
   D. Assist the person to translate defensive thinking into nondefensive, direct thinking; a problem-solving approach to conflicts minimizes the need to use coping mechanisms.

Psychosocial Development Model (Erikson, Maslow, Piaget, Duvall)

I. **Erik Erikson**—*Eight Stages of Man* (1963)
   A. Psychosocial development—interplay of biology with social factors, encompassing total life span, from birth to death, in progressive developmental tasks.
   B. *Stages of life cycle*—life consists of a series of developmental phases (Table 1.2). (See also Table 1.4 for comparison summary.)
      1. Universal sequence of biologic, social, psychological events.
      2. Each person experiences a series of normative conflicts and crises and thus needs to accomplish specific psychosocial tasks.
      3. Two opposing energies (positive and negative forces) coexist and need to be synthesized.

4. How each age-specific task is accomplished influences the developmental progress of the next phase and the ability to deal with life.

II. **Abraham Maslow**—*Hierarchy of Needs* (1962)
   A. Beliefs regarding emotional health based on a comprehensive, multidisciplinary approach to human problems, involving all aspects of functioning.
      1. *Premise:* mental illness cannot be understood without prior knowledge of mental health.
      2. *Focus:* positive aspects of human behavior (e.g., contentment, joy, happiness).
   B. *Hierarchy of needs:* physiologic, safety, love and belonging, self-esteem and recognition, self-actualization, aesthetic. As each stage is mastered, the next stage becomes dominant (Figure 1.1).
   C. *Characteristics of optimal mental health*—keep in mind that wellness is on a continuum with cultural variations.
      1. *Self-esteem:* entails self-confidence and self-acceptance.
      2. *Self-knowledge:* involves accurate self-perception of strengths and limitations.
      3. *Satisfying interpersonal relationships:* able to meet reciprocal emotional needs through collaboration rather than exploitation or power struggles or jealousy; able to make full commitments in close relationships.
      4. *Environmental mastery:* can adapt, change, and solve problems effectively; can make decisions, choose from alternatives, and predict consequences. Actions are conscious, not impulsive.
      5. *Stress management:* can delay seeking gratification and relief; does not blame or dwell on past; assumes self-responsibility; either modifies own expectations, seeks substitutes, or withdraws from stressful situation when cannot reduce stress.

III. **Jean Piaget**—*Cognitive and Intellectual Development* (1963)
   A. **Assumptions**—child development is steered by interaction of environmental and genetic influences; therefore focus is on environmental and social forces (Table 1.3). (See also Table 1.4 for comparison with other theories.)
   B. **Key concepts**
      1. *Assimilation*—process of acquiring new knowledge, skills, and insights by using what they already know and have.
      2. *Accommodation*—adjusts to change by solving previously unsolvable problems because of newly assimilated knowledge.
      3. *Adaptation*—coping process to handle environmental demands.
   C. **Age-specific development levels:** sensorimotor, preconceptual, intuitive, concrete, formal operational thought.

IV. **E. M. Duvall**—*Family Development* (1971)—developmental tasks are family-oriented, presented in eight stages throughout the life cycle:
   A. *Married couple*

TABLE 1.2   ERIKSON'S STAGES OF THE LIFE CYCLE

Age and Stage of Development	Conflict Areas Needing Resolution	Evaluation: Result of Resolution/Nonresolution
Infancy (birth–18 mo)	Trust *vs* Mistrust	Shows affection, gratification, recognition; trusts self and others; begins to tolerate frustrations; develops *hope* Withdrawn, alienated
Early childhood (18 mo–3 yr)	Autonomy *vs* Shame and doubt	Cooperative, self-controlled, self-expressive, can delay gratification; develops *will* Exaggerated self-restraint; defiance; compulsive; overly compliant
Late childhood (3–5 yr)	Initiative *vs* Guilt	Realistic goals; can evaluate self; explorative; imitates adult, shows imagination; tests reality; anticipates roles; develops *purpose*, self-motivation Self-imposed restrictions relative to jealousy, guilt, and denial
School-age (5–12 yr)	Industry *vs* Inferiority	Sense of duty; acquires social and school *competencies;* persevering in real tasks School and social drop-out; social loner; incompetent
Adolescence (12–18 yr)	Identity *vs* Role diffusion	Has ideologic commitments, self-actualizing; sense of self; experiments with roles; experiences sexual polarizations; develops *fidelity* Ambivalent, confused, indecisive; may act out (antisocial acts)
Young adulthood (18–25 yr)	Intimacy, solidarity *vs* Isolation	Makes commitments to love and work relationships; able to sustain mutual *love* relationships Superficial, impersonal, biased
Adulthood (25–60 yr)	Generativity *vs* Self-absorption, stagnation	Productive, creative, procreative, concerned for others; develops *care* Self-indulgent
Late adulthood (60 yr–death)	Ego integrity *vs* Despair	Appreciates past, present, and future; self-acceptance of own contribution to others, of own self-worth, and of changes in life-style and life cycle; can face "not being"; develops *wisdom* Preoccupied with loss of hope, of purpose; contemptuous, fears death

1. Establishing relationship.
2. Defining mutual goals.
3. Developing intimacy: issues of dependence-independence-interdependence.
4. Establishing mutually satisfying relationship.
5. Negotiating boundaries of couple with families.
6. Discussing issue of childbearing.

B. *Childbearing years*
1. Working out authority, responsibility, and caretaker roles.
2. Having children and forming new unit.
3. Facilitating child's trust.
4. Need for personal time and space while sharing with each other and child.

C. *Preschool-age years*
1. Experiencing changes in parent's energy.
2. Continuing development as couple, parents, family.
3. Establishing own family traditions without guilt related to breaks with tradition.

D. *School-age years*
1. Establishing new roles in work.
2. Children's school activities interfering with family activities.

E. *Teenage years*
1. Parents continue to develop roles in community other than with children.
2. Children experience freedom while accepting responsibility for actions.
3. Struggle with parents in emancipation process.
4. Family value system is challenged.
5. Couple relationships may be strong or weak depending on responses to needs.

F. *Families as launching centers*
1. Young adults launched with rites of passage.
2. Changes in couple's relationship due to empty nest and increased leisure time.
3. Changes in relationship with children away from home.

G. *Middle-aged parents:* Dealing with issues of aging of own parents.

H. *Aging family members*

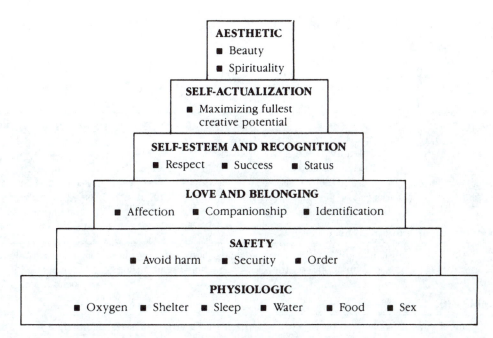

FIGURE 1.1   MASLOW'S HIERARCHY OF NEEDS

TABLE 1.3   PIAGET'S AGE-SPECIFIC DEVELOPMENTAL LEVELS

Age	Stage	Abilities
Infancy–2 yr	Sensorimotor	Preverbal; uses all senses; coordinates simple motor actions
2–4 yr	Preconceptual	Can use language; egocentric; imitation in play, parallel play
4–7 yr	Intuitive	Asks questions; can use symbols and associate subjects with concepts
7–11 yr	Concrete	Sees relationships, aware of viewpoints; understands cause and effect; can make conclusions; solves concrete problems
11 yr and on	Formal operational thought	Abstract and conceptual thinking; can check ideas, thoughts, and beliefs; lives in present and nonpresent; can use formal logic and scientific reasoning

    1. Sense of accomplishment and desire to continue to live fully.
    2. Coping with bereavement and living alone.
V. Comparison of models—Table 1.4 compares four theories of psychosocial development.

Social/Community Mental Health Model (Caplan)— Levels of Prevention

I. Primary prevention involves reducing *risk factors,* to interrupt development of illness; includes:
    A. Patient/family health teaching.
    B. Reduction of stress.
    C. Supportive resources.
II. Secondary prevention focuses on reducing *the effects* of illness; includes:
    A. Health screening.
    B. Crisis intervention/suicide prevention (see pp. 80–83).
    C. Brief counseling.
    D. Short-term hospitalization.
    E. Emergency care.
III. Tertiary prevention involves minimizing long-term *residual effects* of illness; includes:
    A. After-care.
    B. Partial hospitalization.
    C. Vocational training.
    D. Rehabilitation programs.

TABLE 1.4　　SUMMARY OF THEORIES OF PSYCHOSOCIAL DEVELOPMENT THROUGHOUT THE LIFE CYCLE

Freud	*Piaget*	*Sullivan*	*Erikson*
Emphasis on			
Pathology (intrapsychic) Anxiety	*Normal* children *No* emphasis on ego, anxiety, identity, libido	Pathology (interpersonal) Anxiety	Both health and illness
Unconscious, uncontrollable drives	Cognitive development	Unconscious, uncontrollable drives	Problems are manageable and can be solved
Ego needing defense	Tasks can be accomplished through learning process	Self-system needing defense	Need to integrate individual and society
Pathologic Development Influenced by			
Early feelings. Repressed experiences in unconscious mind	Individual differences and social influences on the mind	Unconscious mind *and* interpersonal relationships	Ego, anxiety, identity, libido concepts *combined* with social forces
Change Possible with			
Understanding content and meaning of unconscious	Socialization process to facilitate cognitive development	Improved interpersonal relationships (IPR) and understanding basic good-bad transformations	Integration of attitudes, libido, and social roles for strong ego identity
Age Group			
First five years of life	Middle childhood years	Adolescence	Middle age, old age
Focus on			
Emotional development	Cognitive skills	Emotional and interpersonal development	Emotional, interpersonal, spiritual
Psychosexual aspects	Cognitive, interactive aspects	Psychosocial aspects	Psychosocial aspects
Cause of Conflicts and Problems			
Oral, anal, genital stage problems (especially unresolved Oedipal/castration conflicts)	Faulty adaptation between individual and environment for intellectual development	Threats to self-system. Disturbed communication process; seven stages not complete	Unresolved conflicts, crises in eight successive life cycle stages
Prognosis			
Few changes possible after age 5	Little change in adult cognitive structure after middle adolescence	Change usually possible with improved interpersonal relationships (IPR)	Change not only possible but *expected* throughout life
Sexual problems part of disturbed behavior	Sex as a variable in learning (age, IQ)	Sexual problems are only one type of faulty IPR affecting behavior	Sexual identity as one of many problems solved by interaction of desire and social process

Source: Lagerquist SL. Little, Brown's NCLEX-RN Examination Review. Boston: Little, Brown, 1996. P 315.

Behavioral Model (Pavlov, Watson, Wolpe, Skinner)

I. Assumptions

　A. Roots in neurophysiology.

　B. Stimulus-response learning can be *conditioned* through *reinforcement*.

　C. Behavior is what one does.

　D. Behavior is observable, describable, predictable, and controllable.

　E. Classification of mental disease is clinically useless, only provides legal labels.

II. Aim: change *observable* behavior. There is *no underlying* cause, *no internal* motive.

Communication Model
The Therapeutic Nursing Process

A *therapeutic nursing process* involves an interaction between the nurse and client in which the nurse offers a series of planned, goal-directed activities that are useful to a particular client in relieving discomfort, promoting growth, and satisfying interpersonal relationships.

I. Characteristics of therapeutic nursing:
  A. Movement from first contact through final outcome:
  1. *Eight general phases* occur in a typical unfolding of a natural process of problem solving.
  2. Stages are not always in the same sequence.
  3. Not all stages are present in a relationship.
  B. Phases°
  1. *Beginning* the relationship. *Goal:* build trust. (Table 1.5).
  2. *Formulating* and clarifying a problem and concern. *Goal:* clarify client's statements.
  3. *Setting a contract* or working agreement. *Goal:* decide on terms of the relationship.
  4. *Building* the relationship. *Goal:* increase depth of relationship and degree of commitment.
  5. *Exploring goals* and solutions, gathering data, expressing feelings. *Goals:* (a) maintain and enhance relationship (trust and safety), (b) explore blocks to goal, (c) expand self-awareness, and (d) learn skills necessary to reach goal.
  6. *Developing action plan. Goals:* (a) clarify feelings, (b) focus on and choose between alternative courses of action, and (c) practice new skills.
  7. *Working through* conflicts or disturbing feelings. *Goals:* (a) channel earlier discussions into specific course of action and (b) work through unresolved feelings (Table 1.6).
  8. *Ending* the relationship. *Goals:* (a) evaluation of goal attainment and (b) leave-taking (Table 1.7).

II. Therapeutic nurse-client interactions
  ✉ **A. Plans/goals**
  1. Demonstrate unconditional *acceptance,* interest, concern, and respect.
  2. Develop trust—be *consistent* and *congruent.*
  3. Make *frequent* contacts with the client.
  4. Be *honest* and *direct, authentic* and *spontaneous.*
  5. Offer support, security, and empathy, *not* sympathy.
  6. Focus comments on concerns of client (*client-centered*), not self (social responses). *Refocus* when client changes subject.
  7. Encourage expression of *feelings;* focus on feelings and *here-and-now* behavior.
  8. Give attention to a client who complains.

  9. Give information at client's level of understanding, at appropriate time and place.
  10. Use open-ended questions; ask *how, what, where, who,* and *when* questions; *avoid why* questions; *avoid* questions that can be answered by *yes* or *no.*
  11. Use feedback or reflective listening.
  12. Maintain hope, but *avoid* false reassurances, clichés, and pat responses.
  13. *Avoid* verbalizing value judgments, giving personal opinions, or moralizing.
  14. Do not change the subject *unless* the client is redundant or focusing on physical illness.
  15. Point out *reality;* help the client leave "inner world."
  16. Set *limits* on behavior when client is acting out unacceptable behavior that is self-destructive or harmful to others.
  17. Assist clients in arriving at their own decisions by demonstrating problem solving or involving them in the process.
  18. Do not talk if it is not indicated.
  19. Approach, sit, or walk with agitated clients; stay with the person who is upset, if he or she can tolerate it.
  20. Focus on nonverbal communication.
  21. Remember the *psyche has a soma!* Do not neglect appropriate physical symptoms.

Therapeutic Responses

  ✉ **B.** Examples of **therapeutic** responses as *interventions:*
  1. Being *silent*—being able to sit in silence with a person can connote acceptance and acknowledgment that the person has the right to silence. (**Dangers:** the nurse may wrongly give the client the impression that there is a lack of interest, or the nurse may discourage verbalization if acceptance of this behavior is prolonged; it is not necessarily helpful with acutely psychotic behavior.)
  2. Using *nonverbal communication*—e.g., nodding head, moving closer to the client, and leaning forward; use as a way to encourage client to speak.
  3. Give encouragement to continue with *open-ended leads*—nurse's responses: "Then what?" "Go on," "For instance?" "Tell me more," "Talk about that."
  4. *Accepting, acknowledging*—nurse's responses: "I hear your anger," or "I see that you are sitting in the corner."
  5. *Commenting on nonverbal behavior* of client—nurse's responses: "I notice that you are swinging your leg," "I see that you are tapping your foot," or "I notice that you are wetting your lips." Client may respond with, "So what?" If she does, the nurse needs to reply why the comment was made—for example, "It is distracting," "I am giving the nonverbal behavior meaning," "Swinging your leg makes it difficult

°Adapted from Brammer LM. *The Helping Relationship: Process and Skills.* Englewood Cliffs, NJ: Prentice Hall, 1973. P 55.

TABLE 1.5 ◾ Summary of Beginning (Orientation) Phase of the Therapeutic Nursing Process

Objective	Therapeutic Tasks/Plans	Approaches/Implementation
Establishment of contact in the form of a working relationship with the client	Clarification of purpose of relationship, role of nurse, and responsibilities of client	*Educative:* 1. Provide information regarding purpose, roles, and responsibilities 2. Address misconceptions, fantasies, and fears regarding relationship and/or nurse
	Addressing client's suffering	Use facilitative characteristics, especially emphatic understanding *Avoid* premature reassurance (allow trust to evolve) Be explicit about who has access to client's revelations (degree of confidentiality)
	Negotiation of therapeutic contract (client's definition of personal goals for treatment and nurse's professional responsibilities)	Encourage delineation of goals that: 1. Are specific 2. Address behavioral patterns 3. Designate degree of change necessary for client self-satisfaction Determine place, duration, and time of meeting Consider optional referral sources

Source: Wilson HS, Kneisl CR. *Psychiatric Nursing* (3rd ed). Redwood City, CA: Addison-Wesley, 1988. Reprinted by permission.

for me to concentrate on what you are saying," or "I think when people tap their feet it means they are impatient. Are you impatient?"

6. Encouraging clients to *notice with their senses* what is going on—nurse's responses: "What did you see (or hear)?" or "What did you notice?"

7. Encouraging *recall and description* of details of a particular experience—nurse's responses: "Give me an example," "Please describe the experience further," "Tell me more," or "What did you say then?"

8. *Giving feedback* by *reflecting, restating, and paraphrasing* feelings and content:

   Client: I cried when he didn't come to see me.
   Nurse: You cried. You were expecting him to come and he didn't?

9. Picking up on *latent content* (what is implied) —nurse's response: "You were disappointed. I think it may have hurt when he didn't come."

10. *Focusing, pinpointing*, asking "what" questions:

    Client: They didn't come.
    Nurse: Who are 'they'?
    Client: [Rambling.]
    Nurse: Tell it to me in a sentence or two.

What is your main point? What would you say is your main concern?

11. *Clarifying*—nurse's responses: "What do you mean by 'they'?" "What caused this?" or "I don't understand. Please say it again."

12. *Focusing on reality* by expressing doubt on "unreal" perceptions:

    Client: Run! There are giant ants flying around after us.
    Nurse: That is unusual. I don't see giant ants flying.

13. *Focusing on feelings*, encouraging client to be aware of and describe personal feelings:

    Client: Worms were in my head.
    Nurse: That must have been a frightening feeling. What did you feel at that time? Tell me about that feeling.

14. Helping client to *sort* and *classify impressions, make speculations, abstract* and *generalize* by making connections, seeing common elements and similarities, making comparisons, and placing events in logical sequence—nurse's responses: "What are the common elements in what you just told me?" "How is this similar

TABLE 1.6 **SUMMARY OF MIDDLE (WORKING) PHASE OF THE THERAPEUTIC NURSING PROCESS**

Objective	Therapeutic Tasks/Plans	Approaches/Implementation
Mutual determination of dynamics of client's behavior patterns, especially those considered dysfunctional	Identify and explore important behavior patterns	Explore behavior pattern in depth, including origin, causes, operation, and effect of pattern (intrapersonally and interpersonally)
		Separate environmental factors (familial, political, economic, cultural) from intrapersonal factors
		Link elements of one behavior pattern to other patterns as appropriate, for a gradual unfolding of central life patterns
	Analyze client's mode of conflict resolution	Encourage detailed exploration of how client reacts to reduce anxiety associated with conflict
		Increase awareness of defenses employed to ward off anxiety awakened by such exploration
	Facilitate client self-assessment of growth-producing and growth-inhibiting behavior patterns	Encourage client to evaluate each response pattern to determine which are self-defeating and/or thwart gratification of basic needs
Institution of behavioral change, especially in dysfunctional behavior patterns	Address forces that inhibit desired change (problematic thoughts, feelings, and behaviors)	Assist client in challenging client's personal resistance to change
		Use problem-solving strategies, active decision making, and personal accountability
		Encourage client to assert own needs when external environmental conditions (group, agency, institution) are an inhibiting force
	Create an atmosphere that offers permission for active experimentation to test and assess effectiveness of new behaviors	Allow freedom to make and assess mistakes and blunders
		Avoid parental judgment of any behavioral experimentation—encourage client self-assessment instead
	Facilitate the development of coping skills to deal with anxiety associated with behavioral change	Address, rather than avoid, anxiety and its manifestations
		Strengthen existing growth-promoting coping skills, especially regarding unalterable conditions (e.g., terminal illness, physical deformity, loss of significant other by death)
		Encourage development of new coping skills and their application to actual life experiences

Source: Modified from Wilson HS. *Psychiatric Nursing* (3rd ed). Redwood City, CA: Addison-Wesley, 1988. Reprinted by permission.

TABLE 1.7 ◉ **SUMMARY OF END (RESOLUTION) PHASE OF THE THERAPEUTIC NURSING PROCESS**

Objective	Therapeutic Tasks/Plans	Approaches/Implementation
Termination of contact in a mutually planned, satisfying manner	Assist client evaluation of therapeutic contact and of psychotherapeutic experience in general	Encourage client's appraisal of personal therapeutic goals (motivation, effort, progress, outcome)
		Provide appropriate feedback regarding appraisal of goals
		Underline client's assets and therapeutic gains
		Underline areas for further therapeutic work
	Encourage transference of dependence to other support systems	Encourage client to develop reliance on others in client's immediate environment (spouse, relative, employer, neighbor, friend) for emphatic emotional support
	Participate in explicit therapeutic good-bye with client	Be alert to surfacing of any behavior arising on termination (repression, regression, acting out, anger, withdrawal, acceptance, etc.)
		Assist client in working through feelings associated with these behaviors
		Anticipate own reaction to separation and share in a manner that does not burden client
		Allow "time" and "space" for termination; the longer the duration of the one-to-one relationship, the more time is needed for the resolution phase

Source: Wilson HS, Kneisl CR. *Psychiatric Nursing* (3rd ed). Redwood City, CA: Addison-Wesley, 1988. Reprinted by permission.

to . . ." "What happened just before?" or "What is the connection between this and . . ."

15. *Pointing out discrepancies* between thoughts, feelings, and actions—nurse's response: "You say you were feeling sad when she yelled at you; yet you laughed. Your feelings and actions do not seem to fit together."

16. *Checking perceptions* and *seeking agreement* on how the issue is seen, checking with the client to see if the message sent is the same one that was received—nurse's responses: "Let me restate what I heard you say," "Are you saying that . . ." "Did I hear you correctly?" "Is this what you mean?" or "It seems that you were saying . . ."

17. *Encouraging client to consider alternatives*—nurse's responses: "What else could you say?" or "Instead of hitting him, what else might you do?"

18. *Planning a course of action*—nurse's responses: "Now that we have talked about your on-the-job activities and you have thought of several choices, which are you going to try out?" or "What would you do next time?"

19. *Imparting information*—give additional data as new input to help client; for example, state facts and reality-based data that client may lack.

20. *Summing up*—nurse's response: "Today we have talked about your feelings toward your boss, how you express your anger, and about your fear of being rejected by your family."

21. *Encouraging client to appraise and evaluate* the experience or outcome—nurse's responses: "How did it turn out?" "What was it like?" "What was your part in it?" "What difference did it make?" or "How will this help you later?"

Nontherapeutic Responses

◫ **C.** Examples of **nontherapeutic** responses:

1. *Changing the subject, tangential response,* moves away from problem and/or focuses on incidental, superficial content:

   Client: I hate you.
   Nurse: Would you like to take your shower now?
   Suggested responses reflect, "You hate me; tell me about this," or "You hate me; what does hate mean to you?"

   Client: I want to kill myself today.
   Nurse: Isn't today the day your mother is supposed to come?
   Suggested responses: (a) give open-ended lead, (b) give feedback: "I hear you saying today that you want to kill yourself," or (c) clarify: "Tell me more about this feeling of wanting to kill yourself."

2. *Moralizing:* saying with approval or disapproval that the person's behavior is good or bad, right or wrong; *arguing* with stated belief of person; directly opposing the person:

   Nurse: That's good. It's wrong to shoot yourself.
   Client: I have nothing to live for.
   Nurse: You certainly do have a lot!
   Suggested responses: similar to those in 1. (See above.)

3. *Agreeing with client's autistic inventions:*

   Client: The eggs are flying saucers.
   Nurse: Yes, I see. Go on.
   Suggested response: use clarifying response first: "I don't understand," and then, depending on client's response, use either *accepting and acknowledging, focusing on reality,* or *focusing on feelings.*

4. *Agreeing with client's negative view of self:*

   Client: I have made a mess of my life.
   Nurse: Yes, you have.
   Suggested response: use clarifying response about "mess of my life"—"Give me an example of one time where you feel you messed up in your life."

5. *Complimenting, flattering:*

   Client: I have made a mess of my life.
   Nurse: How could you? You are such an attractive, intelligent, generous person.
   Suggested response: same as in 4. (See above.)

6. *Giving opinions and advice* concerning client's life situation—examples of poor responses include: "In my opinion . . ." "I think you should . . ." or "Why not?"

   Suggested responses: (a) encourage the client to consider alternatives ("What else do you think you could try?"); (b) encourage the client to appraise and evaluate for himself or herself ("What is it like for you?").

7. *Seeking agreement* from client with nurse's personal opinion—examples of poor responses include: "I think . . . Don't you?" and "Isn't that right?"

   Suggested responses: (a) it is best to keep personal opinion to oneself and only to give information that would aid the client's orientation to reality; (b) if you give an opinion as a *model* of orienting to reality, ask client to *state his or her* opinion ("My opinion is . . . What is your opinion?").

8. *Probing* and/or *offering premature solutions and interpretations;* jumping to conclusions:

   Client: I can't find a job.
   Nurse: You could go to an employment agency.
   Client: I'd rather not talk about it.
   Nurse: What are you unconsciously doing when you say that? What you really mean is . . .
   Client: I don't want to live alone.
   Nurse: Are you afraid of starting to drink again?
   Suggested response: use responses that seek clarification and elicit more data.

9. *Changing client's words* without prior validation:

   Client: I am *not feeling well* today.
   Nurse: What makes you feel so *depressed?*
   Suggested response: "In what way are you not feeling well?" Use the same language as the client.

10. *Following vague content* as if understood or *using vague global* pronouns, adverbs, and adjectives:

    Client: People are so *unfair.*
    Nurse: I know what you mean.
    Suggested response: clarify vague referents such as "people" and "unfair."

    Client: I feel sad.
    Nurse: Everyone feels that way at one time or another.
    Suggested response: "What are you sad about?"

11. *Questioning* on different topics *without waiting for a reply:*

    Client: [Remains silent.]
    Nurse: What makes you so silent? Are you angry? Would you like to be alone?

Suggested response: choose one of the above and wait for a response before asking the next question.

12. *Ignoring client's questions or comments:*

Client: Am I crazy, nurse?
Nurse: [Walking away as if he did not hear her.]
Suggested responses: "I can't understand what makes you bring this up at this time," or "Tell me what makes you bring this up at this time." Ignoring questions or comments usually implies that the nurse is feeling uncomfortable. It is important not to "run away" from the client.

13. *Closing off exploration* with questions that can be answered by *yes* or *no:*

Client: I'll never get better.
Nurse: Is something making you feel that way?
Suggested response: "What makes you feel that way?" Use open-ended questions that start with *what, who, when, where,* etc.

14. *Using clichés* or stereotyped expressions:

Client: The doctor took away my weekend pass.
Nurse: The doctor is only doing what's best for you. Doctor knows best. [*Comment:* also an example of moralizing.]
Suggested response: "Tell me what happened when the doctor took away your weekend pass."

15. *Overloading:* giving too much information at one time:

Nurse: Hello, I'm Mr. Brown. I'm a nurse here. I'll be here today, but I'm off tomorrow. Ms. Anderson will assign you another nurse tomorrow. This unit has five RNs, three LVNs, and students from three nursing schools who will all be taking care of you at some time.
Suggested response: "Hello, I'm Mr. Brown, your nurse today." Keep your initial orienting information simple and brief.

16. *Underloading:* not giving enough information so that meaning is not clear; withholding information:

Client: What are visiting hours like here?
Nurse: They are flexible and liberal.
Suggested response: "They are flexible and liberal, from 10 A.M. to 12 noon and from 6 to 8 P.M." Use specific terms and give specific information.

17. *Saying no without saying no:*

Client: Can we go for a walk soon?
Nurse: We'll see. Perhaps. Maybe. Later.
Suggested response: "I will check the schedule in the nursing office and let you know within an hour." Vague, ambiguous responses can be seen as "putting the client off." It is best to be clear, specific, and direct.

18. *Using double-bind communication:* sending conflicting messages that do not have "mutual fit," or are incongruent:

Nurse: [continuing to stay and talk with the client] It's time for you to rest.
Suggested response: "It's time for you to rest and for me to leave [proceeding to leave]."

19. *Protecting:* defending someone else while talking with client; implying client has no right to personal opinions and feelings:

Client: This hospital is no good. No one cares here.
Nurse: This is an excellent hospital. All the staff were chosen for their warmth and concern for people.
Suggested response: focus on feeling tone or on clarifying information.

20. *Asking "why" questions* implies that the person has immediate conscious awareness of the reasons for his or her feelings and behaviors. Examples of this include: "Why don't you?" "Why did you do that?" or "Why do you feel this way?"

Suggested response: ask clarifying questions using *how, what,* etc.

21. *Coercion:* using the interaction between people to force someone to do *your* will, with the implication that if they don't "do it for your sake," you won't love them or stay with them:

Client: I refuse to talk with him.
Nurse: Do it for my sake, before it's too late.
Suggested response: "Something keeps you from wanting to talk with him?"

22. Focusing on *negative* feelings, thoughts, actions:

Client: I can't sleep; I can't eat; I can't think; I can't do anything.
Nurse: How long have you not been sleeping, eating, or thinking well?
Suggested response: "What *do* you do?"

23. *Rejecting* client's behavior or ideas:

Client: Let's talk about incest.
Nurse: Incest is a bad thing to talk about; I don't want to.
Suggested response: "What do you want to say about incest?"

24. *Accusing, belittling:*

Client: I've had to wait 5 minutes for you to change my dressing.
Nurse: Don't be so demanding. Don't you see that I have several people who need me?
Suggested response: "It must have been

hard to wait for me to come when you wanted it to be right away."

25. *Evading a response* by asking a question in return:

Client: I want to know your opinion, nurse. Am I crazy?
Nurse: Do you think you are crazy?
Suggested response: "I don't know. What do you mean by 'crazy'?"

26. *Circumstantiality:* communicating in such a way that the main point is reached only after many side comments, details, and additions:

Client: Will you go out on a date with me?
Nurse: I work every evening. On my day off I usually go out of town. I have a steady boyfriend. Besides that, I am a nurse and you are a client. Thank you for asking me, but no, I will not date you.
Suggested response: abbreviate your response to: "Thank you for asking me, but no, I will not date you."

27. *Making assumptions* without checking them:

Client: [Standing in the kitchen by the sink, peeling onions, with tears in her eyes.]
Nurse: What's making you so sad?
Client: I'm not sad. Peeling onions always makes my eyes water.
Suggested response: use simple acknowledgment and acceptance initially, such as "I notice you have tears in your eyes."

28. *Giving false, premature reassurance:*

Client: I'm scared.
Nurse: Don't worry; everything will be all right. There's nothing to be afraid of.
Suggested response: "I'd like to hear about what you're afraid of, so that together we can see what could be done to help you." Open the way for clarification and exploration, and offer yourself as a helping person—not someone with magic answers.

General Principles of Health Teaching

One key nursing function is to promote and restore health. This involves teaching patients or clients new psychomotor skills, general knowledge, coping attitudes, and social skills related to health and illness (such as proper diet, exercises, colostomy care, wound care, insulin injections, urine testing). The teaching function of the nurse is vital in assisting normal development and helping patients and clients meet health-related needs.

I. Purpose of health teaching
   A. General goal: motivate health-oriented behavior.
   B. Nursing interventions
      1. Fill in *gaps* in information.
      2. *Clarify* misinformation.

   3. Teach necessary *skills.*
   4. *Modify* attitudes.
II. Educational theories on which effective health teaching is based:
   A. Motivation theory
      1. Health-oriented behavior is determined by the degree to which person sees health problem as *threatening,* with *serious consequences, high probability of occurrence,* and *belief in availability of effective course of action.*
      2. Non–health-related motives may *supersede* health-related motives.
      3. Health-related motives may not always give rise to health-related behavior, and vice versa.
      4. Motivation may be influenced by:
         a. *Phases of adaptation* to crisis (poor motivation in early phase).
         b. *Anxiety and awareness of need* to learn. (Mild anxiety is highly motivating.)
         c. *Mutual* versus externally imposed goal setting.
         d. Perceived *meaningfulness* of information and material. (If within client's frame of reference, both meaningfulness and motivation increase.)
   B. Theory of planned change
      1. *Unfreeze* present level of behavior—develop awareness of problem.
      2. Establish *need* for change and relationship of trust and respect.
      3. *Move* toward change—examine alternatives, develop intentions into real efforts.
      4. *Freeze* on a new level—generalize behavior, stabilize change.
   C. Elements of learning theory
      1. *Drive* must be present based on experiencing uncertainty, frustration, concern, or curiosity; hierarchy of needs exists.
      2. *Response* is a learned behavior that is elicited when associated stimulus is present.
      3. *Reward and reinforcement* are necessary for response (behavior) to occur and remain.
      4. *Extinction of response,* that is, elimination of undesirable behavior, can be attained through conditioning.
      5. Memorization is the easiest level of learning, but least effective in changing behavior.
      6. Understanding involves the incorporation of generalizations and specific facts.
      7. After introduction of new material, there is a period of floundering when assimilation and insight occur.
      8. Learning is a two-way process between learner and teacher; defensive behavior in either makes both activities difficult, if not impossible.
      9. Learning flourishes when client feels respected, accepted by enthusiastic nurse; learning occurs best when differing value systems are accepted.
      10. Feedback increases learning.
      11. Successful learning leads to more successes in learning.

12. Teaching and learning should take place in the area where *targeted activity* normally occurs.
13. Priorities for learning are dependent on client's *physical and psychological status*.
14. Decreased visual and auditory perception leads to decreased readiness to learn.
15. Content, terminology, pacing, and spacing of learning need to correspond to client's *capabilities, maturity level, feelings, attitudes, and experiences*.

▶III. **Assessment** of the client-learner
  A. *Characteristics:* age, sex, race, medical diagnosis, prognosis.
  B. *Sociocultural-economic:* ethnic, religious group beliefs and practices; family situation (roles, support); job (type, history, options, stress); financial situation, living situation (facilities).
  C. *Psychological:* own and family's response to illness; premorbid personality; current self-image.
  D. *Educational:*
    1. Client's *perception* of current situation: What is wrong? Cause? How will life-style be affected?
    2. *Past experience:* previous hospitalization and treatment; past compliance.
    3. *Level of knowledge:* What has the client been told? From what source? How accurate? Known others with the same illness?
    4. *Goals:* what the client *wants* to know.
    5. *Needs:* what nurse thinks the client *should* know for self-care.
    6. Readiness for learning.
    7. *Educational* background; ability to read and learn.

▶IV. **Analysis** of factors influencing learning:
  A. *Internal*
    1. Physical condition.
    2. Senses (sight, hearing, touch).
    3. Age.
    4. Anxiety.
    5. Motivation.
    6. Experience.
    7. Values (cultural, religious, personal).
    8. Comprehension.
    9. Education and language deficiency.
  B. *External*
    1. Physical environment (heat, light, noise, comfort).
    2. Timing, duration, interval.
    3. Teaching methods and aids.
    4. Content, vocabulary.

▶ V. **Teaching plan** needs to be:
  A. Compatible with the *three domains of learning*—
    1. *Cognitive* (knowledge, concepts): use written and audiovisual materials, discussion.
    2. *Psychomotor* (skills): use demonstrations, illustrations, role models.
    3. *Affective* (attitudes): use discussions, maintain atmosphere conductive to change; use role models.
  B. Appropriate to educational material.
  C. Related to client's abilities and perceptions.
  D. Related to objectives of teaching.

💡 Study and Memory Aids

Psychosexual developmental stages: Freud—"O APE LG"

Oral	Infancy (0–1 yr)
Anal	1–3 yr
Phallic	Preschool (3–6 yr)
Electra/o**E**dipal	Preschool (3–6 yr)
Latency	School-age (6–12 yr)
Genital	Adolescence and adulthood (12–18 yr)

Source: Rogers PT. *The Medical Student's Guide to Top Board Scores (2nd ed).* Boston: Little, Brown, 1996. P 43.

Anxiety interventions—"CALM"

Calm environment
Activities that provide external outlet for excess energy
Listen
Medications

Erikson's developmental task stages—"TAF⁴I, PI"

Trust vs. mistrust	Infant
Autonomy vs. shame and doubt	Toddler
Four "I's":	
Initiative vs. guilt	Preschool
I Industry vs. inferiority	School-age
Identity vs. role diffusion	Adolescent
Intimacy vs. isolation	Young adult
Productivity vs. stagnation	Later adult
Integrity vs. despair	Old age

Source: Rogers PT. *The Medical Student's Guide to Top Board Scores (2nd ed).* Boston: Little, Brown, 1996. P 43.

Basic to a therapeutic nurse-patient relationship—"TRUST"

Therapeutic communication (e.g., broad openings, open-ended questions)
Reflection used in active listening
Unhurried
Silently sit; set limits
Take time to *allow* and accept

▶ VI. **Implementation**—*teaching guidelines* to use with clients:

A. Select conducive *environment* and best *timing* for activity.

B. Assess the client's *needs*, interests, *perceptions*, motivations, and *readiness* for learning.

C. State purpose and *realistic* goals of planned teaching/learning activity.

D. Actually involve the client by giving him or her the opportunity to *do, react, experience,* and *ask questions.*

E. Make sure that the client views the activity as useful and worthwhile and that it is within the client's grasp.

F. Use comprehensible terminology.

G. Proceed from the *known to the unknown,* from *specific to general* information.

H. Provide opportunity for client to *see results* and progress.

I. Give *feedback* and *positive reinforcement.*

J. Provide opportunities to achieve *success.*

K. Offer repeated practice in *real-life* situations.

L. *Space and distribute* learning sessions over a period of time.

VII. Evaluation/outcome criteria:

A. Client's deficit of knowledge is lessened.

B. Increased compliance to treatment.

C. Length of hospital stay is reduced.

D. Rate of readmission to hospital is reduced.

⚷ Key Points

Anxiety

1. *Interventions:* listen, develop trust, protect ego defenses and coping mechanisms. Help patient to identify and describe feelings.

2. *Environment needed:* calm, quiet, with soft music. Provide motor outlet (e.g., walking) and concrete tasks.

3. *Anxiety relief medications*—"**EVAL**"
   - **E**quanil (meprobamate), **V**alium (diazepam), **A**tarax (hydroxyzine hydrochloride), **L**ibrium (chlordiazepoxide hydrochloride).
   - **EVAL**uate for side effects: *Equanil*—interferes with liver function tests, ↓ PT if on Coumadin; *Librium* and *Valium*—leukopenia and postural hypotension.

Therapeutic Communication

1. Use open-ended questions to focus on feelings when there is no immediate need to get information.

2. Therapeutic nursing process uses an eclectic approach, incorporating the medical/biologic model, psychodynamic and anxiety models, psychosocial and behavioral models

Health Teaching

Assessment of client learners, and analysis of factors influencing learning are based on learning theory and theory of planned change.

Glossary

catharsis Anxiety reduction technique that provides relief when the individual *verbalizes* fears and feelings, and faces problems and events.

cognitive restructuring Relabeling how a situation or event is perceived (e.g., financial failure in one business is seen as an opportunity to try a new venture).

cognitive theory A theory focusing on faulty *thinking* as a basis for emotional problems.

conflict Emotional struggle resulting from *opposing* demands and drives of the id, ego, and superego.

conscious According to Freudian theory, that part of the mind that is aware of reality.

coping mechanisms Any efforts aimed at warding off anxiety or uncomfortable thoughts and feelings. Some involve direct problem solving to cope with the actual *threat;* others are intrapsychic (ego-defensive), aimed at controlling own *emotional* distress, such as an activity of the ego that holds in check impulses that might cause conflict (e.g., repression, regression).

developmental tasks In normal personality development, certain basic behaviors (physical, social, emotional, and intellectual) that need to be mastered at each age/stage of life.

ego According to Freudian theory, that aspect of the psyche (personality) that is mostly *conscious,* operates on the *reality principle,* and can integrate and *mediate* conflicts between the primitive, pleasure-seeking, instinctual drives of the id and the self-critical, prohibitive, restraining forces of the superego. The "I," "self," and "person," as distinguished from "others." The part of the personality that has to make *decisions,* and represents the *thinking/feeling* part of a person. The *compromises* that are worked out by the ego help to resolve intrapsychic conflicts by keeping thoughts, interpretations, judgments, and behaviors practical and efficient.

ego defense mechanisms Coping mechanisms that are aimed at protecting an individual from feelings of worthlessness and awareness of anxiety. Most are unconscious and involve distortion of reality and self-deception.

empathy A therapeutic skill used to experience what another person is experiencing (feelings and thoughts) in order to understand that person's perspective. An objective awareness of another's thoughts, feelings, or behavior and their meaning and significance; intellectual identification *versus* emotional identification (sympathy).

free association A therapy technique used by physicians to elicit unconscious thoughts and memories, by having the patient say what comes to mind, without censorship.

id According to Freudian theory, the source of instincts, needs, and primitive drives that lead to immediate gratification, and dominated by the *pleasure principle;* mainly unconscious. The id wants what it wants when it wants it.

libido A Freudian term for psychic energy (commonly referred to as sexual drive).

maladaptive behavior Unhealthy and ineffective coping mechanisms, by which anxiety is not reduced; these mechanisms may interfere with work and personal goals. Maladaptive behaviors may be inappropriate in frequency, intensity, and duration.

☞ Summary of Key Points

Conceptual Framework for Psychiatric Care—with Relevance for Nursing Application

Conceptual Model	Focus	Therapy	Main Implications for Nursing Intervention
Psychodynamic/psycho-sexual/psychoanalytic (Freud)	*Intrapsychic* factors and *processes* (conflicts, anxiety, defenses, sexual and aggressive drives) *Stages:* oral, anal, phallic, latency, genital *Mental operations:* conscious, preconscious, unconscious Id, ego, superego (pleasure principle, reality principle, and moral principle)	Free association Dream analysis Catharsis Transference	Give attention to patient's anxiety and coping behaviors
Psychosocial (Erikson)	Stages of development		Use developmental stages when doing developmental assessment Apply principles to understanding behavior
Behavioral (Wolpe, Skinner)	Learned, external behavior is changed through classical and operant conditioning Maladaptive behaviors can be modified by changing the environment Focus is on *what* happens, not on internal thoughts and feelings and *why*	Desensitization Aversion Biofeedback Relaxation Assertiveness	Base *limit-setting* techniques on behavioral principles Nurse and patient together need to identify behavior for change Can measure change by objective methods Use as *reinforcement* such privileges as a pass to go out Help patient practice new behaviors, to reinforce them
Interpersonal (Sullivan)	Interpersonal relationships create self-concept ("self system") Social, cultural, and interpersonal factors affect personal development *Two* basic needs act as motivators: need for *satisfaction* (e.g., hunger, rest, loneliness), and need for *security* (e.g., conformity) Anxiety and security operations to minimize, avoid anxiety	A trusting, therapeutic interpersonal relationship as a basis for corrective experience	Interpersonal theory of nursing in anxiety intervention and problem solving Interpersonal relationship between nurse and client is based on here-and-now interpersonal concerns *Roles:* teacher/learner; empathizer/client; counselor/client; resource provider/consumer Healthy, corrective relationship with nurse serves as a model for other successful relationships

Conceptual Framework for Psychiatric Care—with Relevance for Nursing Application (*continued*)

Conceptual Model	Focus	Therapy	Main Implications for Nursing Intervention
Interpersonal (Sullivan) (**continued**)	*Three* views of self can evolve through relationships with significant others: "Good Me," "Bad Me," and "Not Me"		
Biomedical	Disease approach: *Symptoms* that can be classified (e.g., DSM-IV) and treated *Diagnosis* (e.g., CNS dysfunction) *Etiologies* (genetics and environment) Sick role *Biochemical/neurologic* basis of emotions, behavior, thought and mood, and of mental illness	Pharmacotherapy	Base interventions on treatment, recovery, and prevention Administer *treatments* and pharmacotherapy Teach patient how to recognize symptoms, manage the illness, and prevent complications and recurrence
Humanistic (existential, Glasser, Perls, Maslow's hierarchy of needs, Rogers)	Search for meaning and authenticity Conscious human experiences in here-and-now Growth potential Freedom of choice Self-responsibility for behavior	Client-oriented therapy (Rogers) Gestalt therapy (Perls)	Base client-centered interactions on principles of empathy and respect Encourage client to initiate talk in areas of concern Use reflective listening to help client increase self-understanding Help client to see options Use role playing
Cognitive (Ellis)	Long-held beliefs shape thinking patterns, feelings, and behavior Thinking influences feelings and behavior (especially in *depression*); these thinking processes (based on expectations, beliefs, memory) can be altered Causes of disturbed behavior: irrational, illogical beliefs, unrealistic self-appraisal	Rational, emotive, to dispute irrational beliefs Cognitive therapy (cognitive restructuring)	Assess how patient thinks. Encourage patient to practice alternative thinking patterns (e.g., use self-affirmation sentences rather than using self-defeating behaviors)

model   A means of organizing a complex body of knowledge.

primary prevention   A component of the social community health model, through which holistic interventions (biologic, social, and psychological) promote health and well-being, or *reduce the incidence* of illness in a community by *altering risk factors before* illness occurs. Approach includes health teaching and stress reduction.

psyche   Synonymous with mind, or the *mental and emotional "self."*

psychoanalysis   Theory of human development and behavior that is also a method of research and a type of therapeutic approach described by Freud, based on the belief that abnormal behaviors (disorders) are related to unresolved, anxiety-provoking childhood experiences which are pushed out of awareness (*repressed*). The goal is to bring repressed memories into conscious awareness of the origin and effects of unconscious conflict, so that more adaptive means of coping with anxiety can be learned, and conflicts can be eliminated or diminished. Treatment involves *dream interpretation* and *free association.*

psychogenic   Symptoms or physical disorders caused by emotional or mental factors, as opposed to physical (organic) factors.

psychosis   A severe mental disorder, with dysfunctional behavior involving a loss of reality; a disorder of *thinking, feeling,* and *action.*

psychotic disorders   A category of *severe,* dysfunctional emotional illnesses characterized by: personality disintegration, significant reality orientation problems, severe mood disorders, and inability to function.

secondary prevention   A component of the social community health model, with interventions aimed at reducing or minimizing actual illness through *early identification and treatment;* e.g., screening, crisis intervention, suicide prevention, short-term counseling, and hospitalization.

security operations   A term derived from *Sullivan's* interpersonal model of care, referring to processes for coping with anxiety-provoking situations.

soma   The body, or *physical* aspects.

stressors   In *Selye's* theory, these are sources of anxiety that the individual sees as threatening or harmful, and that cause a state of tension.

superego   According to Freudian theory, that part of the personality that has incorporated the parental or societal values, ethics, and standards. It functions as the moral *conscience* and enforces cultural values about good and bad, right and wrong; it guides, restrains, criticizes, and punishes. It is unconscious and learned.

tertiary prevention   A component of the social community health model, utilizing *rehabilitation* measures aimed at *minimizing long-term residual disability* as a result of illness. Aspects include: vocational training, rehabilitation, after-care, partial hospitalization.

therapeutic nurse-patient relationship   Therapeutic tool by which a nurse uses him- or herself to provide a corrective emotional experience to help the patient to change behavior. It is a mutual learning experience; the nurse uses eclectic techniques based on interpersonal theory, communication theory, behavioral theory, existential and social models, as well as the medical model.

transference   Unconscious projection of feelings, attitudes, and wishes that were originally associated with *early* significant others onto persons or events in the *present;* may be positive or negative.

unconscious   According to Freudian theory, that part of the mind that is not directly accessible for awareness, but contains thoughts and memories that can affect behavior.

Questions

1. The nurse needs to be aware that a basic assumption of Freud's psychoanalytic theory about personality is that:
   1. All behavior is meaningful.
   2. All behavior is governed by sexuality.
   3. All behavior is unconscious.
   4. All behavior is learned.

2. The nurse notes that the patient is exhibiting tachycardia, tachypnea, and foot tremors. What stage of anxiety does this suggest?
   1. Panic.
   2. Severe anxiety.
   3. Moderate anxiety.
   4. Mild anxiety.

3. In preparation for teaching a patient newly diagnosed with diabetes about self-administration of insulin, the nurse assesses the patient for readiness to learn. Which level of anxiety is optimal for health teaching to be effective?
   1. Severe anxiety.
   2. Moderate anxiety.
   3. Mild anxiety.
   4. Absence of anxiety.

4. What is the priority nursing action when a patient is exhibiting signs and symptoms of severe anxiety?
   1. Place the patient in temporary seclusion.
   2. Place the patient in a quiet environment.
   3. Administer medication stat.
   4. Engage the patient in "talk-down" 1 : 1 therapy.

5. In which stage of anxiety is the nurse most likely to see the patient exhibit assaultive behavior and pose a danger to self and others?
   1. Mild anxiety.
   2. Moderate anxiety.
   3. Severe anxiety.
   4. Panic.

6. What is the main goal for a patient in therapy to help cope with anxiety?
   1. Limit stressors.
   2. Change life-styles.
   3. Avoid stressors that cause anxiety.
   4. Change response to sources of stress.

7. What concept related to anxiety is important for the nurse to keep in mind when interacting with a patient who is severely anxious?
   1. Anxiety is self-limiting.
   2. Anxiety is not observable.
   3. Anxiety is important for learning to occur.
   4. Anxiety is contagious.

8. While doing an assessment, the nurse notices that the patient is having a problem with remote memory. The patient starts to make up dates and names while trying to answer questions. The nurse should identify this behavior as:

1. Ideas of reference.
2. Confabulation. ✓
3. Flight of ideas.
4. Loose association.

9. Patients who are suspicious tend to use projection. The nurse is aware that the main purpose of this action is to:
   1. Control and manipulate others.
   2. Deny reality.
   3. Handle feelings and thoughts not acceptable to the ego. ✓
   4. Express resentment toward others.

10. The nurse is aware that patients who exhibit reaction formation can be described as:
   1. Using socially acceptable outlets for impulses from the id.
   2. Adopting the feelings and attitudes of a hero.
   3. Keeping unacceptable ideas or feelings from awareness.
   4. Adopting behaviors or attitudes that are the opposite of the original attitude. ✓

11. The nurse is aware that a patient is exhibiting regressive behavior, which is common in physical and emotional illness. Which of the following best explains this mechanism?
   1. When faced with frustration, conflict, and/or anxiety, people may need to return to a previous level of functioning where they felt secure and comfortable. ✓
   2. Immature behavior has secondary benefits.
   3. Childlike behavior is a way of getting away with expressing hostility.
   4. Individuals enjoy the sympathy and attention they received as children when they were ill.

12. When a patient is described as exhibiting fixation, the nurse is aware that this mode of coping is related to:
   1. Reversion to an earlier developmental phase.
   2. Behavior that was appropriate in an earlier developmental phase persisting into later life. ✓
   3. A disturbance in the rate of speech.
   4. A wish to be like another and to assume attributes of the other.

13. An angry person may channel hostilities into competitive sports in which there are many opportunities for combat. The nurse identifies this as:
   1. Sublimation. ✓
   2. Repression.
   3. Rationalization.
   4. Reaction formation.

14. The nurse would determine that a patient who reflects on life and looks to the future is in which of Erikson's developmental stages?
   1. Trust vs. mistrust.
   2. Industry vs. inferiority.
   3. Generativity vs. stagnation and self-absorption.
   4. Ego integrity vs. despair. ✓

15. In assessing an adolescent's psychosocial needs, which factor is most important for the nurse to consider, according to Erikson's theory of personality development?
   1. Grades in school.
   2. Approval of parents.
   3. Criticism by peers.
   4. Self-identity. ✓

16. In assessing a patient's needs, which need would the nurse consider most basic?
   1. Love and belonging.
   2. Self-esteem and recognition.
   3. Self-actualization.
   4. Environmental safety. ✓

17. What is an example of the mental health nurse's role in primary prevention?
   1. Holding prenatal classes for pregnant teenagers. ✓
   2. Leading a postdischarge group for patients who have attempted suicide.
   3. Home visitation to discuss a phenothiazine medication regimen.
   4. Crisis intervention in the mental health center.

18. What is an example of the nurse's role in primary prevention according to the social/community mental health model?
   1. Holding a sex education class for schoolchildren. ✓
   2. Being a group leader in a support group for women with postmastectomy prostheses.
   3. Interviewing a victim of suspected rape who comes into the emergency room.
   4. Visiting a newly discharged patient with diabetes.

19. At the start of a therapeutic nurse-patient relationship, the nurse needs to explain to a patient that the main goal of a 1:1 therapeutic relationship is to:
   1. Ensure that medications are taken.
   2. Remove stress.
   3. Build a trusting relationship.
   4. Help promote change. ✓

20. In establishing a therapeutic nurse-patient relationship, what is the initial goal?
   1. Identify the patient's needs.
   2. Show empathy.
   3. Establish trust. ✓
   4. Clarify the patient's expectations.

21. The nurse would be demonstrating therapeutic skills during the orientation phase of the therapeutic nursing process when the nurse:
   1. Sets goals for the patient.
   2. Offers reassurance from the start.
   3. Convinces the patient of the merits of the therapeutic relationship.
   4. Avoids persuading the patient to go into therapy. ✓

22. What is an essential component of a therapeutic nurse-patient relationship?
   1. Relabeling.
   2. Confrontation.
   3. Empathy. ✓
   4. Catharsis.

23. During an assessment interview in the crowded dayroom, a newly admitted patient starts to pace and breathe rapidly, and has a problem focusing on the nurse's questions. What is the most appropriate approach for the nurse to take at this time?
   1. Reassure the patient that "it's all right."
   2. Stop the assessment interview and ask if going for a walk would be helpful.
   3. Remove the patient to a quiet area. ✓
   4. Tell the patient to sit down and practice controlled breathing.

24. A patient who has a problem with substance abuse asks the nurse for a date. The nurse responds by stating what a therapeutic relationship is. What technique is the nurse using?
    1. Avoidance of the embarrassing situation.
    2. Confrontation.
    ✓ 3. Defining the limits of the relationship.
    4. Rationalization.
25. What communication technique is the nurse using when the nurse says to the patient, "You became tearful when I mentioned your father"?
    1. Reflecting.
    ✓ 2. Making an observation.
    3. Showing acceptance.
    4. Initiating awareness.

Answers/Rationale

1. (1) A basic premise of Freudian theory is that everything a person does has meaning, whether or not that person is aware of it. **No. 2** is false; sexuality does not underlie or drive all behaviors. **No. 3** is incorrect because behavior can be conscious or preconscious, as well as unconscious. **No. 4** is incorrect because this more accurately represents an assumption of *social* theorists. **AN, 7, PsI**

2. (3) Effects of sympathetic stimulation are observed in moderate anxiety; they include foot-swinging, toe-tapping, and other manifestations of muscle tension. GI discomfort and perspiration are also prevalent. Panic (**No. 1**) is characterized by scattered thoughts, feelings of terror, increased distortion, and loss of reality orientation. Severe anxiety (**No. 2**) is characterized by focus on fragmented details, headaches, dizziness, inability to see connections between details, and drastically reduced awareness. Mild anxiety (**No. 4**) is characterized by increased alertness, with increased visual and auditory perceptions and increased awareness of meanings and relationships. **AN, 7, PsI**

3. (2) At the moderate level, the person is able to focus on what is relevant and tune out interferences to learning (such as distracting noises in the surrounding environment). At the severe level (**No. 1**), learning is severely limited. Details are typically blown out of proportion and the ability to recall is diminished. The perceptual field is restricted. Behavior is aimed at getting relief through "fight or flight." At the mild level (**No. 3**), *focused* energy is missing. With absence of anxiety

(**No. 4**), a motivating factor ("keyed up" energy) necessary for learning is lacking. **AS, 7, PsI**

4. (2) Decreased stimulus is needed to reduce confusion associated with scattered thoughts. Seclusion (**No. 1**) is not necessary—just a quiet place away from too many stimuli. Medications (**No. 3**) may be the *next* in order of priority, after removing the patient from excess stimuli. One-to-one interaction (**No. 4**) may *follow* providing a quiet environment (**No. 2**) and medications (**No. 3**) in order of priority. **IMP, 1, SECE**

5. (4) At the panic stage, the patient experiences terror and exhibits distortions. Behavior of others may be misperceived as a threat to the patient, resulting in the patient's striking out. In mild or moderate anxiety (**Nos. 1 and 2**), the patient can still use reason. In severe anxiety (**No. 3**), contact with reality is not yet lost, although awareness is greatly reduced. **AN, 7, PsI**

6. (4) According to "stress theory" (Hans Selye), it is not the stress stimulus or situation (**No. 1**) that is crucial, but rather the individual's *reaction* to the stressor. Changing life-style (**No. 2**) does not address the need to change the patient's reaction to the stress itself. It is not realistic to attempt to *avoid* anxiety-causing stressors (**No. 3**), or even to limit stressors in general (**No. 1**); moreover, it is not the stressors that determine the effect of stress, but rather the patient's reactions. The goal of therapy is to change coping reactions. **PL, 7, PsI**

7. (4) The nurse's ability to intervene effectively can be hampered when a patient's severe anxiety affects the nurse. The nurse's own mild anxiety can be potentiated by the patient's anxiety, and levels of anxiety in both can escalate. Anxiety *can* escalate out of control and is therefore *not* self-limiting (**No. 1**). There *are* observable physical and behavioral manifestations of anxiety (**No. 2**). A *severe* level of anxiety can *interfere* with learning and problem solving (**No. 3**). **AN, 7, PsI**

8. (2) When there are memory gaps, especially for names and events, a person may use confabulation as a coping mechanism, to attempt to fill in these gaps. Ideas of reference (**No. 1**) are usually seen in paranoid behaviors. Flight of ideas (**No. 3**) is usually seen in the manic phase of bipolar disorder or in anxiety disorders. Loose associations (**No. 4**) are common manifestations of thought disorders, such as schizophrenic disorders. **AN, 7, PsI**

9. (3) Projection is a coping mechanism. Most coping mechanisms are aimed at either reducing anxiety or maintaining self-esteem. Although suspicious patients *may in some cases* use projection to deny reality (**No. 2**), this is not the case in *all* instances of projection. The main focus of coping mechanisms is on the *self*, not on others (**Nos. 1 and 4**.) **AN, 7, PsI**

10. (4) Reaction formation is the mechanism of adopting behaviors or attitudes that are the opposite of those normally expected. By definition, **No. 1** describes sublimation, **No. 2** introjection, and **No. 3** repression. **AN, 7, PsI**

11. (1) This option is the most comprehensive, inclusive explanation of the mechanism of regression. **No. 2** and **No. 4** may be *encompassed* by **No. 1**, as aspects of se-

---

Key to Codes

Nursing process: AS = Assessment; **AN** = Analysis; **PL** = Planning; **IMP** = Implementation; **EV** = Evaluation. (See Appendix E for explanation of nursing process steps.)

Category of human function: 1 = Protective; **2** = Sensory-Perceptual; **3** = Comfort, Rest, Activity, and Mobility; **4** = Nutrition; **5** = Growth and Development; **6** = Fluid-Gas Transport; **7** = Psychosocial-Cultural; **8** = Elimination. (See Appendix G for explanation.)

Client need: SECE = Safe, Effective Care Environment; **PhI** = Physiologic Integrity; **PsI** = Psychosocial Integrity; **HPM** = Health Promotion/Maintenance. (See Appendix H for explanation.)

curity and comfort. Since regression is a coping mechanism, we know that the key purpose is to increase self-esteem and/or decrease anxiety; expressing hostility (**No. 3**) does not necessarily increase self-esteem or decrease anxiety, and so does not explain the use of this mechanism. **AN, 7, PsI**

💡 *Test-taking tip:* Choose the option that is more inclusive (here, **No. 1** covers **Nos. 2 and 4**).

12. (2) Fixation involves behavior that *persists* from an earlier developmental phase into later phases. **No. 1** describes regression (key word: *reversion*, as opposed to *persisting*). **No. 3** describes blocking, and **No. 4** describes identification. **AN, 7, PsI**

💡 *Test-taking tip:* In the options, look for synonyms or words with somewhat similar meanings to a key word in the question.

13. (1) By definition, sublimation is the release of energy or impulses into socially acceptable outlets. Repression (**No. 2**) refers to keeping unacceptable ideas or feelings from awareness. Rationalization (**No. 3**) involves offering a socially acceptable or logical explanation to justify feelings or behavior. Reaction formation (**No. 4**) is the mechanism of adopting behaviors or attitudes that are the opposite of those normally expected. **AN, 7, PsI**

14. (4) This behavior (reflection on the past and facing the future) describes successful resolution of the conflict of ego integrity vs. despair. According to Erikson's stages of the life cycle, during late adulthood (60 yr to death), an individual who resolves this conflict is able to appreciate the past, present, and future; to accept his or her own contribution to others as well as accept his or her own self-worth; and can face "not being" (rather than despairing). Trust vs. mistrust (**No. 1**) is the developmental task in the first stage of development (birth to 18 mo); the infant is able to show affection and recognition. Industry vs. inferiority (**No. 2**) is the developmental task of the school-age child (5–12 yr). It is characterized by a sense of duty, acquisition of social and school competencies, and perseverance in real tasks. Generativity vs. stagnation (**No. 3**) is the developmental task in adulthood (25–60 yr). It is characterized by concern for others and development of caring. It is a productive, creative, and procreative stage. **EV, 7, PsI**

15. (4) According to Erikson, the adolescent's chief developmental task is identity vs. role diffusion ("Who am I?"). Academic success (**No. 1**) and approval of parents and peers (**Nos. 2 and 3**) are also concerns of the adolescent, because these issues are *components* of self-identity, the main concern. **AS, 7, HPM**

💡 *Test-taking tip:* When all options are correct, choose the one that covers them all, the "umbrella" answer (in this case, **No. 4**).

16. (4) According to Maslow's hierarchy of needs, the most basic needs are physiologic, specifically safety. **Nos. 1, 2, and 3** cannot be met until the patient *feels* and *is* safe. **AS, 1, PsI**

17. (1) The goal of primary prevention is to provide support and reduce anxiety in order to *prevent* emotional difficulties, for example, those that are associated with teenage parenthood. Leading a postdischarge group (**No. 2**) is an example of *tertiary* prevention. Supervising a medication regimen (**No. 3**) and treatment to *reduce* psychiatric problems (**No. 4**) are examples of *secondary* prevention. **IMP, 7, PsI**

18. (1) Primary prevention involves educational programs designed to *prevent* illness and to identify and work with high-risk populations. A postdischarge support group (**No. 2**) is an example of *tertiary* prevention, in which the focus is on recovery, after-care, and rehabilitation. Interviewing a rape victim (**No. 3**) is an example of *secondary* prevention, in which treatment is aimed at *reducing* problems. Home supervision (**No. 4**) is another example of *secondary* prevention, in which the goal is to reduce problems connected with the medical condition (e.g., through medication and dietary supervision). **IMP, 7, PsI**

19. (4) A basic premise in establishing a 1 : 1 nurse-patient relationship is to help bring about change when a patient is unhappy with the status quo. Medications (**No. 1**) are not the main focus of a 1 : 1 relationship. Removing stress (**No. 2**) is unrealistic. The nurse can help the patient to *reduce* stress, cope more efficiently with stress, and identify stressors, but the nurse cannot *remove* the stress in a patient's life. It is *through* a trusting relationship (**No. 3**) that the nurse can attain the main goal, facilitating change. The relationship itself is not the goal. **PL, 7, PsI**

20. (3) The *first* important goal is to develop trust. Trust must be developed *before* identifying needs (**No. 1**). Empathy (**No. 2**) should be part of *all* phases of the nurse-patient relationship, not only in the first phase. Clarifying expectations (**No. 4**) is characteristic of the *working* phase of the relationship. **PL, 7, PsI**

21. (4) It is not therapeutic to persuade a patient to go ("talk a patient into going") into therapy; for the relationship to be effective, the patient needs to be self-motivated, not other-directed. (Moreover, there is no need to focus on persuasion because the patient presumably has *already entered* into a therapeutic nurse-patient relationship, since the question refers to the *orientation* phase or the *beginning* nurse-patient therapeutic relationship.) The nurse does *not* set the goals *for* the patient (**No. 1**); it is done jointly. Reassurance at the start (**No. 2**) is usually *premature* reassurance, and is therefore inappropriate. Convincing (i.e., persuading) the patient (**No. 3**) is the opposite of the correct response, the therapeutic process of *avoiding* persuasion (**No. 4**). **EV, 7, PsI**

22. (3) Care and concern (empathy) are essential general elements of a therapeutic nurse-patient relationship, as opposed to sympathy (feeling sorry for the patient). Relabeling (**No. 1**), or reframing, is also part of the therapeutic nursing process, but *not* a *basic* component. Relabeling may be an effective approach in working with patients who are depressed. Confrontation (**No. 2**) could be an important component of the *advanced* skills of the psychiatric clinical nurse specialist when working with *certain* problematic behaviors (e.g., substance abuse, manipulative behaviors). Catharsis (**No. 4**) is not a therapeutic nursing component. Catharsis may be the *result* of an effective interaction (e.g., when

a sudden release of emotional energy occurs).
IMP, 7, PsI

23. **(3)** The patient is showing signs of severe anxiety and needs to be moved to a quieter setting away from the dayroom to decrease external stimuli. Reassurance in the form of a cliché (**No. 1**) is inappropriate. Whereas stopping the interview is therapeutic, asking for a decision (**No. 2**) is not when the person is experiencing severe anxiety. **No. 4** is inappropriate because at the severe level of anxiety, the person has little control. **IMP, 7, PsI**

24. **(3)** By defining the therapeutic relationship, the nurse is setting limits. Establishing limits is an important aspect of the therapeutic nursing process, especially when a person with manipulative behaviors (characteristic of patients with a history of substance abuse) tests the limits. Avoidance (**No. 1**) may be manifested by ignoring the patient's behavior; in this case, the nurse is not avoiding but addressing it. Confrontation (**No. 2**) does not describe the limit-setting response of the nurse in this question; an example of confrontation would be if the nurse said, "You are putting me on the spot." Rationalization (**No. 4**) is used as a coping strategy, and would be identified in a response involving a *reason* to justify a reaction or behavior. **IMP, 7, PsI**

25. **(2)** At the most obvious level, observation states what the nurse *saw*. In turn, the patient can acknowledge the correctness of the observation or correct it. Reflection (**No. 1**) involves *repeating* what the nurse hears the patient *say*. Acceptance (**No. 3**) can be conveyed, and perceived by the patient, *through* the nurse's technique of making an observation (**No. 2**). Feeling accepted, rather than challenged, can in turn increase the patient's awareness (**No. 4**), again as a *result* of the observation. **IMP, 7, PsI**

💡 *Test-taking tip:* **Nos. 3 and 4** "fit into" **No. 2,** because they can occur as a result of **No. 2**; **No. 2** would therefore be the "telescope" answer.

Psychosocial Growth and Development— Selected Concepts

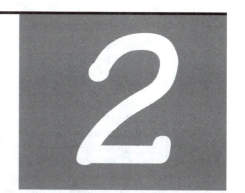

Chapter Outline

Body Image

Development of Body Image Throughout the Life Cycle

I. Definition—"Mental picture of body's appearance; an interrelated phenomenon which includes the surface, depth, internal and postural picture of the body, as well as the attitudes, emotions, and personality reactions of the individual in relation to his body as an object in space, apart from all others."[a]

II. Operational definition[b]
  A. Body image is created by social interaction.
    1. Approval given for "normal" and "proper" appearance, gestures, posture, etc.
    2. Behavioral and physical deviations from normality not given approval.
    3. Body image formed by the person's response to the approval and disapproval of others.

    4. Person's values, attitudes, and feelings about self continually evolving and unconsciously integrated.
  B. Self-image, identity, personality, sense of self, and body image are interdependent.
  C. Behavior is determined by body image.

III. Concepts related to persons with problems of body image:
  A. Image of self changes with *changing posture* (walking, sitting, gestures).
  B. *Mental picture of self* may not correspond with the actual body; subject to continual but slow revision.
  C. The degree to which people like themselves (good self-concept) is directly related to how well defined they perceive their body image to be.
    1. *Vague, indefinite, or distorted body image* correlates with the following personality traits:
      a. Sad, empty, hollow feelings.
      b. Mistrustful of others; poor peer relations.
      c. Low motivation.
      d. Shame, doubt, sense of inferiority, poor self-concept.
      e. Inability to tolerate stress.
    2. *Integrated body image* tends to correlate positively with the following personality traits:
      a. Happy, good self-concept.

[a]From Kolb L. Disturbances in Body Image. In S Arieti (ed), *American Handbook of Psychiatry*. New York: Basic Books, 1959. Pp 749–769.
[b]From Norris C. Body Image. In C Carlson, B Blackwell (eds), *Behavioral Concepts and Nursing Intervention* (2nd ed). Philadelphia: Lippincott, 1978. P 6.

b. Good peer relations.
c. Sense of initiative, industry, autonomy, identity.
d. Able to complete tasks.
e. Assertive.
f. Academically competent; high achievement.
g. Able to cope with stress.

D. Child's concept of body image can indicate degree of *ego strength* and personality integration; vague, distorted self-concept may indicate schizophrenic processes.

E. *Successful* completion of various developmental phases determines body concept and degree of *body boundary definiteness.* (See Table 2.2.)

F. *Physical changes* of height, weight, and body build lead to changes in perception of body appearance and of how body is used.

G. Success in *using* one's body (motor ability) influences the value one places upon self (self-evaluation).

H. *Secondary sex characteristics* are significant aspects of body image (*too much, too little, too early, too late, in the wrong place,* lead to disturbed body image). Sexual differences in body image are in part related to differences in anatomic structure and body function, as well as to contrasts in life-styles and cultural roles.

I. Different *cultures and families* value body traits and body deviations differently.

J. Different *body parts* (e.g., hair, nose, face, stature, shoulders) have varying personal significance; therefore there is variability in degree of threat, personality integrity, and coping behavior.

K. *Attitudes* concerning the self will influence and be influenced by person's physical appearance and ability. Society has developed stereotyped ideas regarding outer body structure (body physique) and inner personalities (temperament). Current stereotypes are:
  1. *Endomorph*—talkative, sympathetic, good natured, trusting, dependent, lazy, fat.
  2. *Mesomorph*—adventuresome, self-reliant, strong, tall.
  3. *Ectomorph*—thin, tense and nervous, suspicious, stubborn, pessimistic, quiet.

L. Person with a *firm ego boundary or body image* is more likely to be independent, striving, goal oriented, influential. Under stress, may develop skin and muscle disease.

M. Person with *weak ego boundary or poorly integrated body image* is more likely to be passive, less goal oriented, less influential, more prone to external pressures. Under stress, may develop heart and GI diseases.

N. Any situation, *illness,* or *injury* that causes a change in body image is a crisis, and the person will go through the *phases of crisis* in an attempt to reintegrate the body image (Table 2.1).

IV. Assessment—Table 2.2.

V. Analysis/nursing diagnosis—*body image development disturbance* may be related to:

A. *Obvious loss* of a major body part—amputation of an extremity, hair, teeth, eye, breast.

B. Surgical procedures in which the relationship of body parts is *visibly* disturbed—colostomy, ileostomy, gastrostomy, ureteroenterostomy.

C. Surgical procedures in which the loss of body parts is *not visible* to others—hysterectomy, lung, gallbladder, stomach.

D. Repair procedures (plastic surgery) that do *not* reconstruct body image as assumed—rhinoplasty, plastic surgery to correct large ears, breasts.

E. *Changes in body size and proportion*—obesity, emaciation, acromegaly, gigantism, pregnancy, pubertal changes (*too early, too late, too big, too small, too tall*).

F. Other changes in *external* body surface—hirsutism in women, mammary glands in men.

G. Skin *color* changes—chronic dermatitis, Addison's disease.

H. Skin *texture* changes—scars, thyroid disease, excoriative dermatitis, acne.

I. *Crippling* changes in bones, joints, muscles—arthritis, multiple sclerosis, Parkinson's.

J. Failure of a body part to *function*—quadriplegia, paraplegia, cerebrovascular accident (CVA).

K. Distorted ideas of structure, function, and significance stemming from *symbolism* of disease seen in terms of *life and death* when heart or lungs are afflicted—heart attacks, asthmatic attacks, pneumonia.

L. *Side effects* of drug therapy—moon face, hirsutism, striated skin, changes in body contours.

M. *Violent attacks* against the body—incest, rape, shooting, knifing, battering.

N. *Mental, emotional disorders*—schizophrenia with depersonalization, somatic delusions, and hallucinations about the body; anorexia nervosa, hypochondriasis; hysteria, malingering.

O. *Diseases requiring isolation* may convey attitude that body is undesirable, unacceptable—tuberculosis, malodorous conditions (e.g., gangrene, cancer).

P. *Women's movement and sexual revolution*—use of body for pleasure, not just procreation, sexual freedom, wide range of normality in sex practices, legalized abortion.

Q. *Medical technology*—organ transplants, lifesaving but scar-producing burn treatment, alive but hopeless, alive but debilitated with chronic illnesses.

VI. General nursing care plan/implementation:

A. *Protect from psychological threat* related to impaired *self-attitudes.*
  1. Emphasize person's *normal* aspects.
  2. Encourage self-performance.

B. *Maintain warm, communicating relationship.*
  1. Encourage awareness of positive responses from others.
  2. Encourage expression of feelings.

C. *Increase reality perception.*
  1. Provide *reliable* information about health status.
  2. Provide *kinesthetic* feedback to paralyzed part; e.g., "I am raising your leg."

TABLE 2.1   FOUR PHASES OF BODY IMAGE CRISIS

Phase	▶ Assessment	▶ Nursing Plan/Implementation
Acute shock	Anxiety, numbness, helplessness	Provide sustained support, be available to listen, express interest and concern
		Allow time for silence and privacy
Denial	Retreat from reality; fantasy about the wholeness and capability of the body; euphoria; rationalization; refusal to participate in self-care	Accept denial without reinforcing it. *Avoid* arguing and overloading with reality. Gradually raise questions, reply with doubt to convey unrealistic ideas
		Follow client's suggestions for personal care routine to help increase feelings of adequacy and to decrease helplessness
Acknowledgment of reality	Grief over loss of valued body part, function, or role; depression, apathy; agitation, bitterness; physical symptoms (insomnia, anorexia, nausea, crying) serve as outlet for feeling; redefinition of body structure and function, with implications for change in life-style; acceptance of and cooperation with realistic goals for care and treatment; preoccupation with body functions	Expect and accept displacement onto nurse of anger, resentment, projection of client's inadequacy
		Examine own behavior to see if client's remarks are justified
		Simply listen if this is the only way the client can handle feelings at this time
		Offer sustained nonjudgmental listening without being defensive or taking remarks personally
		Help dispel anger by encouraging its ventilation
		Encourage self-care activities
		Support family members as they cope with changes in client's health or body image, role changes, treatment plans
Resolution and adaptation	Perceives crisis in new light; increased mastery leads to increased self-worth; can look at, feel, and ask questions regarding altered body part; tests others' reactions to changed body; repetitive talk on painful topic of changed self; concentration on *normal* functions in order to increase sense of control	Teaching and counseling by same nurse in warm, supportive relationship
		Assess level of knowledge; begin at that level
		Consider motivational state
		Provide gradual, nontechnical medical information and specific facts
		Repeat instructions frequently, patiently, consistently
		Support sense of mastery in self-care; draw on inner resources
		Do not discourage dependence while gradually encouraging independence
		Focus on necessary adaptations of life-style due to realistic limitations
		Provide follow-up care via referral to community resources after client is discharged

TABLE 2.2   ⋈ Body Image Development and Disturbance Through the Life Cycle: Assessment

Age Group	Development of Body Image	Developmental Disturbances in Body Image
Infant and toddler	Becomes aware of body boundaries and separateness of own external body from others through sensory stimulation Explores external body parts; handles and controls the environment and body through play, bathing, and eating Experiences pain, shame, fear, and pleasure. Feels doubt or power in mastery of motor skills and strives for autonomy. Learns who one is in relation to the world	*Infant* Inadequate somatosensory stimulation → impaired ego development, increased anxiety level, poor foundation for reality testing Continues to see external objects as extension of self → unrealistic, *distorted* perceptions of significant persons, inability to form normal attachments to others (possessive, engulfing, autistic, withdrawn) *Toddler* If body fails to meet parental expectations → shameful, self-deprecating feelings Failure to master environment and control own body → helplessness, inadequacy, and doubt
Preschool and school-age	Experiences praise, blame, derogation, or criticism for body, its parts, or use (pleasure, pain, doubt, or guilt) Explores genitals—discovers anatomic differences between sexes with joy, pride, or shame Begins awareness of sexual identity Differentiates self as a body and self as a mind Beginning of self-concept; of self as male or female Learns mastery of the body (to *do*, to protect *self*, to protect *others*) and environment (run, skip, skate, swim); feels pleasure, competence, worth, or inadequacy	*Preschool* Distortion of body image of genital area due to conflict over pleasure vs. punishment If body build does not conform to sex-typed expectations and sex role identification → body image confusion *School-age* Physical impairments (speech, poor vision, poor hearing) → feelings of inadequacy and inferiority Overly self-conscious about, and excessive focus on, body changes in puberty
Adolescent	Physical self is of more concern than at any other time except old age Forced body awareness due to physical changes (new senses, proportions, features); feelings of pleasure, power, confidence, or helplessness, pain, inadequacy, doubt, and guilt Adult body proportions emerge Anxiety over ideal self vs. emerging/emerged physical self; body is compared competitively with same-sex peers Use of body (adolescents' values and attitudes) to relate with opposite sex	Growth and changes may produce distorted view of self → overemphasis on defects with compensations; inflated ideas of body ability, beauty, perfection; preoccupation with body appearance or body processes, females more likely than males to see body fatter than it is; egocentrism

TABLE 2.2   (CONTINUED)

Age Group	Development of Body Image	Developmental Disturbances in Body Image
Adolescent (cont.)	Body image crucial for self-concept formation, status achievement, and adequate social relations	
	Physical changes need to be integrated into evolving body image (strong, competent, powerful, or weak and helpless)	
Early adulthood	Learns to accept own body without undue preoccupation with its functions or control of these functions	
	Stability of body image	
Middle age	New challenges due to differential rates of aging in various body parts	Less dependable, less likable body → regression to adolescent behavior and dress due to denial of aging, defeat, depression, self-pity, egocentrism due to fear of loss of sexual identity, withdrawal to early old age
	Body not functioning as well; unresolved fears, misconceptions, and experiences in relation to body image persist and become recognized	Females more likely to judge themselves uglier than do males or younger and older females
Old age	Accelerated physical decline with influence on self-concept and life-style	Ill health → fear of invalidism, hypochondriasis. Denial related to feelings of threatened incapacity and fear of declining functions
	Can accept self and personality as a whole; continued emphasis on physical self, with increased emphasis on inner, emotional self	Despair over loss of beauty, strength, and youthfulness, with self-disgust about body → projection of criticism onto others
		Regression
		Isolation (separation of affect and thought) leads to less intense response to death, disease, aging
		Compartmentalization (focus on one thing at a time) causes narrowing of consciousness, resistance, rigidity, repetitiveness
		Resurgence of egocentrism

3. Provide *perceptual* feedback; e.g., touch, describe, look at scar.
4. Support a realistic assessment of the situation.
5. Explore with the client his or her strengths and resources.

D. *Help achieve positive feelings about self, about adequacy.*
  1. Support strengths *despite* presence of handicaps.
  2. Assist client to look at self in *totality* rather than focus on limitations.

E. *Health teaching:*
  1. Teach client and family about expected changes in functioning.

  2. Explain importance of maintaining a positive self-attitude.
  3. Advise that negative responses from others be regarded with minimum significance.

▶VII. **Evaluation/outcome criteria:**
  A. Able to resume function in activities of daily living rather than prolonging illness.
  B. Able to accept limits imposed by physical or mental conditions and not attempt unrealistic tasks.
  C. Can shift focus from reminiscence about the healthy past to present and future.
  D. Less verbalized discontent with present body; diminished display of self-displeasure, despair, weeping, and irritability.

Body Image Disturbance—Examples

I. **Definition**—a body image disturbance arises when a person is unable to accept the body as is and to adapt to it; a conflict develops between the body as it actually is and the body that is pictured mentally, that is, the ideal self.

II. **Analysis/nursing diagnosis:** *body image disturbance* may be related to:

  A. Sensation of *size change* due to obesity, pregnancy, weight loss.

  B. Feelings of being *dirty*—may be imaginary due to hallucinogenic drugs, psychoses.

  C. Dual change of body *structure and function* due to trauma, amputation, stroke, myocardial infarction, etc.

  D. Progressive *deformities* due to chronic illness, burns, arthritis.

  E. Loss of body boundaries and *depersonalization* due to sensory deprivation, such as blindness, immobility, fatigue, stress, anesthesia. May also be due to psychoses or hallucinogenic drugs.

III. **Assessment**—see Table 2.1.

Body Image and Obesity

I. **Definition:** body weight exceeding 20% above the norm for person's age, sex, and height constitutes obesity. Although a faulty adaptation, obesity may serve as a protection against more severe illness; it represents an effort to function better, be powerful, stay well, or be less sick. The *problem* may *not* be difficulty in losing weight; reducing may *not* be the appropriate *cure*.

II. **Assessment**—characteristics:

  A. Age—one out of three under 30 years of age is more than 10% overweight.

  B. Increased risks of CVA, MI.

  C. Feelings: self-hate, self-derogation, failure, helplessness; tendency to avoid clothes shopping and mirror reflections.

  D. Viewed by others as ugly, repulsive, lacking in will power, weak, unwilling to change, neurotic.

  E. Discrepancy between actual body size (real self) and person's concept of it (ideal self).

  F. Pattern of successful weight loss followed quickly and repetitively by failure, that is, weight gain.

  G. Eating in response to outer environment (e.g., food odor, time of day, food availability, degree of stress, anger), *not inner* environment (hunger, increased gastric motility).

  H. Experiences less pleasure in physical activity; less active than others.

  I. All obese people are *not* the same.

    1. In obese *newborns and infants*, there is an increased *number* of adipocytes via *hyperplastic* process.

    2. In obese *adults*, there may be increased body fat deposits, resulting in increased *size* of adipocytes via *hypertrophic* process.

    3. When an *obese infant becomes an obese adult*, the result may be an increased *number* of cells available for fat *storage*.

  J. Loss of control of own body or eating behavior.

III. **Analysis/nursing diagnosis:** *Defensive coping* related to eating disorder. **Contributing factors:**

  A. Genetic.

  B. Thermodynamic.

  C. Endocrine.

  D. Neuroregulatory.

  E. Biochemical factors in metabolism.

  F. Ethnic and family practices.

  G. *Psychological:*

    1. Compensation for feelings of helplessness and inadequacy.

    2. Maternal overprotection; overfed and forcefed, especially formula-fed infants.

    3. Food offered and used to relieve anxiety, frustration, anger, and rage can lead to difficulty in differentiating between hunger and other needs.

    4. As a child, food offered instead of love.

  H. *Social:*

    1. Food easily available.

    2. Use of motorized transportation and labor-saving devices.

    3. Refined carbohydrates.

    4. Social aspects of eating.

    5. Restaurant meals high in salt, sugar.

IV. **Nursing care plan/implementation:**

  A. Encourage *prevention* of life-long body image problems.

    1. Support *breastfeeding*, where infant determines quantity consumed, not mother; work through her feelings against breastfeeding (fear of intimacy, dependence, feelings of repulsion, concern about confinement, and inability to produce enough milk).

    2. Help mothers to *not overfeed* the baby if formula-fed: suggest water between feedings; do not start solids until 6 months old or 14 pounds; do not enrich the prescribed formula.

    3. Help mothers *differentiate* between hunger and other infant cries; help her to try out different responses to the expressed needs other than offering food.

  B. Use *case findings* of obese infants, young children, and adolescents.

  C. Assess current eating patterns.

  D. Identify need to eat, and relate need to preceding events, hopes, fears, or feelings.

  E. Employ behavior modification techniques.

  F. Encourage outside interests not related to food or eating.

  G. Alleviate guilt, reduce stigma of being obese.

  H. *Health teaching:*

    1. Promote awareness of certain *stressful* periods that can produce maladaptive responses such as obesity—e.g., puberty, postnuptial, postpartum, menopause.

    2. Assist in drawing up a meal plan for slow, steady weight loss.

    3. Advise eating five small meals a day.

V. **Evaluation/outcome criteria:** goal for desired weight is reached; weight-control plan is continued.

Body Image Disturbance Caused by Amputation

I. Assessment:
   A. Loss of self-esteem; feelings of helplessness, worthlessness, shame, and guilt.
   B. Fear of abandonment may lead to appeals for sympathy by exhibiting helplessness and vulnerability.
   C. Feelings of castration (loss of self) and symbolic death; loss of wholeness.
   D. Existence of phantom pain (most clients).
   E. Passivity, lack of responsibility for use of disabled body parts.

II. Nursing care plan/implementation:
   A. *Avoid* stereotyping person as being less competent now than previously by not referring to client as the "amputee."
   B. Foster independence; encourage self-care by assessing what client *can* do for himself or herself.
   C. Help person set *realistic* short-term and long-term goals by exploring with the client his or her strengths and resources.
   D. *Health teaching:*
      1. Encourage family members to work through their feelings, to accept person as he or she presents self.
      2. Teach how to set realistic goals and limitations.
      3. Explain what phantom pain is, that it is a normal experience.
      4. Explain role and function of prosthetic devices, where and how to obtain them, and how to find assistance in their use.

III. Evaluation/outcome criteria:
   A. Can acknowledge the loss and move through three stages of mourning (shock and disbelief, developing awareness, and resolution).
   B. Can discuss fears and concerns about loss of body part, its meaning, the problem of compensating for the loss, and reaction of persons (repulsion, rejection, and sympathy).

Body Image Disturbance in CVA (Stroke)

I. Assessment:
   A. Feelings of shame (personal, private, self-judgment of failure) due to loss of bowel and bladder control, speech function.
   B. Body image boundaries disrupted; contact with environment is hindered by inability to ambulate or manipulate environment physically; may result in personality deterioration due to diminished number of sensory experiences. Loses orientation to body sphere; feels confused, trapped in own body.

II. Nursing care plan/implementation:
   A. Reduce frustration and infantilism due to communication problems by:
      1. Rewarding all speech efforts.
      2. Listening and observing for all nonverbal cues.
      3. Restating verbalizations to see if correct meaning is understood.
      4. Speaking slowly, using two- to three-word sentences.
   B. Assist *reintegration* of body parts and function; help regain awareness of paralyzed side by:
      1. Tactile stimulation.
      2. Verbal reminders of existence of affected parts.
      3. Direct visual contact via mirrors and grooming.
      4. Use of safety features like the Posey belt.
   C. *Health teaching:* control of bowel and bladder function; how to prevent problems of immobility.

III. Evaluation/outcome criteria: dignity is maintained while relearning to control elimination.

Body Image Disturbance in Myocardial Infarction (MI)

Emotional problems (such as anxiety, depression, sleep disturbance, fear of another MI) during convalescence can seriously hamper rehabilitation. The adaptation and convalescence are influenced by the multiple *symbolic* meanings of the heart, for example:

1. Seat of emotions (love, pride, fear, sadness).
2. Center of the body (one-of-a-kind organ).
3. Life itself (can no longer rely on the heart; failure of the heart means failure of life).

I. Assessment:
   A. *Attitude*—overly cautious and restrictive; may result in boredom, weakness, insomnia, exaggerated dependency.
   B. *Acceptance* of illness—Use of denial may result in noncompliance.
   C. *Behavior*—self-destructive.
   D. *Family conflicts*—over activity, diet.
   E. *Effects of MI on:*
      1. *Changes in life-style*—eating, smoking, drinking; activities, employment, sex.
      2. *Family members*—may be anxious, overprotective.
      3. *Role in family*—role reversal may result in loss of incentive for work.
      4. *Dependence-independence*—issues related to family conflicts (especially restrictive attitudes about desirable activity and dietary regimen).
      5. *Job*—social pressure to "slow down" may result in loss of job, reassignment, forced early retirement, "has-been" social status.

II. Nursing care plan/implementation:
   A. Prevent "cardiac cripple" by shaping person's and family's attitude toward damaged organ.
      1. Instill optimism.
      2. Encourage *productive* living rather than inactivity.
   B. Set up a physical and mental activity program with client and mate.
   C. Provide anticipatory guidance regarding expected weakness, fear, uncertainty.
   D. *Health teaching:* nature of coronary disease, interpretation of medical regimen, effect on sexual behavior.

III. Evaluation/outcome criteria:
   A. Adheres to medical regimen.
   B. Modifies life-style without becoming overly dependent on others.

Alterations in Self-Concept

⋈ **I. Assessment:**

A. Self-derision; self-diminution; and criticism.

B. Denies own pleasure due to need to punish self; doomed to failure.

C. Disturbed interpersonal relationships (cruel, demeaning, exploitative of others; passive-dependent).

D. Exaggerates self-worth or rejects personal capabilities.

E. Feels guilty, worries (nightmares, phobias, obsessions).

F. Sets unrealistic goals.

G. Withdraws from reality with intense self-rejection (delusional, suspicious, jealous).

H. Views life as either-or, worst-or-best, wrong-or-right.

I. Postpones decisions due to ambivalence (procrastination).

J. Physical complaints (psychosomatic).

K. Self-destructive (substance abuse or other destructiveness).

⋈ **II. Analysis/nursing diagnosis:** *Altered self-concept* may be related to:

A. *Acute low self-esteem* related to parental rejection, unrealistic parental expectations, repeated failures.

B. *Personal identity disturbance (negative):* self-rejection and self-hate related to unrealistic self-ideals.

C. *Identity confusion* related to role conflict, role overload, and role ambiguity.

D. Feelings of *helplessness, hopelessness,* worthlessness, fear, vulnerability, inadequacy related to extreme *dependency* on others and *lack of personal responsibility.*

E. *Body image disturbance.*

F. Physiologic factors that produce self-concept distortions (e.g., fatigue, oxygen and sensory deprivation, toxic drugs, isolation, biochemical imbalance).

⋈ **III. Nursing care plan/implementation:**

A. Long-term goal: Facilitate client's self-actualization by helping him or her to grow, develop, and realize potential while compensating for impairments.

B. Short-term goals:

1. Expand client's *self-awareness:*

   a. Establish open, trusting relationship to *reduce fear* of interpersonal relationships.

   (1) Offer unconditional acceptance.

   (2) Nonjudgmental response.

   (3) Listen and encourage discussion of thoughts, feelings.

   (4) Convey that client is valued as a person, is responsible for self *and* able to help self.

   b. Strengthen client's capacity for *reality testing, self-control,* and *ego integration.*

   (1) Identify ego strengths.

   (2) Confirm identity.

   (3) Reduce panic level of anxiety.

   (4) Use undemanding approach.

   (5) Accept and clarify communication.

   (6) Prevent isolation.

   (7) Establish simple routine.

   (8) Set limits on inappropriate behavior.

   (9) Orient to reality.

   (10) Activities: increase gradually; provide positive experiences.

   (11) Encourage self-care; assist in grooming.

   c. Maximize *participation in decision making* related to self.

   (1) Gradually increase participation in own care.

   (2) Convey expectation of ultimate self-responsibility.

2. Encourage client's *self-exploration.*

   a. Accept client's feelings and assist *self-acceptance* of emotions, beliefs, behaviors, and thoughts.

   b. Help *clarify* self-concept and relationship to others.

   (1) Elicit client's perception of own strengths and weaknesses.

   (2) Ask client to describe: ideal self, how client believes he or she relates to other people and events.

   c. Nurse needs to be aware of *own* feelings as a model of behavior and to limit countertransference.

   (1) Accept own positive and negative feelings.

   (2) Share own perception of client's feelings.

   d. Respond with *empathy,* not sympathy, with the belief that client is subject to own control.

   (1) Monitor sympathy and self-pity by client.

   (2) Reaffirm that client is *not* helpless or powerless but is responsible for own choice of maladaptive or adaptive coping responses.

   (3) Discuss: alternatives, areas of ego *strength,* available coping resources.

   (4) Utilize family and group support system for self-exploration of client's conflicts and maladaptive coping responses.

3. Assist client in *self-evaluation.*

   a. Help to clearly *define* problem.

   (1) Identify relevant stressors.

   (2) Mutually identify: faulty beliefs, misperceptions, distortions, unrealistic goals, areas of strength.

   b. Explore use of adaptive *and* maladaptive coping responses and their positive and negative *consequences.*

4. Assist client to formulate a *realistic action plan.*
  a. Identify alternative solutions to client's *inconsistent perceptions* by helping him or her to change:
    (1) Own beliefs, ideals—to bring closer to reality.
    (2) Environment—to make consistent with beliefs.
  b. Identify alternative solutions to client's *self-concept not consistent with his or her behavior* by helping him or her to change:
    (1) Own behavior to conform to self-concept.
    (2) Underlying beliefs.
    (3) Self-ideal.
  ☞ **c.** Help client set and clearly define *goals* with *expected concrete* changes. Use role rehearsal, role modeling, and role playing to see practical, reality-based, emotional consequences of each goal.
5. Assist client to become committed to decision to *take necessary action* to replace maladaptive coping responses and maintain adaptive responses.
  a. Provide opportunity for success and give assistance (vocational, financial, and social support).
  b. Provide positive reinforcement; strengths, skills, healthy aspects of client's personality.
  c. Allow enough time for change.
6. *Health teaching:* how to focus on strengths rather than limitations; how to apply reality-oriented approach.

✉ **IV. Evaluation/outcome criteria:**
  A. Client able to discuss perception of self and accept aspects of own personality.
  B. Client assumes increased responsibility for own behavior.
  C. Client able to transfer new perceptions into possible solutions, alternative behavior.

Human Sexuality Throughout the Life Cycle

Human sexuality refers to all the characteristics of an individual (social, personal, and emotional) that are manifest in his or her relationships with others and that reflect gender-genital orientation.

Growth and Development

I. Components of sexual system
  A. *Biologic sexuality*—refers to chromosomes, hormones, primary and secondary sex characteristics, and anatomic structure.
  B. *Sexual identity*—based on own feelings and perceptions of how well traits correspond with own feelings and concepts of maleness and femaleness; also includes gender identity.

  C. *Gender identity*—a sense of masculinity and femininity shaped by biologic, environmental, and intrapsychic forces as well as cultural traditions and education.
  D. *Sex role behavior*—includes components of both sexual identity and gender identity. Aim: sexual fulfillment through masturbation, heterosexual, and/or homosexual experiences. Selection of behavior is influenced by personal value system and sexual, gender, and biologic identity. Gender identity and roles are learned and constantly reinforced by input and feedback regarding social expectations and demands (Table 2.3).
II. Concepts and principles of human sexual response
  A. Human sexual response involves not only the genitals but the total body.
  B. Factors in early postnatal and childhood periods influence gender identity, gender role, sex typing, and sexual responses in later life.
  C. Cultural and personally subjective variables influence ways of sexual expression and perception of what is satisfying.
  D. Healthy sexual expressions vary widely.
  E. Requirements for human sexual response:
    1. Intact central and peripheral nervous system to provide *sensory* perception, *motor* reaction.
    2. Intact circulatory system to produce *vasocongestive* response.
    3. Desirable and interested partner, if sex outlet involves mutuality.
    4. *Freedom* from guilt, anxiety, misconceptions, and interfering conditioned responses.
    5. Acceptable physical *setting*, usually private.
  💊 **F.** Medications may affect sexual performance (Table 2.4).

Sexual Health Counseling
General Issues

I. Issues in sexual practices with implications for counseling:
  A. *Sex education*—need to provide accurate and complete information on all aspects of sexuality to all people.
  B. *Sexual health care*—should be part of total health care planning for all.
  C. *Sexual orientation*—need to avoid discrimination based on sexual orientation (such as homosexuality); the right to satisfying, nonexploitative relationships with others, regardless of gender.
  D. *Sex and the law*—sex between consenting adults not a legal concern.
  E. *Explicit sexual material* (pornography)—can be useful in fulfilling various needs in life, as in quadriplegia.
  F. *Masturbation*—a natural behavior at all ages; can fulfill a variety of needs. (See **I. Masturbation,** p. 37.)
  G. Availability of *contraception* for minors—the right of access to medical contraceptive care should be available to all ages.

TABLE 2.3   SEXUAL BEHAVIOR THROUGHOUT THE LIFE CYCLE

Age	*Development of Sexual Behavior*
First 18 mo	Major source of pleasure from touch and oral exploration
18 mo–3 yr	Pleasurable and sexual feelings are associated with genitals (acts of urination and defecation). Masturbation without fantasy or eroticism
3–6 yr	Beginning resolution of Oedipal and Electra complexes; foundation for heterosexual relationships; masturbation with curiosity about genitals of opposite sex
6–12 yr	Peer relations with same sex; onset of sex play; morality and sexual attitudes taught and learned; phase of sexual tranquility
12–18 yr (adolescence)	Onset of puberty with biologic development of secondary sex characteristics; menstruation and ejaculation occur. Frequent masturbation. Intense anxiety and guilt may occur over heterosexual or homosexual behavior (petting, coitus, masturbation, STD, pregnancy, genital size)
18–23 yr (early adulthood)	Maximum interpersonal and intrapsychic self-consciousness about sexuality. Issues: premarital coitus, sexual freedom. Anxiety about: sexual competency, genital size, impotence, fear of pregnancy, rejection. Peak sexuality for men
23–30 yr	Focus on sexual activity in coupling and parenthood; mutual masturbation
30–45 yr (middle adulthood)	For women–peak sexuality without new sexual experiences. Conflict regarding extramarital sex may increase

Purpose of Intercourse
Need for body contact (and procreation until age 35 +)
Physical expression of trust, love, and affection
Reaffirmation of self-concept as sexually desirable and sexually competent due to worry about effects of aging

Sexual Dysfunctions
Men: impotence, premature ejaculation, decreasing libido
Women: intermittent lack of orgasmic response, vaginismus, dyspareunia
For either or both: changes or divergences in degree of sexual interest

Causes of Sexual Dysfunction (Men)
Overindulgence in food or drink
Preoccupation with career and economic pursuits
Mental or physical fatigue
Boredom with monotony of relationship
Drug dependency: alcohol, tobacco, certain medications
Fear of failure
Chronic illness: diabetes, alcoholism → peripheral neuropathy → impotence; (smoking and drinking may result in decreased testosterone production) excessive smoking → vascular constriction → decreased libido; spinal cord injuries
Self-devaluation due to accumulation of role function losses, sexual self-image, and body image
Past history of lack of sexual enjoyment in younger years

Causes of Sexual Dysfunction (Women)
Belief in myths regarding "shoulds and should nots" of frequency, variations, and enjoyment
Widowhood: inhibition and loyalty to deceased

45–60 yr (later adulthood)	Menopause occurs
	Little or no fear of pregnancy; evidence of sexual activity differences in male and female: women may have increased pleasure, men take longer to reach orgasm; may prefer less strenuous mutual masturbation
Over 60 yr (old age)	Activity depends on earlier sexual attitude
	May suffer guilt and shame when engaging in sex
	Can have active and enjoyable sex life with continuing sex needs
	Age is not a barrier provided there is opportunity for sexual activity with a partner or for sublimated activities. Women in this age group outnumber men; single women outnumber single men by an even larger margin

Table 2.4	MEDICATIONS THAT MAY AFFECT SEXUAL PERFORMANCE
Drug Category	**Effect**
Antidepressants	Loss of desire due to confusion
Antiemetics	Impotence, restlessness
Antihypertensives	Loss of desire
Cimetidine	Impotence, headaches, dizziness, nausea
Diuretics	Headaches, dizziness, weakness
Ranitidine	Impotence, headaches, dizziness, nausea
Steroids	Mood changes, headaches, weakness
Tranquilizers	Loss of desire, drowsiness, confusion

H. *Abortion*—confidentiality for minors (in selected states).

I. *Treatment for STD*—naming of partners as part of STD control.

J. *Sex and the elderly*—need opportunity for sexual expression; need privacy when in communal living setting.

K. *Sex and the disabled*—need to have possible means available for rewarding sexual expressions.

II. Sexual myths

Ignorance and myths are threats to both psychological and physiologic health (Table 2.5). Examples of the effects of misinformation:

A. Fear related to early sexual experiences, based on myths and lack of knowledge, may affect individual's sexual responses later in life.

B. Myths such as "masturbation causes mental illness/pimples/blindness" may lead to guilt over a normal and appropriate sexual outlet.

C. Misinformation such as "you can't get pregnant the first time you have sex/before you start getting your period/during your period" could lead to unplanned teenage pregnancy.

D. Myths such as "if he doesn't use a condom, it means he really loves me" or "condoms can be washed and reused" could lead to transmission of HIV or other STDs.

III. Basic principles of sexual health counseling

A. There is no universal consensus about acceptable values in human sexuality. Each social group has definite values regarding sex.

B. Counselors need to examine own feelings, attitudes, values, biases, knowledge base.

C. Help reduce fear, guilt, ignorance.

D. Offer guidance and education rather than indoctrination or pressure to conform.

E. Each person needs to be helped to make personal choices regarding sexual conduct.

IV. Counseling in sexual health

A. **General considerations**

1. Create atmosphere of *trust and acceptance* for objective, nonjudgmental dialogue.

2. Use *language* related to sexual behavior that is mutually comfortable and understood between client and nurse.
   a. Use alternative terms for definitions.
   b. Determine exact meaning of words and phrases since sexual words and expressions have different meanings to people with different backgrounds and experiences.

3. *Desensitize* own stress reaction to the emotional component of taboo topics.
   a. Increase awareness of own sexual values, biases, prejudices, stereotypes, and fears.
   b. *Avoid* overreacting, underreacting.

4. Become sensitively aware of *interrelationships* between sexual needs, fears, and behaviors and other aspects of living.

5. Begin with *commonly* discussed areas (such as menstruation) and progress to discussion of individual sexual experiences (such as masturbation). Move from areas where there is less voluntary control (nocturnal emissions) to more responsibility and voluntary behavior (premature ejaculation).

6. Offer *educational information* to dispel fears, myths; give tacit permission to explore sensitive areas.

7. Bring into awareness possibly *repressed* feelings of guilt, anger, denial, and suppressed sexual feelings.

8. Explore possible *alternatives* of sexual expression.

9. Determine *interrelationships* among mental, social, physical, and sexual well-being.

B. **Assessment parameters**

1. Self-awareness of body image, values, and attitudes toward human sexuality; comfort with own sexuality.

2. Ability to identify sex problems on basis of own satisfaction or dissatisfaction.

3. Developmental history, sex education, family relationships, cultural and ethnic values, and available support resources.

4. Type and frequency of sexual behavior.

5. Nature and quality of sex relations with others.

6. Attitude toward and satisfaction with sexual activity.

7. Expectations and goals. Table 2.6 suggests guidelines for conducting an *assessment* interview.

C. **Nursing care plan/implementation:**

1. *Long-term goals*
   a. Increase knowledge of reproductive system and types of sex behavior.
   b. Promote positive view of body and sex needs.

Table 2.5   COMMON SEXUAL MYTHS

Myth	Fact
A woman's role is to please her partner; women have lesser needs for sexual gratification	Men and women have equal rights to sexual freedom and expression. Sexual expression meets the needs of both men and women, including needs for communication, companionship, and intimacy; it also helps affirm identity
Contraception is the responsibility of the woman	Both partners have the *right* to and the *responsibility* for contraception (and protection from transmission of STDs)
With menopause, the female sex drive drops off and sex is no longer pleasurable	Sexual interest may *increase* with menopause, as the action of androgen becomes more pronounced (and when concern about contraception is no longer a stressor). Research suggests that regular sexual activity helps prevent reduction in sexual capacity ("disuse atrophy")
Older men become impotent	As a man ages, the time required to achieve erection increases; however, erection *is* possible (assuming no physical or psychological disorder). Again, regular activity may help preserve sexual function
Certain sexual preferences and practices (such as homosexuality) can indicate a personality disturbance	No one behavior or preference is "correct"; each individual has the right to determine what type of sexual expression is most satisfactory

TABLE 2.6   SUGGESTED FORMAT FOR SEXUAL ASSESSMENT INTERVIEW

Interview Step	Rationale
1. Open the discussion of sexual matters subtly with an open-ended question: "People with your illness or stresses often experience other difficulties, sometimes with sexual functioning."	This gentle opening lets the client know that other people have difficulties too. It gives the client permission to talk with the nurse about sexual matters without labeling these matters as problems
2. Follow up with another open-ended question about the client's current status: "Has your illness or stresses made any difference in what it's like for you to be a wife or husband (lover, boyfriend, girlfriend, sexual partner)?"	The phrasing of this question enables the client to acknowledge a problem without admitting a shortcoming
3. If the client speaks of having a dysfunction, ask about its effect: "How does this affect you?" or "How do you feel about it?"	This indicates that the nurse is willing to explore sexual matters more completely
4. Ask about the severity and duration of the dysfunction: "Is it always difficult to control your ejaculation?" "Tell me when you first noticed this."	These questions are directed at identifying the specific problem
5. Ask about the effects on the client's sexual partner: "Has this affected your relationship with your partner?"	This question is directed toward exploring the interactional aspects of the identified problem
6. Ask what the client has already done to alleviate the situation: "Have you made any adjustments in your sexual activity?"	This question yields data that will help the nurse to formulate an intervention plan
7. Ask the client if and how he or she would like the situation changed. "How would you like to change the situation to make it more satisfying?"	This question conveys the negotiated nature of the therapeutic relationship, in which the client's own goals play an important part

Source: Adapted from Whitley MP, Willingham W. Adding a sexual assessment to the health interview. *J Psychiatr Nurs and Ment Health Servs,* 16(4):17–27, 1978.

c. Integrate sex needs into self-identity.
d. Develop adaptive and satisfying patterns of sexual expression.
e. Understand effects of physical illness on sexual performance.

2. *Primary sexual health interventions*
   a. Goals: minimize stress factors, strengthen sexual integrity.
   b. Provide education to uninformed or misinformed.
   c. Identify stress factors (myths, stereotypes, negative parental attitudes).

3. *Secondary sexual health interventions:* identify sexual problems early and refer for treatment.

D. Evaluation/outcome criteria:
1. Reduced impairment or dysfunction from acute sex problem or chronic, unresolved sex problem.
2. Evaluate how client's goals were achieved in terms of *positive* thoughts, feelings, and *satisfying* sexual behaviors.

Specific Situations

I. Masturbation

A. Definition—act of achieving sexual arousal and orgasm through manual or mechanical stimulation of the sex organs.

B. Characteristics
1. Can be an interpersonal as well as a solitary activity.
2. "It is a healthy and appropriate sexual activity, playing an important role in ultimate consolidation of one's sexual identity."°
3. Accompanied by fantasies that are important for:
   a. Physically disabled.
   b. Fatigued.
   c. Compensation for unreachable goals and unfulfilled wishes.
   d. Rehearsal for future sexual relations.
   e. Absence or impersonal action of partner.
4. Can help release tension harmlessly.

C. Concepts and principles related to masturbation
1. Staff's feelings and reactions influence their responses to client and affect continuation of masturbation (that is, negative staff actions increase client's frustration, which increases masturbation).
2. Masturbation is normal and universal, *not* physically or psychologically harmful in itself.
3. Pleasurable genital sensations important for increasing *self-pride*, finding *gratification* in *own* body, increasing sense of *personal value* of being lovable, helping to *prepare for adult* sexual role.
4. Excessive masturbation—some needs not being met through interpersonal relations; may use behavior to *avoid* interpersonal relations.

5. Activity may be related to:
   a. Curiosity, experimentation.
   b. Tension reduction, pleasure.
   c. Enhanced interest in sexual development.
   d. Fear and avoidance of social relationships.

D. Nursing care plan:
1. *Long-term goals*
   a. Gain insight into *preference* for masturbation.
   b. Relieve accompanying guilt, worry, self-devaluation (Figure 2.1).
2. *Short-term goals*
   a. Clarify myths regarding masturbation.
   b. Help client see masturbation as an acceptable sexual activity for individuals of all ages.
   c. Set limits on masturbation in inappropriate settings.

E. Nursing implementation:
1. Examine, control nurse's own negative feelings; show respect.
2. *Avoid* reinforcement of guilt and self-devaluation; scorn; threats, punishment, anger, alarm reaction; use of masturbation for rebellion in power struggle between staff and client.
3. *Identify* client's unmet needs; consider purpose served by masturbation (may be useful behavior).
4. *Examine* pattern in which behavior occurs.
5. Intervene when degree of functioning in other daily life activities is *impaired*.
   a. Remain calm, accepting, but nonsanctioning.
   b. Promptly help clarify client's feelings, thoughts, at stressful time.
   c. Review precipitating events.
   d. Be a neutral "sounding board"; *avoid* evasiveness.
   e. If unable to handle situation, find someone who can.
6. For clients who masturbate at *inappropriate* times or in inappropriate places:
   a. Give special attention when they are not masturbating.
   b. Encourage new interests and activities, but not immediately after observing masturbation.
   c. Keep clients distracted, occupied with interesting activities.
7. *Health teaching:* explain myths and teach facts regarding cause and effects.

F. Evaluation/outcome criteria:
1. Acknowledges function of own sexual organs.
2. States sexual experience is satisfying.
3. Views sexuality as pleasurable and wholesome.
4. Views sex organs as acceptable, enjoyable, and valued part of body image.
5. Self-image as fully functioning person is restored and maintained.

II. Homosexuality

°Marcus IM, Francis JJ. *Masturbation from Infancy to Senescence.* New York: International Universities Press, 1975.

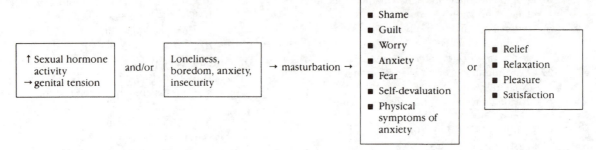

FIGURE 2.1   OPERATIONALIZATION OF THE BEHAVIORAL CONCEPT OF MASTURBATION

A. Definition—alternative sexual behavior; applied to sexual relations between persons of the same sex.

B. Theories regarding causes
1. Hereditary tendencies.
2. Imbalance of sex hormones.
3. Environmental influences and conditioning factors, related to learning and psychodynamic theories.
   a. Defense against unsatisfying relationship with father.
   b. Unsatisfactory and threatening early relationships with opposite sex.
   c. Oedipal attachment to parent.
   d. Seductive parent (incest).
   e. Castration fear.
   f. Labeling and guilt leading to sexual acting out.
   g. Faulty sex education.
4. Preferred choice as a life-style.

C. Nursing care plan/implementation:
1. Nurse needs to be aware of and work through own attitudes that may interfere with providing care.
2. Accept and respect life-style of gay (male homosexual) or lesbian (female homosexual) client.
3. Assess and treat for possible sexually transmitted diseases and hepatitis.
4. *Health teaching:* assess and add to knowledge base alternatives in sexual behavior. Teach specific assessment measures related to sexual activities.

D. Evaluation/outcome criteria: expresses self-confidence and positive self-image; able to sustain satisfying sexual behavior with chosen partner.

III. Sex and the person who is disabled
A. Assessment parameters
1. Previous level of sex functioning and conflict.
2. Client's view of sex activity (self and mutual pleasure, tension release, procreation, control).
3. Cultural environment (influence on body image).
4. Degree of acceptance of illness.
5. Support system (partner, family, support group).
6. Body image and self-esteem.
7. Outlook on future.

B. Analysis/nursing diagnosis: *Sexual dysfunction* associated with physical illness related to:
1. Disinterest in sexual activity.
2. Fear of precipitating or aggravating physical illness through sexual activity.
3. Use of illness as excuse to avoid feared or undesired sex.
4. Physical inability or discomfort during sexual activity.

C. Nursing care plan/implementation:
1. Approach with nonjudgmental attitude.
2. Elicit concerns about current physical state and perceptions of changes in sexuality.
3. Observe nonverbal clues of concern.
4. Identify genital assets.
5. Support client and partner during adjustment to current state.
6. Explore culturally acceptable sublimation activities.
7. Promote adjustment to body image change.
8. *Health teaching:*
   a. Teach self-help skills.
   b. Teach partner to care for client's physical needs.
   c. Teach alternative sex behaviors and acceptable sublimation (e.g., touching).

D. Evaluation/outcome criteria: attains satisfaction with adaptive alternatives of sexual expressions; has a positive attitude toward self, body, and sexual activity.

IV. Inappropriate sexual behavior
A. Assessment: public exhibitions of sexual behaviors that are offensive to others; making sexual advances to other clients or staff.

B. Analysis/nursing diagnosis: *Conflict with social order* related to:
1. Acting out angry and hostile feelings.
2. Lack of awareness of hospital and agency rules regarding acceptable public behavior.
3. Variation in cultural interpretations of what is acceptable public behavior.
4. Reaction to unintended seductiveness of nurse's attire, posture, tone, or choice of terminology.

C. Nursing care plan/implementation:
1. Maintain calm, nonjudgmental attitude.

2. Set firm limits on unacceptable behavior.
3. Encourage verbalization of feelings rather than unacceptable physical expression.
4. Reinforce appropriate behavior.
5. Provide constructive diversional activity for clients or patients.
6. *Health teaching:* explain rules regarding public behavior; teach acceptable ways to express anger.

✉ **D. Evaluation/outcome criteria:** verbalizes anger rather than acting out; accepts rules regarding behavior in public.

Death and Dying, Grief
Concept of Death Throughout the Life Cycle

I. Ages 1–3
 A. No concept per se, but experiences *separation anxiety and abandonment anxiety* any time significant other disappears from view for a period of time.
 B. *Coping* means: fear, resentment, anger, aggression, regression, withdrawal.
 ✉ **C. Nursing care plan/implementation**—Help the family:
  1. Facilitate transfer of affectional ties to another nurturing adult.
  2. Decrease separation anxiety of hospitalized child by encouraging family visits and by reassuring child that she or he will not be alone.
  3. Provide stable environment through consistent staff assignment.

II. Ages 3–5
 A. Least anxious about death.
 B. Denial of death as inevitable and final process.
 C. Death is separation, being alone.
 D. Death is *sleep* and sleep is death.
 E. "Death" is part of vocabulary; seen as real, gradual, *temporary,* not permanent.
 F. Dead person is seen as alive, but in altered form, that is, lacks movement.
 G. There are *degrees* of death.
 H. Death means not being here anymore.
 I. "Living" and "lifeless" are not yet distinguished.
 J. Illness and death seen as *punishment* for "badness"; fear and guilt about sexual and aggressive impulses.
 K. Death happens, but only to others.
 ✉ **L. Nursing care plan/implementation** (in addition to above):
  1. Encourage play for expression of feelings; use clay, dolls, etc.
  2. Encourage verbal expression of feelings using children's books.
  3. Model appropriate grieving behavior.
  4. Protect child from the overstimulation of hysterical adult reactions by limiting contact.
  5. Clearly state what death is—death is final, no

breathing, eating, awakening—and that death is *not* sleep.
  6. Check child at night and provide support through holding and staying with child.
  7. Allow a choice of attending the funeral and, if child decides to attend, describe what will take place.
  8. If parents are grieving, have other family or friends attend to child's needs.

III. Ages 5–10
 A. Death is cessation of life; question of what happens after death.
 B. Death seen as definitive, *universal,* inevitable, *irreversible.*
 C. Death occurs to all living things, including self; may express, "It isn't fair."
 D. Death is distant from self (an eventuality).
 E. Believe death occurs by accident, happens only to the very *old* or very sick.
 F. Death is personified (as a separate person) in fantasies and magical thinking.
 G. Death anxiety handled by *nightmares, rituals,* and *superstitions* (related to fear of darkness and sleeping alone because death is an external person, like a skeleton, who comes and takes people away at night).
 H. Dissolution of bodily life seen as a perceptible result.
 I. Fear of body mutilation.
 ✉ **J. Nursing care plan/implementation** (in addition to above):
  1. Allow child to experience the loss of pets, friends, and family members.
  2. Help child talk it out and experience the appropriate emotional reactions.
  3. Understand need for increase in play, especially competitive play.
  4. Involve child in funeral preparation and rituals.
  5. Understand and accept regressive or protest behaviors.
  6. Rechannel protest behaviors into constructive outlets.

IV. Adolescence
 A. Death seen as inevitable, *personal,* universal, and *permanent;* corporal life stops; body decomposes.
 B. Does not fear death, but concerned with: how to *live now,* what death feels like, *body changes.*
 C. Experiences *anger, frustration, and despair* over lack of future, lack of fulfillment of adult roles.
 D. Openly asks *difficult,* honest, *direct* questions.
 E. Anger at healthy peers.
 F. Conflict between *developing* body vs. *deteriorating* body, *independent* identity vs. *dependency.*
 ✉ **G. Nursing care plan/implementation** (in addition to above):
  1. Facilitate full expression of grief by answering direct questions.
  2. Help let out feelings, especially through creative and aesthetic pursuits.
  3. Encourage participation in funeral ritual.

    4. Encourage full use of peer group support system by providing opportunities for group talks.

V. Young adulthood

    A. Death seen as *unwelcome* intrusion, *interruption* of what might have been.

    B. Reaction: *rage, frustration, disappointment.*

    ▶ **C. Nursing care plan/implementation:** all of above, especially peer group support.

VI. Middle age

    A. Concerned with *consequences* of own death and that of significant others.

    B. Death seen as disruption of involvement, responsibility, and *obligations.*

    C. End of plans, projects, experiences.

    D. Death is *pain.*

    ▶ **E. Nursing care plan/implementation** (in addition to above): assess need for counseling when also in midlife crisis.

VII. Old age

    A. *Philosophic* rationalizations: death as inevitable, final process of life, when "time runs out."

    B. *Religious* view: death represents only the dissolution of life and is a doorway to a new life (a preparatory stage for another life).

    C. Time of rest and peace, supreme refuge from turmoil of life.

    ▶ **D. Nursing care plan/implementation** (in addition to above):

        1. Help person prepare for own death by helping with funeral prearrangements, wills, and sharing of mementos.

        2. Facilitate life review and reinforce positive aspects.

        3. Provide care and comfort.

        4. Be present at death.

Death and Dying—Stages and Phases

Too often the process of death has had such frightening aspects that people have suffered alone. Today there has been a vast change in attitudes; death and dying are no longer taboo topics. There is a growing realization that we need to accept death as a natural process. Elisabeth Kübler-Ross has written extensively on the process of dying, describing the stages of *denial* ("not me!"), *anger* ("why me?"), *bargaining* ("yes me —but"), *depression* ("yes, me"), and *acceptance* ("my time is close now, it's all right"), with implications for the helping person.

  I. Concepts and principles related to death and dying

    A. Persons may know or *suspect* they are dying and may want to talk about it; often they look for someone to share their fears and the process of dying.

    B. Fear of death can be reduced by helping clients feel that they are *not alone.*

    C. The dying need the opportunity to live their final experiences to the fullest, in their *own* way.

    D. People who are dying remain more or less the *same* as they were during life; their approaches to death are consistent with their approaches to life.

    E. Dying persons' need to review their lives may be a purposeful attempt to reconcile themselves to what "was" and "what could have been."

    F. *Three ways* of facing death are (1) quiet acceptance with inner strength and peace of mind, (2) restlessness, impatience, anger, and hostility, and (3) depression, withdrawal, and fearfulness.

    G. *Four tasks* facing a dying person are (1) reviewing life, (2) coping with physical symptoms in the end stage of life, (3) making a transition from known to unknown state, (4) reaction to separation from loved ones.

    H. Crying and tears are an important aspect of the grief process.

    I. There are many *blocks* to providing a helping relationship with the dying and bereaved:

        1. Nurses' unwillingness to share the process of dying—minimizing their contacts and blocking out their own feelings.

        2. Forgetting that a dying person may be feeling lonely, abandoned, and afraid of dying.

        3. Reacting with irritation and hostility to the person's frequent calls.

        4. Nurses' failure to seek help and support from team members when feeling afraid, uneasy, and frustrated in caring for a dying person.

        5. Not allowing client to talk about death and dying.

        6. Nurses' use of technical language or social chitchat as a defense against their own anxieties.

  ▶ **II. Assessment** of death and dying:

    A. Physical

        1. Observable deterioration of physical and mental capacities—person is unable to fulfill physiologic needs, such as eating and elimination.

        2. Circulatory collapse (blood pressure and pulse).

        3. Renal or hepatic failure.

        4. Respiratory decline.

    B. Psychosocial

        1. Fear of death is signaled by agitation, restlessness, and sleep disturbances at night.

        2. Anger, agitation, blaming.

        3. Morbid self-pity with feelings of defeat and failure.

        4. Depression and withdrawal.

        5. Introspectiveness and calm acceptance of the inevitable.

        6. Variable attitudes toward death and dying based on ethnic beliefs and cultural practices.

  ▶ **III. Analysis/nursing diagnosis:**

    A. Terminal illness response

    B. *Altered feeling states* related to fear of being alone.

    C. *Altered comfort patterns* related to pain.

    D. *Altered meaningfulness* related to depression, hopelessness, helplessness, powerlessness.

    E. *Altered social interaction* related to withdrawal.

  ▶ **IV. Nursing care plan/implementation:**

    A. *Long-term goal:* foster environment where person and family can experience dying with dignity.

B. *Short-term goals*
1. Express feelings (person and family).
2. Support person and family.
3. Minimize physical discomfort.

C. Explore your own feelings about death and dying with team members; form support groups.

D. Be aware of the *normal grief* process.
1. *Allow* person and family to do the work of grieving and mourning.
2. Allow crying and mood swings, anger, demands.
3. Permit yourself to cry.

E. Allow person to *express* feelings, fears, and concerns.
1. *Avoid* pat answers to questions about "why."
2. Pick up symbolic communication.

F. Provide care and comfort with *relief from pain;* do not isolate person.

G. Stay *physically close.*
1. Use touch.
2. Be available to form a consistent relationship.

H. *Reduce isolation and abandonment* by assigning person to room in which it is less likely to occur and by allowing flexible visiting hours.

I. Keep activities in room as *near normal* and *constant* as possible.

J. Speak in *audible* tones, not whispers.

K. Be alert to cues when person needs to be alone *(disengagement process).*

L. Leave room for *hope.*

M. Help person die with peace of mind by lending support and providing opportunities to express anger, pain, and fears to someone who will accept her or him and not censor verbalization.

N. *Health teaching:* teach grief process to family and friends; teach methods to relieve pain.

▶ V. Evaluation/outcome criteria:
A. Remains comfortable and free of pain as long as possible.
B. Dies with dignity.

Grief/Bereavement Stages

Grief is a typical reaction to the loss of a source of psychological gratification. It is a syndrome with somatic and psychological symptoms that diminish when grief is resolved. Grief processes have been extensively described by Erich Lindemann and George Engle.°

I. Concepts and principles related to grief:
A. Cause of grief: reaction to loss (real or imaginary, actual or pending).
B. Healing process can be interrupted.
C. Grief is universal.
D. Uncomplicated grief is a self-limiting process.
E. Grief responses may vary in degree and kind (e.g., absence of grief, delayed grief, and unresolved grief).
F. People go through stages similar to stages of death

described by Elisabeth Kübler-Ross. (See Death and Dying—Stages and Phases, p. 40.)

G. Many factors influence successful outcome of grieving process:
1. The more *dependent* the person on the lost relationship, the greater the difficulty in resolving the loss.
2. A *child* has greater difficulty resolving loss.
3. A person with *few meaningful relationships* also has greater difficulty.
4. The *more losses* the person has had in the past, the most affected that person will be, as losses tend to be cumulative.
5. The more *sudden* the loss, the greater the difficulty in resolving it.
6. The more *ambivalence* (love-hate feelings, with guilt) there was toward the dead, the more difficult the resolution.
7. *Loss of a child* is harder to resolve than loss of an older person.

▶ II. Assessment—characteristic stages of grief responses:
A. Shock and disbelief (initial and recurrent stage)
1. *Denial* of reality. ("No, it can't be.")
2. Stunned, *numb* feeling.
3. Feelings of loss, *helplessness*, impotence.
4. Intellectual acceptance.

B. Developing awareness
1. Anguish about loss.
   a. *Somatic* distress.
   b. Feelings of emptiness.
2. *Anger* and hostility toward person or circumstances held responsible.
3. Guild feelings—may lead to self-destructive actions.
4. Tears (inwardly, alone; or inability to cry).

C. Restitution
1. Funeral *rituals* are an aid to grief resolution by emphasizing the reality of death.
2. Expression and sharing of feelings by gathered family and friends are a source of acknowledgment of grief and support for the bereaved.

D. Resolving the loss
1. Inreased *dependency* on others as an attempt to deal with painful void.
2. More aware of own *bodily sensations*—may be identical with symptoms of the deceased.
3. Complete *preoccupation* with thoughts and memories of the dead person.

E. Idealization
1. All hostile and negative feelings about the dead are *repressed.*
2. Mourner may *assume* qualities and attributes of the dead.
3. Gradual lessening of preoccupation with the dead; *reinvesting* in others.

▶ III. Analysis/nursing diagnosis—Table 2.7
▶ IV. Nursing care plan/implementation in grief states:
A. *Apply crisis theory and interventions.*
B. *Demonstrate unconditional respect* for cultural, religious, and social mourning customs.

°Adapted from Engle G. Grief and grieving. *Am J Nurs* 9(64):93–98, 1964.

TABLE 2.7 ◄ ANALYSIS/NURSING DIAGNOSIS: *ALTERED FEELING STATES* RELATED TO GRIEF

Problem Classification	Characteristics
1. Somatic distress	Occurs in waves lasting from 20 min to 1 hr
	Deep, sighing respirations most common when discussing grief
	Lack of strength
	Loss of appetite and sense of taste
	Tightness in throat
	Choking sensation accompanied by shortness of breath
2. Preoccupation with image of deceased	Similar to daydreaming
	May mistake others for deceased person
	May be oblivious to surroundings
	Slight sense of unreality
	Fear that he or she is becoming "insane"
3. Feelings of guilt	Accuses self of negligence
	Exaggerates existence and importance of negative thoughts, feelings, and actions toward deceased
	Views self as having failed deceased—"If I had only . . ."
4. Feelings of hostility	Irritability, anger, and loss of warmth toward others
	May attempt to handle feelings of hostility in formalized and stiff manner of social interaction
5. Loss of patterns of conduct	Inability to initiate or maintain organized patterns of activity
	Restlessness, with aimless movements
	Loss of zest—tasks and activities are carried on as though with great effort
	Activities formerly carried on in company of deceased have lost their significance
	May become strongly dependent on whoever stimulates him or her to activity

Source: Wilson HS, Kneisl CR. *Psychiatric Nursing* (3rd ed). Redwood City, CA: Addison-Wesley, 1988. Reprinted by permission.

C. *Utilize knowledge of the stages of grief* to anticipate reactions and facilitate the grief process.
   1. Anticipate and permit expression of different manifestations of shock, disbelief, and denial.
      a. News of impending death is best communicated to a family group (rather than an individual) in a private setting.
      b. *Let mourners see the dead or dying*, to help them accept reality.
      c. Encourage description of circumstances and nature of loss.
   2. *Accept guilt, anger, and rage* as a common response to coping with guilt and helplessness.
      a. Be aware of potential suicide by the bereaved.
   3. Mobilize social support system; promote hospital policy that allows gathering of friends and family in a private setting.
   4. Allow dependency on staff for initial decision making while person is attempting to resolve loss.
   5. Respond to somatic complaints.
   6. Permit reminiscence.
   7. Encourge mourner to relate accounts connected with the lost relationship that reflect positive and negative feelings and remembrances; *place loss in perspective.*
   8. Begin to encourage and reinforce new interests and social relations with others by the end of the idealization stage, loosen bonds of attachment.
   9. Identify high-risk persons for maladaptive responses. (Many factors influence successful outcome of grieving process; see **I(G),** p. 41.)
   10. *Health teaching:*

a. Explain that emotional response is appropriate and common.
b. Explain and offer hope that emotional pain will diminish with time.
c. Describe normal grief stages.

 V. Evaluation/outcome criteria: outcome may take 1 year or more—can remember comfortably and realistically both pleasurable and disappointing aspects of the lost relationship.
  A. Can express feelings of sorrow caused by loss.
  B. Can describe ambivalence (love, anger) toward lost person, relationship.
  C. Able to review relationship, including pleasures, regrets, etc.
  D. Bonds of attachment are loosened and new object relationships are established.

💡 Study and Memory Aid

Stages of dying—"DAB DA"

Denial
Anger
Bargaining

Depression
Acceptance

Source: Rogers PT. *The Medical Student's Guide to Top Board Scores.* Boston: Little, Brown, 1996. P 44.

🔑 Summary of Key Points

Body Image

An individual's body image can indicate degree of *ego strength* and personality integration; vague, distorted self-concept may indicate schizophrenic processes. Any situation, *illness,* or *injury* that causes a change in body image is a crisis; the person will go through the *phases of crisis* in an attempt to reintegrate the body image.

Alterations in Self-Concept

Self-concept problems can result in *disturbed interpersonal relationships* (e.g., passive-dependent, exploitative, demeaning), *phobias, obsessions, withdrawal* from reality (delusional, suspicious), *ambivalence* (procrastination), physical complaints (*psychosomatic*), and *self-destructive behaviors* (e.g., substance abuse).

Glossary

Alterations in Self-Concept

body image The internalized perception of past and current (conscious and unconscious) views, attitudes, and feelings that an individual has toward the size, appearance, and function of own body and its parts.

depersonalization A disintegration of self-concept, in which the individual has a feeling of unreality and strangeness about his or her body.

identity confusion Unclear and inconsistent view of self.

narcissism Self-absorption, with exaggerated self-importance.

role conflict Incompatible, incongruent, confusing demands about appropriate behavior, which cause frustration.

self-actualization The process of reaching one's own potential.

self-concept A composite of all views, ideas, attitudes, and beliefs an individual has about him- or herself, based on value systems that develop primarily as a result of responses from significant others, which in turn affect interpersonal relationships.

self-esteem An individual's own view of self-worth based on how closely behavior approximates the "ideal self."

self-system A term from Sullivan's interpersonal theory that refers to the self as seen by the individual.

Sexuality

bisexuality Sexual attraction to both sexes.

dyspareunia Painful intercourse, often due to physical causes (e.g., pelvic disorders, infections, lack of lubrication). Pain may be recurrent or persistent before, during, or after intercourse.

Sexuality/Sexual Health Counseling

Nursing focus:

- Decrease fear, guilt, and ignorance.
- Minimize stress factors (myths, stereotypes, negative attitudes) to help develop adaptive and satisfying patterns of sexual expression.
- Understand effects of physical illness on sexual performance.

Death and Dying, Bereavement

Nursing implications:

- *Unconditional* respect for cultural, religious, social, and personal expressions of grief.
- Utilize knowledge of stages of dying/grief to *anticipate* reactions and *facilitate grief process.*

gender identity   The sex role assigned at birth; a sense of personal identity that is feminine, masculine, or ambivalent.

heterosexuality   Erotic attraction to the opposite sex.

homosexuality   Erotic attraction to the same sex; may be an emotional preference; is part of one's identity.

masturbation   Obtaining sexual satisfaction from manual stimulation of the genitals, in either sex. The act may be for the purpose of erotic stimulation, a conscious expression of hostility, or an expression of anxiety.

sexual response cycle   Cycle involving *five phases:* sexual desire, excitement, plateau, orgasm, and resolution (refractory period).

transsexualism   Discomfort with one's sex, with feelings of "being trapped in the wrong body."

vaginismus   An alteration in sexual functioning; recurrent or persistent involuntary vaginal muscle spasm (outer third of the vagina), making intercourse painful or impossible.

Death and Dying

grief   A universal response of sadness to loss (real or imagined, actual or impending); e.g., loss of a body part, relationship, employment, object, or concept.

mourning   All of the psychological processes used to resolve a loss.

unresolved grief   Delayed or prolonged reaction to loss. May result in depression.

Questions

1. A young adult accident victim with a T-5 injury had a laminectomy with a spinal fusion. When told by the doctor that she will need supportive devices in order to walk, the patient reacted with verbal abuse and uncooperativeness. How would the nurse explain this behavior to a colleague who finds it difficult to care for this patient?
   1. The patient is blaming others for her problems.
   2. The patient is trying to get others angry with her as a form of punishment for her injury.
   3. The patient cannot handle the lengthy rehabilitation ahead.
   4. The patient is beginning to exhibit early stages of adjustment to a body image crisis.

2. The nurse bases a nursing care plan on the knowledge that body image is the:
   1. Conscious attitude the individual has toward his or her body.
   2. Sum of the conscious and unconscious attitudes the person has toward his or her body.
   3. Image the person sees of himself or herself in the mirror.
   4. Attitude others have about an individual's body.

3. Several days after admission to the chemical dependency unit, the patient is scheduled to attend group therapy. The patient says, "I'm not going. I know everyone thinks I'm a basket case already." Which type of alteration in self-concept best describes this patient's problem?
   1. Depersonalization.

2. Distorted body image.
3. Low self-esteem.
4. Role ambiguity.

4. In primary sex health intervention, what is the nurse's major task?
   1. Identifying sexual problems.
   2. Referring patients to other health care providers.
   3. Providing education to individuals who are uninformed or misinformed about the nature of human sexuality.
   4. Providing follow-up therapy after initial treatment for sexual dysfunction.

5. In conducting a nursing history of a preadolescent or adolescent, what consideration should the nurse give to masturbation?
   1. Masturbation is indicative of homosexual behavior.
   2. Masturbation is abnormal.
   3. Masturbation is harmful to self-image.
   4. Masturbation is normal.

6. In doing a complete assessment of an elderly patient, the nurse would include assessing sexual activity. What would be an accurate statement regarding sexual activity in the elderly?
   1. Activity and interest decrease faster in men than women.
   2. Activity and interest decrease after 50 years of age.
   3. Activity and interest are continuous.
   4. Activity and interest are dependent on what others consider normal and age-appropriate.

7. In response to a colleague's concern about masturbation, which statement by the nurse is most accurate?
   1. It is unhealthy because it prevents a person from acknowledging the function of his or her sexual organs.
   2. It is a healthy and appropriate sexual activity that enables a person to consolidate his or her own sexual identity.
   3. It prevents a person from enjoying heterosexual sexual activity.
   4. It is an unhealthy and inappropriate sexual activity that confuses a person's sexual identity.

8. What is the most important priority in providing nursing care for a patient with a terminal illness?
   1. Physical comfort.
   2. Medications to reduce pain.
   3. Prevention of pressure sores.
   4. Encouraging unlimited visits from family and friends.

9. The nurse would determine that grief counseling with a patient following the death of a spouse was not effective when the patient makes which comment at the last session?
   1. "I would like to continue with these interesting sessions."
   2. "I like trying to do different things to feel better."
   3. "I don't like to sleep too much any more."
   4. "I went to the movies with my neighbor."

Answers/Rationale

1. **(1)** Noncompliance and anger are characteristic stages of reactions to changes in mobility, which is an important

part of body image. There are insufficient data to support **Nos. 3** and **4. No. 2** is inappropriate because it is an interpretation that is too analytical, without validation. **AN, 7, PsI**

2. **(2)** This is the *most complete* description of body image. The others (**Nos. 1, 3,** and **4**) are only *partial* descriptions. **AN, 2, HPM**

💡 *Test-taking tip:* **No. 2** is an example of an "umbrella" answer, which covers all the other partial answers.

3. **(3)** The patient is projecting his or her own feelings of worthlessness. Depersonalization (**No. 1**) refers to feelings of unreality about one's body. Distorted body image (**No. 2**) refers to distorted perceptions about one's body. Role ambiguity (**No. 4**) is the lack of knowledge of specific role expectations. **AN, 7, PsI**

4. **(3)** Providing information is the *primary* sex health intervention. **Nos. 1** and **2** are *secondary* health interventions. **No. 4** is a *tertiary* intervention. **PL, 7, HPM**

💡 *Test-taking tip:* Note the key word in the question: "primary"; this question asks for the *primary* intervention (**No. 3**).

5. **(4)** Masturbation is a normal process by which tension is released and sexual discovery occurs. Masturbation can be part of both homosexual (**No. 1**) *and* heterosexual behaviors. Abnormal (**No. 2**) and harmful (**No. 3**) are op-

---

Key to Codes

Nursing process: AS = Assessment; **AN** = Analysis; **PL** = Planning; **IMP** = Implementation; **EV** = Evaluation. (See Appendix E for explanation of nursing process steps.)

Category of human function: 1 = Protective; **2** = Sensory-Perceptual; **3** = Comfort, Rest, Activity, and Mobility; **4** = Nutrition; **5** = Growth and Development; **6** = Fluid-Gas Transport; **7** = Psychosocial-Cultural; **8** = Elimination. (See Appendix G for explanation.)

Client need: SECE = Safe, Effective Care Environment; **PhI** = Physiologic Integrity; **PsI** = Psychosocial Integrity; **HPM** = Health Promotion/Maintenance. (See Appendix H for explanation.)

posites of the correct answer, and are therefore incorrect. **EV, 7, HPM**

6. **(3)** Studies support the fact that some form of sexual activity, and certainly interest, continue in the elderly, into the 80s or 90s. There are no research data to support **Nos. 1** and **2**. While sexual activity *may* be influenced by the reactions of others (peers and community) as to what is age-appropriate (**No. 4**), the elderly individual's sexual interest and activity are more realistically dependent on *opportunities* for sexual expression and age-related *physical limitations.* **AS, 7, HPM**

7. **(2)** Masturbation is an appropriate sexual activity that enables a person to become comfortable with his or her sexual identity. Masturbation *can* be healthy (**No. 1**) and *can enhance* heterosexual activity (**No. 3**). **No. 4** is the *opposite* of the correct response. **IMP, 7, HPM**

💡 *Test-taking tip:* Look at patterns: in this case, three options are "unhealthy"; one option (**No. 2**) is "healthy." When in doubt, consider the option that is not like the others.

8. **(1)** Physical comfort is the priority in nursing care of a terminally ill patient. Other important aspects of care are covered by providing physical comfort: giving pain medications (**No. 2**) is one way to enhance physical comfort; skin care and positioning to prevent pressure sores (**No. 3**) is another. Encouraging visitors (**No. 4**) is not always appropriate. The terminally ill patient may not want unlimited visitors, especially during the disengagement phase of dying. **PL, 5, HPM**

9. **(1)** For an intervention to be effective, the patient needs to be self-reliant in coping with problems; this statement is an example of continuing *dependence* on the nurse. To help the person handle anxiety and cope with problems on his or her own; the nurse needs to explore the patient's feelings of dependence. The other statements (**Nos. 2, 3,** and **4**) are examples of *desired* self-reliance, *not* trying out new coping behaviors for self-help. **EV, 7, HPM**

Assessment Tools

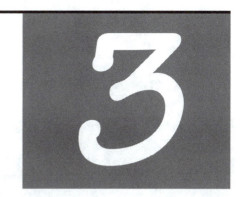

Chapter Outline

Mental Status Assessment

I. Components of mental status exam
  A. Appearance—appropriate dress, grooming, facial expression, stereotyped movements, mannerisms, rigidity.
  B. Behavior—anxiety level, congruence with situation, cooperativeness, openness, hostility, reaction to interview, consistency.
  C. Speech characteristics—relevance (*circumstantiality*), coherence, meaning (e.g., *neologism*), repetitiveness, qualitative (*what* is said), quantitative (*how much* is said), abnormalities, inflections, affectations, congruence with level of education, impediments, tone quality.
  D. Mood or affect—appropriateness, intensity, hostility turned inward or toward others, duration, swings.
  E. Thought content—delusions (e.g., *nihilistic*), hallucinations, obsessive ideas, phobic ideas, themes, areas of concern, self-concept.
  F. Thought processes—organization and association of ideas (e.g., *blocking, flight of ideas, word salad*), coherence, ability to abstract and understand symbols.
  G. Sensorium
    1. *Orientation* to person, time and place, situation.
    2. *Memory*—immediate, rote, remote, and recent.
    3. *Attention and concentration*—susceptibility to distraction.
    4. *Information and intelligence*—account of general knowledge, history, and reasoning powers.
    5. *Comprehension*—concrete and abstract.
    6. *Stage of consciousness*—alert/awake, somnolent, lethargic, delirious, stuporous, comatose.
  H. Insight and judgment
    1. Extent to which client sees self as having problems, needing treatment.
    2. Client awareness of intrapsychic nature of own difficulties.
    3. Soundness of judgment.

Individual Assessment

Consider the following (Table 3.1):

  I. Physical and intellectual factors.
  II. Socioeconomic factors.
  III. Personal values and goals.
  IV. Adaptive functioning and response to present involvement.
  V. Developmental factors.

Family Assessment: Response to Chronic Illness

See also Chap. 4, Family Therapy, III. Family assessment, p. 60.

Table 3.1   ⋈ Individual Assessment

Physical and Intellectual Factors

1. Presence of physical illness and/or disability
2. Appearance and energy level
3. Current and potential levels of intellectual functioning
4. How client sees personal world, translates events around self; client's perceptual abilities
5. Cause and effect reasoning, ability to focus

Socioeconomic Factors

1. Economic factors—level of income, adequacy of subsistence; how this affects life-style, sense of adequacy, self-worth
2. Employment and attitudes about it
3. Racial, cultural, and ethnic identification; sense of identity and belonging
4. Religious identification and link to significant value systems, norms, and practices

Personal Values and Goals

1. Presence or absence of congruence between values and their expression in action; meaning of values to individual
2. Congruence between individual's values and goals and the immediate systems with which client interacts
3. Congruence between individual's values and assessor's values; meaning of this for intervention process

Adaptive Functioning and Response to Present Involvement

1. Manner in which individual presents self to others—grooming, appearance, posture
2. Emotional tone and change or constancy of levels
3. Style of communication—verbal and nonverbal; ability to express appropriate emotion, follow train of thought; factors of dissonance, confusion, uncertainty
4. Symptoms or symptomatic behavior
5. Quality of relationship individual seeks to establish—direction, purposes, and uses of such relationships for individual
6. Perception of self
7. Social roles that are assumed or ascribed; competence in fulfilling these roles
8. Relational behavior:
   a. Capacity for intimacy
   b. Dependence-independence balance
   c. Power and control conflicts
   d. Exploitiveness
   e. Openness

Developmental Factors

1. Role performance equated with life stage
2. How developmental experiences have been interpreted and used
3. How individual has dealt with past conflicts, tasks, and problems (premorbid personality)
4. Uniqueness of present problem in life experience

Source: Wilson HS, Kneisl CR. *Psychiatric Nursing* (2nd ed). Menlo Park, CA: Addison-Wesley, 1983. Pp 204–205. Reprinted by permission.

⋈ **I. Assessment:** Accurate assessment is basic to helping families and children cope with *chronic illness*. The assessment model presented here will help the nurse to identify strengths and deficiencies in order to develop intervention strategies.
  A. Feelings generated, and how they are dealt with; e.g., fears about permanent loss.
  B. Adequacy of adaptive resources and support for all members.
  C. Ability to cope with changes in life-style, financial demands, and alterations in *roles* and *relationships*.
  D. Reactions:
    1. *Denial*—to cushion feelings related to loss: to protect from confronting full implication of the diagnosis all at once.
    2. *Depression* and *despair*—as reality replaces denial, and family becomes overburdened by extra responsibilities.
    3. *Anger* and *protest*—related to understanding the ramifications of the illness, deprivation,

fears, inconveniences, and burdens imposed by the illness and its treatment.
    4. *Guilt*—related to the anger and the cause of illness; blame may be placed on other family members.
    5. *Helplessness*—related to inability to alleviate suffering.
    6. *Frustration*—related to abandoned dreams.
⋈ **II. Analysis/nursing diagnosis:** *Ineffective family coping* related to illness/disability of a family member, with difficulty in seeing entire situation objectively.
⋈ **III. Nursing care plan:**
  A. Assist patient and family to cope effectively with the grieving process (loss).
  B. Determine how each family member *perceives* and is affected by the illness; the areas of strength; and the areas of weakness in which each family member needs support and intervention in trying to cope.
  C. Assist the patient and family to develop ways of

coping effectively with the change in body image, roles, relationships, and life-style.

  D. Help patient and family participate actively in the treatment, without guilt, possessiveness, overprotectiveness, or withdrawal.

  E. Help patient and family integrate the *loss* of:
1. Well-being (health).
2. Independence (dependency conflict).
3. Familiar surroundings (frequent hospitalizations).
4. Comfort (e.g., pain, immobility).
5. Physical function (e.g., weakness, sexual dysfunction).
6. Mental function (e.g., cognitive and affective dysfunction, memory and language impairment, confusion).
7. Familiar appearance (change in body image).
8. Roles in society and family.
9. Self-concept.

  F. Increase communication.

  G. Decrease isolation, guilt, depression, and anxiety.

IV. Implementation:

  A. Assess interaction between patient and family, being alert for potentially destructive behaviors (e.g., withdrawal, neglect, abuse, overprotectiveness).

  B. Encourage verbalization of feelings in appropriate ways.

  C. Encourage family to participate in patient's care; teach family the skills required for care.

  D. Implement counseling for the family as a system in:
1. Allocation of resources (money, space, time).
2. Rearranging division of labor among family members.
3. Giving and receiving affection.
4. Limit-setting and consistency.
5. Understanding feelings generated by disruption of family life.
   a. How various members express these feelings, especially children's fears and fantasies.
   b. How each may be supported in their resolution.
6. Conflict resolution.

V. Evaluation/outcome criteria:

  A. Family members acknowledge change in family roles.

  B. Family members identify coping patterns.

  C. Family members participate in decision-making processes.

  D. The chronically disabled person who is well-adjusted (i.e., has successfully coped) is more likely to:
1. Develop feelings of competence (rather than withdrawing).
2. Be as independent as possible.
3. Be optimistic (rather than negativistic and irritable).
4. Adhere to treatment plan (rather than "giving up").

5. Have an accepting attitude toward the illness (as opposed to seeing self as different and blaming others for the illness).

Cultural Assessment*

I. Knowledge of ethnic beliefs and cultural practices can assist the nurse in the planning and implementation of holistic care.

II. Consider the following aspects of cultural assessment (highlighted in Table 3.2):

  A. *Demographic data:* Is this an "ethnic neighborhood"?

  B. *Socioeconomic status:* occupation, education (formal and informal), income level; who is employed?

  C. *Ethnic/racial orientation:* ethnic identity, value orientation (see Table 3.2).

  D. *Country of origin:* date of immigration; where were the family members born? Where has the family lived?

  E. *Languages spoken:* does family speak English? Language and dialect preferences (see Table 3.2).

  F. *Communication patterns:* social customs, nonverbal behaviors.

  G. Communication barriers between nurse and client:
1. Differences in language.
2. Technical languages.
3. Inappropriate place for discussion.
4. Personality or gender of the nurse.
5. Distrust of the nurse.
6. Time-orientation differences.
7. Differences in pain perception and expression.
8. Variable attitudes toward death and dying.

  H. *Family relationships:* What are the formal roles? Who makes the decisions within the family? What are the family life-style and living arrangements?

  I. *Degree of acculturation* of family members: How are the family customs and beliefs similar to or different from the dominant culture?

  J. *Religious preferences:* What role do beliefs, rituals, and taboos play in health and illness? Is there a significant religious person who is influential (e.g., priest, rabbi, nun, pastor, etc.)? Are there any dietary symbolisms or preferences or restrictions due to religious beliefs?

  K. *Cultural practices related to health and illness* (see Table 3.2): Does the family use folk medicine practices or a folk healer? Are there specific dietary practices related to health and illness?

  L. *Support systems:* Do extended family members provide support?

  M. *Health beliefs:* response to pain and hospitalization; disease predisposition and resistance.

  N. Other significant factors related to ethnic identity: What health care facilities does the family use?

*Adapted from Ross B, Cobb KL. *Family Nursing.* Redwood City, CA: Addison-Wesley, 1990. Reprinted by permission.

Table 3.2 ⋈ Family Assessment: Cultural Profile

Communication Style

1. Language and dialect preference (understand concept, meaning of pain, fever, nausea)
2. Nonverbal behaviors (meaning of bowing, touching, speaking softly, smiling, gestures)
3. Social customs (acting agreeable or pleasant to avoid the unpleasant, embarrassing)

Orientation

1. Ethnic identity and adherence to traditional habits and values
2. Acculturation: extent
3. Value orientations—variables:
   a. *Human nature:* evil, good, or both
   b. *Relationship between humans and nature:* subjugated, harmony, or mastery
   c. *Time:* past, present, future
   d. *Purpose of life:* being, becoming, or doing
   e. *Relationship to one another:* lineal, collateral, or individualistic

Nutrition

1. Symbolism of food
2. Preferences, taboos

Family Relationships

1. Role and position of women, men, aged, boys, girls
2. Decision-making styles/areas: finances, childrearing, health care
3. Family: nuclear, extended, or tribal
4. Matriarchal or patriarchal
5. Life-style, living arrangements (crowded; urban/rural; ethnic neighborhood or mixed)

Health Beliefs

1. Alternative *health care:* self-care, folk medicine; cultural healer: herbalist, medicine man, curandero
2. Health crisis and illness beliefs concerning *causation:* germ theory, maladaptation, stress, evil spirits, ying/yang imbalance, envy and hate
3. *Response to pain, hospitalization:* stoic endurance, loud cries, quiet withdrawal
4. Disease predisposition—selected examples:
   a. *African Americans:* sickle cell anemia, CVD/CVA and hypertension; high infant mortality, diabetes
   b. *Asians:* lactose intolerance, myopia
   c. *Hispanics:* cardiovascular, diabetes, cancer, obesity, substance abuse, TB, AIDS, suicide, homicide
   d. *Native Americans:* high infant and maternal mortality, cirrhosis, fetal alcohol abnormalities, pancreatitis, malnutrition, TB, alcoholism
   e. *Jews:* Tay-Sachs

Key: CVD/CVA = cerebrovascular disease/cerebrovascular accident; TB = tuberculosis.

Adapted from Fong C. Ethnicity and nursing practice. *Topics in Clinical Nursing* 7(3):4, 1985. Pp 1–10. With permission of Aspen Publishers, Inc., Aspen Systems Corp., Rockville, MD. Copyright © 1985 Aspen Publishers, Inc.

Interviewing

I. **Definition:** Interviewing is a goal-directed method of communicating facts, feelings, and meanings. For interviewing to be successful, interaction between the two persons involved must be effective.

II. **Nine principles for verbal interaction**
   A. *Client's initiative*—let client begin the discussion.
   B. *Indirect approach*—move from the periphery to the core.
   C. *Open-ended* statements—use open-ended statements (incomplete forms of statements such as "You were saying . . .") to prompt rather than close off an exchange.
   D. *Minimal verbal activity*—limit speaking in order not to obstruct thought process and client's responses.
   E. *Spontaneity*—be flexible and let content direct flow of interview rather than having fixed interview topics; may bring out much more relevant data.

   F. *Facilitate expression of feelings* to help assess events and reactions by asking, for example, "What was that like for you?"
   G. *Focus on emotional areas* about which client may be in conflict, as noted by repetitive themes.
   H. *Pick up cues, clues, and signals* from client, such as facial expressions and gestures, behavior, emphatic tones, and flushed face.
   I. *Introduce material related to content* already brought up by client; do not bring in a tangential focus from "left field."

III. **Purpose and goals of interviewing**
   A. *Initiate and maintain a positive nurse-client relationship,* which can decrease symptoms, lessen demands, and move client toward optimum health when nurse demonstrates understanding and sharing of client's concerns.
   B. *Determine client's view of nurse's role* in order to utilize it or change it.
   C. *Collect information on emotional crisis* to plan goals and approaches in order to increase effectiveness of nursing interventions.

D. *Identify and resolve crisis;* the act of eliciting cause or antecedent event may in itself be therapeutic.

E. *Channel feelings directly* by exploring interrelated events, feelings, and behaviors in order to discourage displacement of feelings onto somatic and behavioral symptoms.

F. *Channel communication* and transfer significant information to the physician and other team members.

G. *Prepare for health teaching* in order to help the client function as effectively as possible.

 ## Study and Memory Aid

Mental status exam

Primary: judgment, orientation, memory; then **"STA⁴T":**

Speech **"RATE"** $\begin{cases} \textbf{R}\text{ate} \\ \textbf{A}\text{mount} \\ \textbf{T}\text{one} \\ \textbf{E}\text{cholalia} \end{cases}$

Thought processes (flight of ideas, loose associations, tangential, circumstantiality, blocking)

A⁴ $\begin{cases} \textbf{A}\text{ttitude} \\ \textbf{A}\text{ppearance} \\ \textbf{A}\text{ctivity} \\ \textbf{A}\text{ffect} \end{cases}$

Thought content (suicidal, homicidal, obsessive, delusional)

Source: Adapted from Rogers PT. *The Medical Student's Guide to Top Board Scores.* Boston: Little, Brown, 1996. P 42.

Summary of Key Points

Mental Status Assessment

Six major categories of data to collect:

• General observations (e.g., appearance)
• Sensorium and intelligence (e.g., level of consciousness (LOC), orientation, memory, judgment, intellectual function, comprehension)
• Thought processes (e.g., form, content)
• Affect (e.g., appropriateness, intensity)
• Mood (e.g., suicidal or homicidal ideation or plan)
• Insight (e.g., client aware of own problems and difficulties?)

Individual Assessment

Categories:

• Physical and *intellectual* factors
• Socioeconomic factors (life-style, identification and belonging)
• Personal values and goals (assess for congruency)
• *Adaptive functioning and response* (most emphasis)
• Developmental factors

Family Assessment: Response to Chronic Illness

Nursing implications:

• Identify ethnic and cultural beliefs and practices.

• Assess family "rules," roles, and relationships (e.g., subsystems like coalitions and triangles), family communication styles, patterns, and themes.
• Assess perception of problems and solutions.
• View family as a system.

Cultural Assessment

Nursing implications:

• *Avoid:* polysyllabic or overly technical words; overload (too much information; speaking too fast) or "underload" (will lose attention if too slow); "buzz words" or jargon; loud or slurred speech.
• *Use* gestures with shared meanings; drawings. Observe and validate meaning of client's gestures.

Interviewing

• Purpose is to establish rapport and get data about patient; prepare for health teaching.
• Review principles for verbal interview (patient-focused; move from periphery to core; open-ended; minimal speaking by nurse; spontaneity; focus on expression of feelings and emotional areas; pick up clues from patient; avoid tangents).

Glossary

Mental Status Assessment

affect   Mood tone, feeling, emotion (e.g., labile, flat, blunt, inappropriate).

blocking   Sudden, inexplicable interruption in a stream of thought that may be a result of delusional, hallucinatory, or conflict-producing experience.

circumstantiality   A pattern of extraneous thinking and speaking, involving too many unnecessary details and digressions before getting to the main point. In some cases, it may serve to avoid an emotionally charged area.

delusion   False *belief* system that cannot be refuted by logic or dispelled by humor (e.g., persistent belief that one's phone lines are tapped without objective proof); may be delusions of *grandeur* ("I am famous") or delusions of *persecution* ("Everyone is out to get me").

disorientation   Loss of awareness of the position of self in relation to time, place, or person.

flight of ideas   A thought disorder in which one topic moves rapidly to another without reaching a main idea or point, as in manic behavior. The next sentence may be triggered by a word in the previous sentence or by something in the environment; phrases may also be connected by rhymes.

hallucination   A false impression that affects the *senses,* without external stimuli; can be auditory, visual, tactile, olfactory, or gustatory (e.g., hearing voices, seeing snakes, feeling creepy spiders, smelling rotting flesh, tasting excreta).

illusion   Misinterpretation of a real, external sensory stimulus (e.g., seeing a shadow on the floor and thinking it is a hole).

labile   Unstable and rapidly shifting (used to describe emotions).

neologism   A made-up word or expression that does not have shared meaning with other people.

nihilistic delusion   False belief of nonexistence of self, part of self, or someone else (e.g., "I have no cranium").

premorbid personality   State of an individual's personality *before* the onset of illness.

word salad   Nonsensical linkage of words and phrases.

Questions

1. As part of a psychiatric nursing assessment, the nurse asks the patient to subtract 7 from 100. What aspect of the mental status examination is being tested?
   1. Ability to concentrate. ✓
   2. Abstract thinking.
   3. General intellectual level.
   4. Memory.
2. The nurse uses the proverb, "Don't cry over spilled milk," to evaluate the patient's ability to think abstractly. Which explanation by the patient would best demonstrate this ability?
   1. "Even if you spill your milk, you shouldn't cry."
   2. "What's done is done; don't get hung up on what's ended or gone." ✓
   3. "Crying won't keep the milk from spilling."
   4. "You can't keep the milk from spilling."
3. An elderly patient calls a lamp "Albert." The nurse knows that this is an example of:
   1. Hallucination.
   2. Delusion.
   3. Illusion. ✓
   4. Sensory overload.
4. During an assessment interview, the patient frequently switches topics while giving a chronology related to his psychiatric illness, although the nurse can still follow the patient's thought pattern. The nurse should assess this pattern of thinking as:
   1. Tangential thinking.
   2. Circumstantiality.
   3. Flight of ideas.
   4. Word salad.
5. During an assessment interview, the patient seems preoccupied, has an inappropriate affect, grimaces, and does not maintain eye contact. What might these behaviors indicate to the nurse?
   1. Auditory hallucinations.
   2. Loose associations.
   3. Phobic behavior.
   4. Flight of ideas.
6. What is most important to assess in a patient who is depressed?
   1. Plans for self-destruction. ✓
   2. Depth of the depression.
   3. Current medication regimen.
   4. History of previous episodes of depression.
7. What characteristic of dysfunctional families should the nurse look for during the assessment interview?
   1. Discussion of conflictual issues.
   2. Definition of family members' roles (who does what, when, where, and how).
   3. Enmeshment or disengagement. ✓
   4. Synergy.
8. In doing a cultural assessment, what are the most important data that the nurse needs to obtain?
   1. The patient's perception of cultural beliefs and values. ✓
   2. The beliefs and values held by the patient's family.
   3. The beliefs and values inherent in the patient's religious group affiliation.
   4. The beliefs and values of the patient's sociocultural group.

Answers/Rationale

1. **(1)** The ability to subtract 7 from 100, and to continue subtracting 7 from the result as long as possible, is called the "serial 7s test," which is used to assess the ability to concentrate. Abstract thinking (**No. 2**) is often assessed by asking the patient to explain a proverb (e.g., "A rolling stone gathers no moss"). General intellectual level (**No. 3**) is assessed by the person's: ability to *grasp facts* and answer general knowledge questions (e.g., "Name five countries in Europe"); ability to do *calculations* involving simple arithmetic problems; and ability to use *reasoning and judgment* in answering such questions as, "If you had $20,000, what would you do?" A test for

memory (**No. 4**) would include assessing the ability to recall the *recent past* and *remote past, recall and retain details,* and recall themes *immediately* after reading a short story. **AN, 7, PsI**

2. (**2**) This shows the ability to apply a specific image (spilled milk) to a more general concept (implications for coping with the concept of loss). **Nos. 1, 3,** and **4** are all examples of concrete or literal interpretations of the proverb. **AS, 7, PsI**

3. (**3**) By definition, an illusion is a misinterpretation of a *real* external sensory stimulus (e.g., a person may see a shadow on the floor and think it is a hole). Hallucinations (**No. 1**) are altered perceptions that occur when there are no external stimuli. They may be due to chemicals or inner needs, and may affect any of the five senses. A delusion (**No. 2**) refers to a false, fixed *belief* or idea rather than misinterpretation of one's environment. The belief or idea is maintained in spite of evidence or facts, and cannot be changed by logic. **No. 4** is not correct because there is no information in the question to suggest that the distortion of reality is due to excessive stimulation of the visual or auditory senses. **AN, 2, PsI**

4. (**3**) The behavior describes loose thought patterns that still have some connections. In tangential thinking (**No. 1**), the thoughts appear to be related, but the main point is not easy to discern. With circumstantial thought patterns (**No. 2**), the person talks all around the topic, with inclusion of a great deal of irrelevant information. Word

salad (**No. 4**) describes a pattern in which there are no apparent logical connections. **AS, 7, PsI**

5. (**1**) The behaviors described indicate that the patient is probably hearing voices; the nurse must next validate this by checking with the patient. Loose associations (**No. 2**) are characterized by speech patterns in which one thought does not relate to another. Phobic behavior (**No. 3**) is driven by severe anxiety, as a response to a specific stressor/stimulus. Flight of ideas (**No. 4**) is characterized by speech patterns in which the patient jumps from one thought to another. **AN, 7, PsI**

6. (**1**) A *direct* approach is needed, in order to be able to intervene in possible plans for suicide. **No. 2** is of a lesser importance, and may also be covered in **No. 1**: in response to the nurse's assessment of any plans for self-destruction, the extent of hopeless, helpless, and worthless feelings may come through. **No. 3** is a *part* of assessing the patient's current status, but it is not an active, direct intervention for a suicide risk. **No. 4** focuses on the *past* (note the words, "history" and "previous"). In assessing depression and possible suicide risk, the focus needs to be on the *here and now.* **AS, 7, PsI**

Test-taking tip: Look for a "telescope" answer—one that incorporates another. In this case, **No. 2** can be included in **No. 1**.

7. (**3**) The definition of enmeshment is *over*involvement of family members, interfering with development of each member's autonomy. Disengagement means *under*involvement of family members, leading to isolation of individual members. **Nos. 1, 2,** and **4** are all characteristics of *functional* families. Synergy (**No. 4**) means cooperative action among family members. **AS, 7, PsI**

8. (**1**) The patient's perceptions are the most significant because they have the most direct, *ultimate* influence on behavior. **Nos. 2, 3,** and **4** all *play a role* in the patient's *perception.* **AS, 7, PsI**

Test-taking tip: This is an example of a "telescope" answer; when several options are subsumed by (or lead to) another option, choose the most inclusive option (i.e., the ultimate result or, in this case, the ultimate influence).

Key to Codes

Nursing process: AS = Assessment; **AN** = Analysis; **PL** = Planning; **IMP** = Implementation; **EV** = Evaluation. (See Appendix E for explanation of nursing process steps.)

Category of human function: 1 = Protective; **2** = Sensory-Perceptual; **3** = Comfort, Rest, Activity, and Mobility; **4** = Nutrition; **5** = Growth and Development; **6** = Fluid-Gas Transport; **7** = Psychosocial-Cultural; **8** = Elimination. (See Appendix G for explanation.)

Client need: SECE = Safe, Effective Care Environment; **PhI** = Physiologic Integrity; **PsI** = Psychosocial Integrity; **HPM** = Health Promotion/Maintenance. (See Appendix H for explanation.)

Psychosocial Treatment Modes

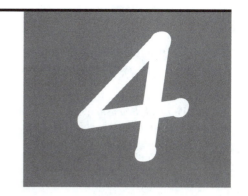

Milieu Therapy

Milieu therapy consists of treatment by means of controlled modification of the client's environment to promote positive living experiences.

I. Concepts and principles related to milieu therapy:
  A. Everything that happens to clients from the time they are admitted to the hospital or treatment setting has a potential that is either therapeutic or antitherapeutic.
    1. Not only the therapists but all who come in contact with the clients in the treatment setting are important to the clients' recovery.
    2. Emphasis is on the social, economic, and cultural dimension, the interpersonal climate, as well as the physical environment.
  B. Clients have the right, privilege, and responsibility to make decisions about daily living activities in the treatment setting.
  C. Indications for milieu therapy: clients with chronic mental illness.

II. Characteristics of milieu therapy:
  A. Friendly, warm, trusting, secure, supportive, comforting atmosphere throughout the unit.
  B. An optimistic attitude about prognosis of illness.
  C. Attention to comfort, food, and daily living needs; help with resolving difficulties related to tasks of daily living.
  D. Opportunity for clients to take responsibility for themselves and for the welfare of the unit in gradual steps.
    1. Client government.
    2. Client-planned and client-directed social activities.
  E. Maximum individualization in dealing with clients, especially regarding treatment and privileges in accordance with clients' needs.
  F. Opportunity to live through and test out situations in a realistic way by providing a setting that is a microcosm of the larger world outside.
  G. Opportunity to discuss interpersonal relationships in the unit among clients and between clients and staff (decreased social distance between staff and clients).
  H. Program of carefully selected resocialization activities to prevent regression.

III. Nursing care plan/implementation in milieu therapy:
  A. *New structured relationships*—allow clients to develop new abilities and use past skills; support them through new experiences as needed; help build liaisons with others; set limits; help clients modify destructive behavior; encourage group solutions to daily living problems.
  B. *Managerial*—inform clients about expectations; preserve orderliness of events.
  C. *Environmental manipulation*—regulate the outside environment to alter daily surroundings.
    1. Move clients to units more conducive to their needs.
    2. Work with families, clergy, employers, etc.

3. Control visitors for the benefit of the client.
   D. *Team approach* uses the milieu to meet each client's needs.
▷ IV. **Evaluation/outcome criteria:**
   A. *Physical dimension:* order, organization.
   B. *Social dimension:* clarity of expectations, practical orientation.
   C. *Emotional dimension:* involvement, support, responsibility, openness, valuing, accepting.

Activity Therapy

Activity therapy consists of a variety of recreational and vocational activities (recreational therapy [RT]; occupational therapy [OT]; music, art, and dance therapy) designed to test and examine social skills and serve as adjunctive therapies.

I. **Concepts and principles** related to activity therapy:
   A. Socialization counters the regressive aspects of illness.
   B. Activities need to be selected for specific psychosocial reasons to achieve specific effects.
   C. Nonverbal means of expression as an additional behavioral outlet add a new dimension to treatment.
   D. Sublimation of sexual drives is possible through activities.
   E. Indications for activity therapy: clients with low self-esteem who are socially unresponsive.
II. **Characteristics** of activity therapy:
   A. Usually planned and coordinated by various team members, e.g., the recreational therapists or music therapists.
   B. Goals:
      1. Encourage socialization in community and social activities.
      2. Provide pleasurable activities.
      3. Help client release tensions and express feelings.
      4. Teach new skills, help client find new hobbies.
      5. Offer graded series of experiences, from passive spectator role and vicarious experiences to more direct and active experiences.
      6. Free and/or strengthen physical and creative abilities.
      7. Increase self-esteem.
▷ III. **Nursing care plan/implementation** in activity therapy:
   A. Encourage, support, and cooperate in client's participation in activities planned by the adjunct therapists.
   B. Share knowledge of client's illness, talents, interests, and abilities with others on the team.
   C. *Health teaching:* teach client necessary skills for each activity (e.g., sports, games, crafts).
▷ IV. **Evaluation/outcome criteria:** client develops occupational and leisure-time skills that will help provide a smoother transition back to the community.

Behavior Modification

Behavior modification is a therapeutic approach involving the application of learning principles so as to change maladaptive behavior.

I. **Definitions:**
   conditioned avoidance (also *aversion* or *aversive therapy*) A technique whereby there is a purposeful and systematic production of strongly unpleasant responses in situations to which the client has been previously attracted but now wishes to avoid.
   desensitization Frequent exposure in small but gradually increasing doses of anxiety-evoking stimuli until undesirable behavior disappears or is lessened (as in phobias).
   operant conditioning A method designed to elicit and reinforce desirable behavior (especially useful in mental retardation).
   positive reinforcement Giving rewards to elicit or strengthen selected behavior or behaviors.
   token economy Desired behavior is reinforced by rewards (e.g., candy, money, verbal approval), used as tokens.

II. **Objectives and process of treatment** in behavior modification:
   A. Emphasis is on changing unacceptable, overt, and observable behavior to that which is acceptable; emphasis is on changed way of *acting* first, not of *thinking.*
   B. Mental health team determines behavior to change and treatment plan to use.
   C. Therapy is based on the knowledge and application of *learning* principles, that is, *stimulus-response;* the unlearning, or *extinction,* of undesirable behavior; and the *reinforcement* of desirable behavior.
   D. Therapist identifies what events are important in the life history of the client and arranges situations in which the client is therapeutically confronted with them.
   E. Two primary aspects of behavior modification:
      1. *Eliminating* unwanted behavior by *negative reinforcement* (removal of an aversive stimulus, which acts to reinforce the behavior that results in removal of the aversive stimulus) and *ignoring* (withholding positive reinforcement).
      2. *Create* acceptable new responses to an environmental stimulus by *positive* reinforcement.
   F. *Useful* with: disturbed children, rape victims, dependent and manipulative behaviors, eating disorders, obsessive-compulsive disorders, sexual dysfunction.
III. **Assumptions** of behavioral therapy:
   A. Behavior is what an organism does.
   B. Behavior can be observed, described, and recorded.
   C. It is possible to predict the conditions under which the same behavior may recur.
   D. Undesirable social behavior is not a symptom of mental illness but is behavior that can be modified.
   E. Undesirable behaviors are learned disorders that relate to acute anxiety in a given situation.
   F. Maladaptive behavior is learned in the same way as adaptive behavior.
   G. People tend to behave in ways that "pay off."

H. *Three ways* in which behavior can be reinforced:
  1. *Positive* reinforcer (adding something pleasurable).
  2. *Negative* reinforcer (removing something unpleasant).
  3. *Adverse* stimuli (punishing).

I. If an undesired behavior is ignored, it will be extinguished.

J. Learning process is the same for all; therefore, all conditions (except organic) are accepted for treatment.

▶ **IV. Nursing care plan/implementation** in behavior modification:
  A. Find out what is a "reward" for the person.
  B. Break the goal down into small, successive *steps*.
  C. Maintain *close* and continual observation of the selected behavior or behaviors.
  D. Be *consistent* with on-the-spot, immediate intervention and correction of undesirable behavior.
  E. Record focused observations of behavior frequently.
  F. Participate in close teamwork with the *entire* staff.
  G. Evaluate procedures and results continually.
  H. *Health teaching*: teach above steps to colleagues and family.

▶ **V. Evaluation/outcome criteria:** acceptable behavior is increased and maintained; undesirable behavior is decreased or eliminated.

Reality Orientation and Resocialization

Table 4.1 outlines the differences between these two modes of therapy.

Group Therapy

Group therapy is a treatment modality in which three or more clients and one or more therapists interact in a helping process to relieve emotional difficulties, increase self-esteem and insight, and improve behavior in relations with others.

I. Concepts and principles related to group therapy:
  A. People's problems usually occur in a social setting; thus they can best be evaluated and corrected in a social setting (Table 4.2).
  B. *Not* all are amenable to group therapies. For example:
    1. Brain-damaged.
    2. Acutely suicidal.
    3. Acutely psychotic.
    4. Persons with very passive-dependent behavior patterns.
    5. Acutely manic.
  C. It is best to match group members not for *complementarity in behaviors* (verbal with nonverbal, withdrawn with outgoing) but for *similarity in problems* (obesity, predischarge group, cancer patients, prenatal group) to facilitate empathy in the

sharing of experiences and to heighten group identification and cohesiveness.

D. Feelings of *acceptance*, belonging, respect, and comfort develop in the group and facilitate change and health.

E. In a group, members can *test reality* by giving and receiving *feedback*.

F. Clients have a chance to experience in the group that they are not alone (concept of *universality*).

G. Expression and *ventilation* of strong emotional feelings (anger, anxiety, fear, and guilt) in the safe setting of a group are an important aspect of the group process aimed at health and change.

H. The group setting and the *interactions* of its members may provide *corrective emotional experiences* for its members. A key mechanism operating in groups is *transference* (strong emotional attachment of one member to another member, to the therapist, and/or to the entire group).

I. To the degree that people modify their behavior through corrective experiences and identification with others rather than through personal-insight analysis, group therapy may be of special advantage over individual therapy in that the possible number of interactions is greater in the group and the patterns of behavior are more readily observable.

J. There is a higher client-to-staff ratio, and it is thus less expensive.

▶ **II. General group goals:**
  A. Provide opportunity for self-expression of ideas and feelings.
  B. Provide a setting for a variety of relationships through group interaction.
  C. Explore current behavioral patterns with others and observe dynamics.
  D. Provide peer and therapist support and source of strength for the individuals to modify present behavior and try out new behaviors; made possible through development of identity and group identification.
  E. Provide on-the-spot, multiple feedback (that is, incorporate others' reactions to behavior), as well as give feedback to others.
  F. Resolve dynamics and provide insight.

▶ **III. Nursing care plan/implementation** in group setting:
  A. Nurses need to fill different roles and functions in the group, depending on the type of group, its size, its aims, and the stage in the group's life cycle. The multifaceted roles may include:
    1. Catalyst.
    2. Transference object.
    3. Clarifier.
    4. Interpreter of "here and now."
    5. Role model and resource person.
    6. Supporter.
  B. During the *first sessions* (orientation phase), explain the purpose of the group, go over the "contract" (structure, format, and goals of sessions), and facilitate introductions of group members.
  C. In *subsequent sessions* (working phase), promote greater group cohesiveness.

TABLE 4.1   DIFFERENCES BETWEEN REALITY ORIENTATION AND RESOCIALIZATION

	Reality Orientation	*Resocialization*
1. Goal	Maximum use of assets	Reality living situation in a community
2. Format	Structured	Unstructured
3. Incentive	Refreshments *may* be served	Refreshments served
4. Focus	Constant reminders of who the clients are, where they are and why, and what is expected of them	Reliving happy experiences; encouragement to participate in home activities
5. Group size	3–5, depending on degree and level of confusion or disorientation	5–17, depending on mental and physical capabilities
6. Meeting frequency and length	30 min daily, same time and place	3 times per week for 30–60 min
7. Structure	Planned topics: reality-centered objects	No planned topic; group-centered feelings
8. Role of leader	Eliciting response of participants	Clarification and interpretation
9. Evaluation of progress	Periodic reality orientation test of participants' level of confusion	Periodic progress note of participants' enjoyment and improvements
10. Emphasis/topics	Time, place, person orientation	Any topic freely discussed
11. Reliance on:	Use of mind function still intact	Memories and experiences
12. Mode of greeting/acknowledging patient	Participant is greeted *by name*, thanked for coming, extended a handshake and/or physical contact	Participant greeted on arrival, thanked, extended a handshake on leaving
13. Leadership	Conducted by trained aides and activity assistants	Conducted by RN, LPN/LVN, aides, program assistants

Source: Adapted with permission from Barns E, Sack A, Shore H. *The Gerontologist* 13:513, 1973.

TABLE 4.2   CURATIVE FACTORS OF GROUP THERAPY

Factor	*Definition*
Instilling of hope	Imbuing the client with optimism for the success of the group therapy experience
Universality	Disconfirming the client's sense of aloneness or uniqueness in misery or hurt
Imparting of information	Giving didactic instruction, advice, or suggestions
Altruism	Finding that the client can be of importance to others; having something of value to give
Corrective recapitulation of the primary family group	Reviewing and correctively reliving early familial conflicts and growth-inhibiting relationships
Development of socializing techniques	Acquiring sophisticated social skills, such as being attuned to process, resolving conflicts, and being facilitative toward others
Imitative behavior	Trying out bits and pieces of the behavior of others and experimenting with those that fit well
Interpersonal learning	Learning that the client is the author of his or her interpersonal world and moving to alter it
Group cohesiveness	Being attracted to the group and the other members with a sense of "we"-ness rather than "I"-ness
Catharsis	Being able to express feelings
Existential factors	Being able to "be" with others; to be a part of a group

Source: Wilson HS, Kneisl CR. *Psychiatric Nursing* (3rd ed). Redwood City, CA: Addison-Wesley, 1988.

1. Focus on *group concerns* and group process rather than on intrapsychic dynamics of individuals.
2. Demonstrate nonjudgmental acceptance of behaviors within the limits of the group contract.
3. Help group members handle their anxiety, especially during the initial phase.
4. Encourage silent members to interact at their level of comfort.
5. Encourage members to interact verbally without dominating the group discussion.
6. Keep the focus of discussion on related themes; *set limits* and *interpret group rules.*
7. Facilitate sharing and *communication* among members.
8. Provide *support* to members as they attempt to work through anxiety-provoking ideas and feelings.
9. Set the expectation that the members are to take responsibility for carrying the group discussion and exploring issues on their own.
   D. *Termination phase:*
   1. Make early preparation for group termination (end point should be announced at the first meeting).
   2. Anticipate common reactions from group members to separation anxiety and help each member to work through these reactions:
      a. Anger.
      b. Acting-out.
      c. Regressive behavior.
      d. Repression.
      e. Feelings of abandonment.
      f. Sadness.
 IV. **Evaluation/outcome criteria:**
   A. *Physical:* shows improvement in daily life activities (eating, rest, work, exercise, recreation).
   B. *Emotional:* asks for and accepts feedback; states that he or she feels good about self and others.
   C. *Intellectual:* is reality-oriented; greater awareness of self, others, environment.
   D. *Social:* willing to take a risk in trusting others; sharing self; reaching out to others.

Family Therapy

Family therapy is a process, method, and technique of psychotherapy in which the focus is not on an individual but on the total family as an interactional system.

 I. **Developmental tasks of North American family** (Duvall, 1971):
   A. *Physical maintenance*—provide food, shelter, clothing, health care.
   B. *Resource allocation*—(physical and emotional) allocate material goods, space, and facilities; give affection, respect, and authority.
   C. *Division of labor*—decide who earns money, manages household, cares for family.
   D. *Socialization*—guidelines to control food intake, elimination, sleep, sexual drives, and aggression.

   E. *Reproduction, recruitment, release of family members*—give birth to, or adopt, children; rear children; incorporate in-laws, friends, etc.
   F. *Maintenance of order*—ensure conformity to norms.
   G. *Placement of members in larger society*—interaction in school, community, etc.
   H. *Maintenance of motivation and morale*—reward achievements, develop philosophy for living; create rituals and celebrations to develop family loyalty. Show acceptance, encouragement, affection; meet crises of individuals and family.
 II. **Basic theoretical concepts** related to family therapy:
   A. The ill family member (called the *identified patient,* or *IP*), through symptoms, sends a message about the "illness" of the family as a *unit.*
   B. *Family homeostasis* is the means by which families attempt to maintain the status quo.
   C. *Scapegoating* is found in disturbed families and is usually focused on one family member at a time, with the intent to keep the family in line.
   D. Communication and behavior by some family members bring out communication and behavior in other family members.
      1. Mental illness in the IP is almost always accompanied by emotional illness and disturbance in other family members.
      2. Changes occurring in one member will produce changes in another; that is, if the IP improves, another IP may emerge, or family may try to place original person back into IP role.
   E. Human communication is a key to emotional stability and instability—to normal and abnormal health. *Conjoint family therapy* is a communication-centered approach that looks at interactions between family members.
   F. *Double-bind* is a "damned-if-you-do, damned-if-you-don't" situation; it results in helplessness, insecurity, anxiety, fear, frustration, and rage.
   G. *Symbiotic tie* usually occurs between one parent and a child, hampering individual ego development and fostering strong dependence and identification with the parent (usually the mother).
   H. *Three basic premises* of communication:[*]
      1. One cannot *not* communicate; that is, silence is a form of communication.
      2. Communication is a *multilevel* phenomenon (e.g., overt, covert, symbolic, verbal, nonverbal).
      3. The message sent is *not* necessarily the *same* message that is received.
   I. Indications for family therapy:
      1. Marital conflicts.
      2. Severe sibling conflicts.
      3. Cross-generational conflicts.
      4. Difficulties related to a transitional stage of family life cycle (e.g., retirement, new baby, death).
      5. *Dysfunctional family patterns:* overprotective mother and distant father, with timid or de-

[*]Adapted from Watzlawick P. *An Anthology of Human Communication.* Palo Alto, CA: Science and Behavior Books, 1964.

structive child, acting-out teenager; overfunctioning "super wife" or "super husband" and the underfunctioning, passive, dependent, and compliant spouse; child with poor peer relationships or academic difficulties.

III. Family assessment (see **Family Assessment: Response to Chronic Illness** in Chap. 3, pp. 47–49) should consider the following factors:

A. Family as a social system:
1. Family as responsive and contributing unit within network of other social units.
   a. Family boundaries—permeability or rigidity.
   b. Nature of input from other social units.
   c. Extent to which family fits into cultural mold and expectations of larger system.
   d. Degree to which family is considered deviant.
2. *Roles* of family members:
   a. Formal roles and role performance (father, child, etc.).
   b. Informal roles and role performance (scapegoat, controller, follower, decision maker).
   c. Degree of family agreement on assignment of roles and their performance.
   d. Interrelationship of various roles—degree of "fit" within total family.
3. Family *rules:*
   a. Family rules that foster stability and maintenance.
   b. Family rules that foster maladaptation.
   c. Conformity of rules to family's life-style.
   d. How rules are modified; respect for difference.
4. *Communication network:*
   a. How family communicates and provides information to members.
   b. Channels of communication—who speaks to whom.
   c. Quality of messages—clarity or ambiguity.

B. Developmental stage of family:
1. Chronologic stage of family.
2. Problems and adaptations of transition.
3. Shifts in role responsibility over time.
4. Ways and means of solving problems at earlier stages.

C. Subsystems operating within family:
1. Function of family alliances in family stability.
2. Conflict or support of other family subsystems and family as a whole.

D. Physical and emotional needs:
1. Level at which family meets essential physical needs.
2. Level at which family meets social and emotional needs.
3. Resources within family to meet physical and emotional needs.
4. Disparities between individual needs and family's willingness or ability to meet them.

E. Goals, values, and aspirations:
1. Extent to which family members' goals and values are articulated and understood by all members.
2. Extent to which family values reflect resignation or compromise.

3. Extent to which family will permit pursuit of individual goals and values.

F. Socioeconomic factors (see list in Chap. 3, Table 3.1, p. 48).

G. Summary: characteristics of a dysfunctional family:
1. *Communication:*
   a. Unclear, indirect messages; indirect intended recipient of messages.
   b. *Incongruence* (i.e., verbal communication does not match nonverbal communication).
   c. Use of *double-bind* ("no-win") situations.
2. *Scapegoating*—one member is blamed for problems of family.
3. *Labeling*—giving members a singular identity (e.g., "the smart one," "the sick one").
4. Relationships: existence of *coalitions* and *triangles.*
5. *Boundaries:* unclear, diffuse, or rigid rules.
6. Individuation: not encouraged; instead, have problems with *enmeshment* (overinvolvement of members) or *disengagement* (underinvolvement and estrangement).
7. *Belief patterns:* based on myths, biases, stereotypes.
8. *Schisms* in couple relationships—forcing children to take sides.
9. *Roles and responsibilities:* unclear as to who does what, when, where, and how.
10. *Change:* resistance to change; inflexible.

IV. Nursing care plan/implementation in family therapy:

A. Establish a family *contract* (who attends, when, duration of sessions, length of therapy, fee, and other expectations).

B. Encourage family members to identify and clarify own *goals.*

C. *Set ground rules:*
1. Focus is on the family as a whole unit, not on the IP.
2. No scapegoating or punishment of members who "reveal all" should be allowed.
3. Therapists should not align themselves with issues or individual family members.

D. *Use self* to empathetically respond to family's problems; share own emotions openly and directly; function as a role model of interaction.

E. Point out and encourage the family to *clarify* unclear, inefficient, and ambiguous family communication patterns.

F. Identify family *strengths.*

G. Listen for repetitive interpersonal *themes, patterns,* and attitudes.

H. *Attempt to reduce guilt and blame* (important to neutralize the scapegoat phenomenon).

I. Present possibility of *alternating* roles and rules in family interaction styles.

J. *Health teaching:* teach clear communication to all family members.

V. Evaluation/outcome criteria: each person clearly speaks for self; asks for and receives feedback; communication patterns are clarified; family problems are delineated; members more aware of each other's needs.

🔑 Summary of Key Points

Milieu Therapy

Benefits: focus on *everyday* living difficulties and learning to take responsibility in gradual steps in an optimistic, supportive environment that is a microcosm of the "outside world."

Activity Therapy

Benefits: provides for *socialization* and *nonverbal* expression of feelings, and a behavioral *outlet* (of tension) through recreational and vocational activities; provides *pleasurable* activities; teaches new skills; increases *self-esteem.*

Behavior Modification

Benefits: eliminates unwanted behavior, *creates* new responses.

Reality Orientation Groups

Benefits: emphasis on time, place, person orientation for disoriented, confused patients; *planned* topics by staff on *reality*-centered *objects.*

Resocialization Groups

Benefits: emphasis on enjoyment and participation in group living activities for patients who have been institutionalized and disengaged from outside world (i.e., regressed behaviors).

Group Therapy

- There are many types of group therapies; composition may be homogeneous (same age, sex, problem) or heterogeneous (varying ages, sex, problems, etc.).
- *Goals:* 11 curative factors (see Table 4.2); provides on-the-spot, multiple feedback; provides an opportunity to express thoughts, feelings in a setting where there are a variety of relationships.

Family Therapy

- Based on family systems theory and on the premise that the whole (family) is more than the sum of its parts (the individual family members).
- Indications: a family member (the identified patient) presents with symptoms, which are symptoms of pain or dysfunction within the whole family.
- *Nursing aim:* help family members identify and express thoughts and feelings, define family roles and rules, try out new ways of relating, and restore family strengths.

💡 Study and Memory Aids

Types of treatment in which behavior modification approach is used

Assertiveness training (for dependency)
Aversion therapy (e.g., Antabuse)
Biofeedback (to control physiologic response, e.g., headache, pulse, respiration, pain)
Relaxation techniques (for anxiety)
Systematic desensitization therapy (for phobias)

Nursing role in group therapy

Orientation phase:	directive, active
Working phase:	consultative, facilitative
Termination phase:	directive, supportive

Glossary

Behavior Therapy

aversion therapy An example of the behavioral model of psychiatric care, in which a painful stimulus is introduced to bring about an avoidance of another stimulus, with the result of a desired change in behavior.

behavior modification A method of treatment derived from learning theory (Pavlov and Skinner), with interventions that are designed to change an individual's behavior patterns and responses through use of techniques that manipulate stimuli. Focus is on the effects rather than the cause of behavior. Commonly used in treatment of phobic and obsessive-compulsive disorders.

Group Treatment

group dynamics Relationships and interactions between members of a group.

group norms Rules for behavior; may be explicit or implicit.

group therapy Three or more individuals who meet on a regular basis with a professional group leader or therapist to focus on self-awareness, problem solving, remotivation, and support.

milieu therapy Purposeful use of people, resources, and events that take place in the patient's therapeutic environment; working with the environment to help produce changes in a patient's behavior, e.g., promoting optimal functioning in activities of daily living, interpersonal interactions, and the ability to manage self-care.

reality orientation A therapeutic approach to help the patient become and remain aware of time, place, and person.

self-help group Homogeneous group led by group members; composed of participants with similar problems (e.g., substance abuse), who provide support and guidance ("It takes one to know [and help] one"). Aim: to improve behavior, reduce stress, boost self-esteem, and assist with social integration.

transference An unconscious phenomenon in which the patient projects onto the nurse or therapist attitudes, feelings, and desires previously connected with significant people earlier in life.

Family Therapy

double-bind A "no-win" situation in which there are incongruent messages (e.g., "you should live at home—but be an independent adult").

homeostasis Maintaining balance (equilibrium), continuity of status quo, and constancy.

incongruence Conflicting, simultaneous messages (e.g., verbal communication says "I'm happy to see you," while nonverbal posture and flat tone say "I wish you weren't here").

individuation The process of developing autonomy and separate self-identity.

nonverbal communication Communication conveyed by methods other than words; includes voice tone, gestures, posture, body language.

Questions

1. What is a main goal or purpose of milieu therapy?
   1. Inclusion of the family in the treatment process.
   2. Permissiveness.
   3. Patient-planned, patient-led activities.
   4. Staff's nonparticipation in decision making.
2. When a colleague is confused about the purpose of a therapeutic environment, the nurse explains to the colleague that in a therapeutic environment, rules and regulations:
   1. Need to be kept to a minimum.
   2. Serve as solutions for commonly occurring problems.
   3. Teach patients self-control.
   4. Should be rigidly enforced.
3. A patient in a therapeutic community setting approaches the nurse one weekend evening, complains of being bored, and requests that some activity be provided. Which response by the nurse would be consistent with a milieu-therapy approach?

1. "All right, I'm not busy. How about playing cards with me?"
2. "I'll go ask the head nurse and see if we can come up with something."
3. "Why don't you ask another patient to play cards with you?"
4. "Let's get the patients and staff together and discuss this."

4. Milieu activities that are initially therapeutic for the schizophrenic patient are:
   1. Basketball, punching bag, and bingo.
   2. Bridge, checkers, and puzzles.
   3. Music, painting, and writing.
   4. Scrabble, Monopoly, and shuffleboard.
5. To improve the table manners of a chronically ill patient with severe regressive behavior, a behavior modification program will probably be most helpful because its main goal is to:
   1. Protect the patient from embarrassment about his table manners.
   2. Offer the patient an incentive for improving his behavior.
   3. Help the patient achieve socially acceptable behavior.
   4. Permit the patient to examine his own behavior without further loss of self-esteem.
6. A middle-aged, long-term patient in a state mental facility upsets other patients with unkempt appearance and avoidance of bathing. Which action will probably be most therapeutic when this patient is started on behavior modification?
   1. Accepting her appearance without comment.
   2. Urging her to bathe and dress like the other patients.
   3. Offering her a reward for each improvement in her appearance and hygiene.
   4. Pointing out to her that her appearance distresses the other patients.
7. In their role in a behavior therapy program, it is essential that nurses:
   1. Ask patients about the content of their dreams.
   2. Interact only with patients who are verbal.
   3. Continually observe patients' behavior and immediately intervene if necessary.
   4. Obtain a detailed account of each patient's growth and development.
8. In group therapy, which role would be inappropriate for the nurse?
   1. Role model and catalyst.
   2. Transference object.
   3. Participant, observer, and facilitator.
   4. Directive.
9. An adolescent has been attending group therapy twice a week for 3 weeks. He is still fairly quiet during group therapy and speaks only when questioned. The nurse should assume that he:
   1. Feels comfortable within the group.
   2. Is threatened by the group.
   3. Does not feel the need to verbalize.
   4. Is progressing as expected.
10. In family therapy sessions, the nurse should:

1. Serve as an arbitrator during disputes.
2. Focus on the person with the presenting problem.
3. Neutralize the scapegoating phenomenon.
4. Use paradoxical communication.

11. The nurse explains to a colleague that the main goal of group therapy is to:
1. Give the therapist a chance to supply authoritative answers common to group problems.
2. Give the patient an opportunity for feedback from several people regarding problems discussed in the group.
3. Give the patient an opportunity to hear other people's problems.
4. Give the therapist the chance to interact with many patients.

12. What is an appropriate goal in group therapy for a patient with an antisocial personality disorder?
1. To obtain feedback about the effect the patient's behavior has on others.
2. To serve as a role model for effective communication.
3. To be a catalyst for interaction among others.
4. To get advice from others.

13. When family therapy is prescribed for a patient with schizophrenic disorder, what is the best explanation for the nurse to give about the focus of the therapy?
1. The focus will be up to the family.
2. The family needs to help the patient change.
3. The focus will be on the need for a change in family interaction.
4. The primary focus will be on the patient with the disturbed behavior.

14. A family with three adolescent children starts family therapy once a week, and the parents begin individual and marital counseling. The mother has a history of alcoholism, suicide attempts, and depression. A 14-year-old son has a history of setting fires and combative behavior. One of the primary goals of therapy with this family system is to provide:
1. A forum in which familial conflicts can be verbalized.
2. Individual therapy for each family member.
3. Treatment for the identified problem child.
4. Crisis intervention for the family system.

15. The parents of an adolescent who is the identified patient are a biracial couple. They are reluctant to discuss the issue of race during family therapy sessions, or even during marital counseling sessions. The nurse therapist's best response to this hesitancy would be to:
1. Confront the couple's resistance to discussing the issue.
2. Avoid the issue unless the couple raises it.
3. Encourage a trusting relationship between the therapist and the couple.
4. Refer the couple to individual psychotherapy.

Answers/Rationale

1. (3) In milieu therapy, patients plan and lead activities rather than staff. Although families and significant others are brought in when needed, *family* therapy (**No. 1**) is neither a key feature nor an emphasis in milieu therapy. Permissiveness (**No. 2**) is not a *main* goal, and while permissiveness should be promoted to the extent possible, some structure is still needed. Staff do participate *with* patients in discussing plans for activities (**No. 4**), although they do not dominate. **PL, 7, SECE**

2. (1) If rules and regulations are at a minimum, patients can work out their own solutions. Imposed solutions in the form of rules do not allow trial-and-error for exploration and personal growth (**No. 2**). Adults do not learn self-control (**No. 3**) from imposed rules, but rather from working out their *own* rules. It is important to teach people to reason and solve problems about rules, rather than responding rigidly (**No. 4**). **IMP, 7, SECE**

3. (4) Milieu therapy calls for *joint* patient-staff planning and decision making in such a situation. The others (**Nos. 1, 2, and 3**) suggest a high degree of direction by the staff, with patients in the passive-dependent role. **IMP, 7, PsI**

4. (3) These are usually *solitary* activities; patients with schizophrenia need activities that do *not* require interaction, cooperation, competition. The activities in **No. 1** require high energy, as well as interaction and competition, and would not be therapeutic. Activities that require instant recall and abstract thinking, such as a puzzle (**No. 2**) and Scrabble (**No. 4**), are not the *initial* activities that are therapeutic for a patient with symptoms of schizophrenia. (*Recall the five As of Bleuler*: associative looseness, autism, ambivalence, inappropriate affect, auditory hallucinations.) **IMP, 3, HPM**

💡 *Test-taking tip:* Look for a pattern. Three options refer to games, but one option lists *only* solitary activities. When you need to guess, choose the one that is different (in this case, **No. 3**).

5. (2) One principal goal of behavior modification is to reward behavior. **Nos. 1, 3, and 4** are not suitable reinforcers for a regressed patient. **PL, 7, PsI**

6. (3) A technique of behavior modification is to use positive reinforcement (such as praise or reward) to increase the probability of a desired behavioral response. **No. 1** allows the patient to continue with unacceptable behavior. **Nos. 2 and 4** are not suitable reinforcers because if she could bathe and dress like others, without external reinforcement, she would; it is doubtful that she is concerned about others' distress. **PL, 2, PsI**

Key to Codes

Nursing process: AS = Assessment; **AN** = Analysis; **PL** = Planning; **IMP** = Implementation; **EV** = Evaluation. (See Appendix E for explanation of nursing process steps.)

Category of human function: 1 = Protective; 2 = Sensory-Perceptual; 3 = Comfort, Rest, Activity, and Mobility; 4 = Nutrition; 5 = Growth and Development; 6 = Fluid-Gas Transport; 7 = Psychosocial-Cultural; 8 = Elimination.

Client need: SECE = Safe, Effective Care Environment; **PhI** = Physiologic Integrity; **PsI** = Psychosocial Integrity; **HPM** = Health Promotion/Maintenance.

7. **(3)** On-the-spot observation and intervention are key. Focus on dreams (**No. 1**) is part of Freudian analysis, not behavior therapy. **No. 2** is incorrect because behavior modification is used in the treatment of *mute* patients also. The emphasis of behavioral therapy is on the present (**No. 3**), *not* the past developmental history (**No. 4**). **IMP, 7, SECE**

8. **(4)** The directive role decreases responsibility and independence in the patient, and is therefore inappropriate. All of the other roles (**Nos. 1, 2, and 3**) are *appropriate* for the nurse. **PL, 7, SECE**

💡 *Test-taking tip:* Focus on key word—*inappropriate.*

9. **(4)** Since the adolescent has only attended six sessions of group therapy, it is expected that he would only speak when questioned. He is probably still unsure of his own feelings and is in the preinteraction phase of trusting other group members. **Nos. 1, 2, and 3** are probably not true at this point. **EV, 7, PsI**

10. **(3)** A contract early in therapy is essential to make expectations clear. These expectations include no scapegoating or blaming of one family member by another. It is crucial that the nurse not take sides or try to referee a family fight (**No. 1**). The *opposites* of **Nos. 2 and 4** are important to practice: focusing on the dynamics of the *family* (**No. 2**), and communicating in a clear and *straightforward* manner (**No. 4**). **PL, 7, SECE**

11. **(2)** One of the main purposes of group therapy is for the patient to discover a universality of problems and a diversity of solutions. Most people do not respond well to authoritative answers (**No. 1**), and authoritative answers lessen learning. While hearing others' problems (**No. 3**) is one aspect of group therapy, this option is not as complete or significant as **No. 2**. The goal of therapy is to assist *patients*, not the therapist (**No. 4**). **PL, 7, PsI**

💡 *Test-taking tip:* The best answers are focused on the *patient,* not on the therapist (**Nos. 1 and 2**).

12. **(1)** A chief goal of group therapy is for each patient to have the opportunity to gain insight from observing and obtaining input from others about the effect of self on others. Serving as a role model (**No. 2**) and catalyst (**No. 3**) are desired *nursing* roles in group therapy, *not* the roles of participants. Giving advice (**No. 4**) is neither a therapeutic role nor a goal. **PL, 7, PsI**

13. **(3)** In order for the patient to improve, the entire family must be willing to look at and alter *family* dynamics, not just the patient. **No. 1** is too open-ended; a goal is needed (i.e., to alter family dynamics). Focusing on the patient (**Nos. 2 and 4**) is the opposite of the correct response—focusing on the family. **IMP, 7, PsI**

💡 *Test-taking tip:* Look for patterns: two options (**Nos. 2 and 4**) focus on the patient, and two options focus on the family (**Nos. 1 and 3**). Note the word "family" in the question; this means that you can *eliminate* **Nos. 2 and 4,** and concentrate on the two options that focus on the family (**Nos. 1 and 3**). You can then *eliminate* **No. 1,** as it is too vague.

14. **(1)** Family therapy should promote the expression of feelings. Intragroup dynamics of the family system should be assessed, and appropriate coping strategies identified. The objective of family therapy is *not* primarily to provide individual therapy for each family member (**No. 2**). If a family member needs one-to-one therapy, individual therapy is usually provided in conjunction with, but at a separate time from, family therapy sessions. The identified patient is treated in individual and family therapy sessions; however, the primary focus of family therapy is treatment of the *family,* not just of this particular individual (**No. 3**). Crisis intervention (**No. 4**) may be *one* aspect of family therapy, used initially to assist in returning a family system to a steady state of functioning, but it is not the primary goal in this case. **PL, 7, PsI**

15. **(3)** Establishing trust between the therapist and the couple is essential to facilitating effective therapy and possible resolution of the marital and familial conflicts. Confrontation (**No. 1**) may prove threatening in this situation, and the couple may leave therapy to avoid feelings of anxiety. Avoidance (**No. 2**) is nontherapeutic in this situation because it does not help resolve the conflict. A referral (**No. 4**) may be appropriate; however, the nurse should *initially* use all therapeutic techniques in assisting the couple to identify relevant issues and possibly to resolve conflicts before making a referral. **PL, 7, PsI**

💡 *Test-taking tip:* "Trust-building" is a key therapeutic intervention.

Somatic Treatment Modes

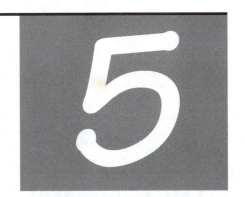

Chapter Outline

- Electroconvulsive Therapy
- Psychopharmacology: Common Psychotropic Drugs
  - Antipsychotics (Also Called Neuroleptics, Major Tranquilizers)
    Neuroleptic malignant syndrome
  - Antidepressants
  - Antianxiety Agents
    - Antimanic Agents
    - Anti-Parkinson Agents
- Use of Restraints
- Study and Memory Aids
- Summary of Key Points
- Glossary
- Questions
- Answers/Rationale

Electroconvulsive Therapy

Electroconvulsive therapy (ECT) is a physical treatment that induces grand mal convulsions by applying electric current to the head. It is also called electroshock therapy (EST).

I. **Characteristics** of electroconvulsive therapy:
   A. Usually used in treating major depression with severe suicide risk, extreme hyperactivity, severe catatonic stupor; or in treating those with bipolar affective disorders not responsive to psychotropic medication.
   B. Consists of a series of treatments (6–25) over a period of time (e.g., 3 times a wk).
   C. Person is asleep through the procedure and for 20–30 min afterward.
   D. Convulsion may be seen as a series of minor, jerking motions in extremities (e.g., toes). Spasms are reduced by use of muscle-paralyzing drugs.
   E. Confusion is present for 30 min after treatment.
   F. Induces loss of memory for *recent* events.

II. **Views concerning success** of electroconvulsive therapy:
   A. Posttreatment sleep is the "curative" factor.
   B. Shock treatment is seen as punishment, with an accompanying feeling of absolution from guilt.
   C. Chemical alteration of thought patterns results in memory loss, with decrease in redundancy and awareness of painful memories.

III. **Nursing care plan/implementation** in electroconvulsive therapy:
   A. Always tell the client of the treatment.
   B. Inform client about temporary memory loss for recent events after the treatment.

C. *Pretreatment care:*
   1. Take vital signs.
   2. Be sure the client has used the toilet.
   3. Remove client's dentures, eyeglasses or contact lenses, and jewelry.
   4. NPO for 8 hr beforehand.
   5. *Atropine sulfate* subcutaneously (Sc) 30 min before treatment to decrease bronchial and tracheal secretions.
   6. Anesthetist gives anesthetic and short-acting muscle relaxant IV (succinylcholine chloride [*Anectine*]) and oxygen for 2–3 min and inserts airway. Often all three are given close together—anesthetic first, followed by another syringe with *Anectine* and *atropine sulfate*. Electrodes and treatment must be given within 2 min of injections, as *Anectine* is very short acting (2 min).
   D. *During the convulsion* the nurse needs to make sure the person is in a safe anatomic position, to *avoid* dislocation and compression fractures (although *Anectine* is given to prevent this).
   E. *Care during recovery stage:*
   1. Put up side rails while client is confused; side position.
   2. Take BP and respirations.
   3. Stay until person awakens, responds to questions, and can care for self.
   4. Orient client to time and place and inform that treatment is over.
   5. Offer support to help client feel more secure and relaxed as the confusion and anxiety decrease.

☞ **6.** Medication for nausea and headache.

F. *Health teaching:* teach family members what to expect of client after ECT (confusion, headache, nausea); how to reorient the client.

◄ **IV. Evaluation/outcome criteria:** feelings of worthlessness, helplessness, and hopelessness seem diminished.

Psychopharmacology: Common Psychotropic Drugs

💊 Antipsychotics (Also Called Neuroleptics, Major Tranquilizers)

I. Phenothiazines (prochlorperazine maleate [*Compazine*], promazine hydrochloride [*Sparine*], chlorpromazine hydrochloride [*Thorazine*], thioridazine hydrochloride [*Melaril*], trifluoperazine hydrochloride [*Stelazine*], perphenazine [*Trilafon*], triflupromazine [*Vesprin*], fluphenazine hydrochloride [*Prolixin*], fluphenazine decanoate [*Prolixin decanoate*], fluphenazine enanthate [*Prolixin enanthate*])

II. Butyrophenones (haloperidol [*Haldol*], droperidol [*Innovar*])

III. Thioxanthenes (chlorprothixene [*Taractan*], thiothixene [*Navane*])

IV. Dibenzoxazepines—atypical antipsychotics (clozapine [*Clozaril*], loxapine succinate [*Loxitane*])

  A. *Use*—those who do not respond to other neuroleptic antipsychotic drugs; offers relief from schizophrenic symptoms: hallucinations, delusions, flat affect, apathy.

  ◄ **B. Assessment**—*side effects:*

    1. Most serious is *agranulocytosis* (potentially fatal; reversible if diagnosed within 1–2 wk of onset).

      a. *Symptoms* of agranulocytosis: infection, high fever, chills, sore throat, malaise, ulceration of mucous membranes.

      b. Lab value: Discontinue drug with WBC < 2000 µl or granulocyte < 1000 µl.

    2. Other side effects: seizures, tachycardia, orthostatic hypotension.

    3. *Caution:* must have weekly blood tests for WBC; do *not* resume clozapine once it is discontinued, due to side effects.

V. Benzisoxazole derivative—risperidone (*Risperdal*)

  A. *Use*—incremental increases for first 3d to manage psychotic symptoms. *Benefit:* less incidence of extrapyramidal symptoms (EPS).

  ◄ **B. Assessment**—*side effects:* same as for phenothiazines (see **General assessment, VII.**).

VI. *General use*—acute and chronic psychoses; most useful in cases of disorganization of thought or behavior; to decrease panic, fear, hostility, restlessness, aggression, and withdrawal.

◄ **VII. General assessment**—*side effects* of antipsychotic drugs:

  A. *Hypersensitivity* effects

    1. *Blood dyscrasia*—agranulocytosis, leukopenia, granulocytopenia.

    2. *Skin reactions*—solar sensitivity, allergic dermatitis, flushing, blue-gray skin.

    3. Obstructive *jaundice.*

  B. *Extrapyramidal symptoms (EPS)* affecting voluntary movement and skeletal muscles

    1. *Akathisia*—motor restlessness, pacing, foot-tapping, inner tremulousness, and agitation.

    2. *Dystonia*—limb and neck spasms (torticollis), extensive rigidity of back muscles (opisthotonus), oculogyric crisis, speech and swallowing difficulties, and tongue protrusion.

    3. *Parkinsonian symptoms (also called Parkinson-like, pseudo-Parkinsonism)*—tremors, cogwheel rigidity, shuffling gait, pill-rolling, masklike facies, salivation, and difficulty starting muscular movement (dyskinesia).

    4. *Tardive dyskinesia (TD)*—excessive blinking; vermiform tongue movement; stereotyped, abnormal, involuntary sucking, chewing, licking, and pursing movements of tongue and mouth; grimacing, blinking, frowning, rocking.

      a. *Cause*—long-term use of high doses of antipsychotic drugs.

      b. *Predisposing factors*—age, women, dementia; history of ECT or use of tricyclics or anti-Parkinson drugs.

  C. *Potentiates* CNS depressants.

  D. *Orthostatic hypotension* (less with butyrophenones).

  E. *Anticholinergic effects* (atropinelike)—dry mouth, stuffy nose, blurred vision, urinary retention, and constipation.

  F. *Pigment retinopathy*—ocular changes (lens and corneal opacity).

  G. Neuroleptic malignant syndrome (NMS)

    1. *Description:* A rare complication of antipsychotic drugs, with a rapid onset (1–2 d) and a 20% mortality rate. It is a serious medical emergency for which early recognition of symptoms is critical.

  ◄ **2. Assessment**

      a. ↑ vital signs: extreme temperature (leading to diaphoresis and confusion), BP.

      b. Lab values: ↑ CPK (creatine phosphokinase), ↑ K (potassium), leukocytosis

      c. Renal failure.

      d. Muscular: rigidity (lead pipe skeletal muscle rigidity) that leads to dyspnea and dysphagia, tremors.

      e. *At risk:* patients with organic brain disorders and severe dehydration.

    3. Medical treatment

      a. Discontinue all drugs

      b. Institute supportive care.

      c. Administer dopamine function-enhancing

substances (e.g., levodopa, carbidopa, bromocriptine, or amantadine)

VIII. General nursing care plan/implementation for antipsychotic drugs:

A. Goal: *anticipate, observe for, and check for side effects.*

  1. Protect the person's skin from *sunburn* when outside.

  ☞ 2. For *hypotension*: take BP and have person lie down for 30 min, especially after an injection.

  3. Watch for signs of *blood dyscrasia*: sore throat, fever, malaise.

  4. Observe for symptoms of *hypo-* or *hyperthermic* reaction due to effect on heat-regulating mechanism.

  5. Observe for, withhold drug for, and report early symptoms of *jaundice* and bile tract obstruction, high fever, upper abdominal pain, nausea, diarrhea, rash; monitor *liver function tests*.

  6. Relieve excessive *mouth dryness*: mouth rinse, increase fluid intake, give gum or hard candy.

  7. Relieve gastric irritation, *constipation*: take with and *increase fluids* and *roughage* in diet.

  8. Observe for and report changes in *carbohydrate* metabolism (glycosuria, weight gain, polyphagia): change diet.

B. Goal: *health teaching.*

  1. Dangers of drug potentiation with alcohol or sleeping pills.

  2. Advise about driving or occupations where blurred vision may be a problem.

  3. Caution against abrupt cessation at high doses.

  4. Warn regarding dark urine.

  5. Have client with respiratory disorder breathe deeply and cough as drug is a cough depressant.

  6. Need for continuous use of drug and follow-up care.

  7. Prompt reporting of hypersensitivity symptoms: fever, laryngeal edema; abdominal distention (constipation, urinary retention); jaundice; blood dyscrasia.

IX. General evaluation/outcome criteria

A. Behavior is less agitated.

B. Knows side effects to observe for, lessen, and/or prevent.

C. Continues to use drug.

🙵 Antidepressants

I. **Tricyclic (also called TCAs)** (imipramine hydrochloride [*Tofranil*], desipramine hydrochloride [*Norpramin*], nortriptyline [*Pamelor*], trimipramine [*Surmontil*], amitriptyline hydrochloride [*Elavil*], perphenazine, amitriptyline HCl [*Triavil*], nortriptyline hydrochloride [*Aventyl*], protriptyline hydrochloride

[*Vivactil*], doxepin hydrochloride [*Sinequan*])—effective in 2–4 wk.

A. *Use*—elevate mood in depression, increase physical activity and mental alertness; may bring relief of symptoms of depression so that client can attend individual or group therapy; bipolar disorder, depressed; dysthmic disorder.

B. **Assessment**—*side effects:*

  1. *Behavioral*—activation of latent schizophrenia; hypomania; suicide attempts; mental confusion. Withhold drug if observed.

  2. *Central nervous system* (CNS)—tremors, ataxia, jitteriness.

  3. *Autonomic nervous system* (ANS)—dry mouth, nasal congestion, aggravation of glaucoma, constipation, urinary retention, edema, paralysis, ECG changes (flattened T waves; arrhythmia severe in overdose).

C. **Nursing care plan/implementation**

  1. Goal: *assess risk of suicide during initial improvement:* careful, close observation.

  ☞ 2. Goal: *prevent risk of cardiac arrhythmias and hypotension.* Use caution with client with hyperthyroidism, having ECT or surgery (gradually discontinue 2–3 d *prior* to surgery). Monitor BP, 2 times per d; ECGs, 2–3 per wk until dose adjusted.

  3. Goal: *observe for signs of urinary retention, constipation:* monitor I&O and weight gain.

  4. Goal: *cautious drug use with glaucoma or history of seizures.* Observe seizure precautions due to lowered seizure threshold.

  5. Goal: *health teaching.*

    a. Advise against driving car or participating in activities requiring mental alertness, due to *sedative* effects.

    b. Encourage increased fluid intake and frequent mouth rinsing to combat dry mouth.

    c. *Avoid* smoking, which decreases drug effects.

    d. *Avoid* use of alcohol and other drugs, due to adverse interactions, especially over-the-counter (OTC) drugs (e.g., antihistamines).

    e. Advise of delay in desired effect (2–4 wk).

    f. Instruct gradual discontinuance to *avoid* withdrawal symptoms.

D. **Evaluation/outcome criteria:** diminished symptoms of agitated depression and anxiety.

II. **Monoamine-oxidase inhibitors** (MAOIs)—phenelzine hydrochloride (*Nardil*), isocarboxazid (*Marplan*), tranylcypromine sulfate (*Parnate*), pargyline hydrochloride (*Eutonyl*), nialamide (*Niamid*).

A. **Assessment**—*side effects:*

  1. *Behavioral*—may activate latent schizophrenia, mania, excitement.

  2. *CNS*—tremors; *hypertensive crisis* (avoid foods listed in B.3.b., p. 68); *intracerebral hemorrhage; hyperpyrexia.*

  3. *ANS*—dry mouth, aggravation of glaucoma,

bowel and bladder control problems; edema, paralysis, ECG changes (arrhythmia severe in overdose).

    4. *Allergic* hepatocellular jaundice.

B. Nursing care plan/implementation

    1. Goal: *reduce risk of hypertensive crisis:* diet restrictions of foods high in *tyramine* content.

    2. Goal: *observe for urinary retention:* measure I&O.

    3. Goal: *health teaching.*

      a. Therapeutic response takes 2–3 wk.

      b. *Food and alcohol restrictions:* avocado, bananas, raisins, licorice, yogurt, sour cream, soy sauce, meat tenderizers. *Avoid* foods with high tyramine: aged cheese, cola, caffeine, red wine, beer, yeast, chocolate, liver, herring.

      c. Change position gradually to prevent postural hypotension.

      d. Report any stiff neck, palpitations, chest pain, headaches because of possible hypertensive crises (can be fatal).

      e. Take *no nonprescribed* drugs.

C. Evaluation/outcome criteria

    1. Improvement in: sleep, appetite, activity, interest in self and surroundings.

    2. Lessening of anxiety and complaints.

● Antianxiety Agents
See Table 5.1

I. Chlordiazepoxide (*Librium*)

    A. *Use*—alcoholism, tension, and irrational fears; has muscle relaxant and anticonvulsant properties.

    B. Assessment—*side effects:* hypotension, drowsiness, motor uncoordination, confusion, skin eruptions, edema, menstrual irregularities, constipation, extrapyramidal symptoms, blurred vision, lethargy; ↑ or ↓ libido.

    C. Nursing care plan/implementation

      1. Goal: *administer cautiously, as drug may:*

        a. Be habituating (causing withdrawal convulsions; therefore gradual withdrawal necessary).

        b. Potentiate CNS depressants.

        c. Have adverse effect on pregnancy.

        d. Be dangerous for those with suicidal tendencies or severe psychoses.

      2. Goal: *reduce GI effects:* crush tablet or take with meals or milk; give *antacids* 1 hr before.

      3. Goal: *monitor effect on liver:* Periodic liver function tests and blood counts, especially with upper respiratory infection.

      4. Goal: *health teaching.*

        a. Advise against suddenly stopping drug (withdrawal symptoms begin in 5–7 d).

        b. Talk with physician if plans to be or is pregnant.

        c. Drink *fluids.*

        d. *Avoid:* alcohol, over-the-counter drugs, and heavy smoking.

D. Evaluation/outcome criteria: decreased alcohol withdrawal symptoms or preoperative anxiety.

II. Diazepam (*Valium*)

    A. *Use*—muscle relaxant; *not* used for psychotics.

    B. Assessment—*side effects:* same as for *Librium,* plus double or blurred vision, difficult speech, headache, hypotension, incontinence, tremor, and urinary retention, liver damage.

    C. Nursing care plan/implementation

      1. Goal: *anticipate, observe for, and check for side effects,* especially depression, suicidal risk, and constipation.

      2. Goal: *reduce risk of hypotension, respiratory depression, phlebitis, venous thrombosis.* Give: IM, in large muscles, slowly, and rotate sites, have client lie down; IV: over 1-min period.

      3. Goal: *observe for psychological and physical dependence: avoid* abrupt discontinuation.

      4. Goal: *health teaching:* sedative effects, potentiation of other CNS-depressant drugs and alcohol, and problem of habituation.

    D. Evaluation/outcome criteria: relief of tension, anxiety, skeletal muscle spasm.

Antimanic Agents

I. *Lithium*—effect occurs 1–3 wk after first dose.

    A. *Use*—acute manic attack and prevention of recurrence of cyclic manic-depressive episodes of bipolar disorders.

    B. Assessment—*side effects:* levels from 1.6–2.0 mEq/L may cause tremors, nausea and vomiting, diarrhea, polyuria, polydipsia; levels *above 2* mEq/L may cause motor weakness, headache, edema, and lethargy; *signs of severe toxicity:* neurologic, e.g., twitching, marked drowsiness, slurred speech, dysarthria, athetotic movements. Convulsions, delirium, stupor, coma may occur with levels above 2.5 mEq/L.

      1. *Precautions*—cautious use with clients: on *diuretics;* with disturbed *electrolytes* (sweating, dehydrated, and postoperative clients); with *thyroid* problems, on *low-salt diets;* with congestive *heart failure;* and with impaired *renal function.* Risk of suicide.

      2. *Dosage*—*therapeutic* level 0.8–1.6 mEq/L; dose for maintenance 300–1500 mEq/d; *toxic* level > 2.0 mEq/L; blood sample drawn in acute phase 10–14 hr after last dose, taken tid.

    C. Nursing care plan/implementation:

      1. Goal: *anticipate, observe for, and check for signs and symptoms of toxicity.*

        a. Reduce GI symptoms: take *with meals.*

        b. Check for edema: daily weight.

        c. Monitor blood levels (1.6–2.0 mEq/L) for signs of *toxicity:* nausea, vomiting, diarrhea, anorexia, ataxia, weakness, drowsiness, tremors or muscle-twitching, slurred speech.

TABLE 5.1 ANTIANXIETY AGENTS

Drug	Use	Side Effects/Cautions
Benzodiazepines *Librium* (chlordiazepoxide) *Valium* (diazepam)	Short-term, for specific stress	Drowsiness Lethal overdose with alcohol High risk for dependency with long-term use Symptoms with abrupt withdrawal: irritability, dizziness Do not use in pregnancy
Propanediol Carbamates *Equanil* (meprobamate, a sedative-hypnotic)	Rarely used	Drowsiness High risk for tolerance, addiction, and overdose *Withdrawal symptoms:* insomnia, anxiety, hallucination, seizures CNS depressant
Acetylinic Alcohol *Placidyl* (ethclorvynol, a sedative-hypnotic)		*See* Propanediol Carbamates; also: Confusion Ataxia Hypotension Exaggerated depression (muscle weakness and deep sleep)
Diphenylmethane Antihistamine *Atarax* (hydroxyzine hydrochloride) *Vistaril* (hydroxyzine pamoate)	Safe for long-term use	No risk of physical dependency or abuse; minimal toxicity May cause drowsiness
Buspirone Hydrochloride *BuSpar*	Long-term use	Less sedation; no risk of dependence Delayed effect (3 wk)
Beta-Adrenergic Blocker *Inderal* (propranolol hydrochloride)	Stage fright Relief of physical signs of anxiety (tachycardia)	Hypotension Bradycardia No risk of dependence or abuse
Tricyclic Antidepressants (TCAs) *Anafranil* (clomipramine) *Tofranil* (imipramine)	Prevention of panic attacks Severe obsessive-compulsive disorder	Dry mouth Blurred vision Constipation Weight gain Abrupt withdrawal may cause seizures, cardiac arrhythmias

   d. Monitor results with repeat thyroid and kidney function tests.
   2. Goal: *report fever* right away.
   3. Goal: *monitor effect* (therapeutic and toxic) through blood samples taken:
      a. 10–14 hr after last dose.
      b. Every 2–3 d until 1.6 mEq/L is reached.
      c. Once a week while in hospital.
      d. Every 2–3 mo to maintain blood levels under 1 mEq/L.
   4. Goal: *health teaching*.
      a. Advise client of 1–3 wk lag time for effect.
      b. Urge to drink adequate *liquids (2–3 L/d)*.
      c. Report: polyuria and polydypsia.

   d. *Diet: avoid* caffeine, crash diets, diet pills, self-prescribed low-salt diet, antacids, high-sodium foods (which increase lithium excretion and reduce drug effect); take *with meals.*
   e. Caution against driving, operating machinery that requires mental alertness until drug is effective.
   f. Warn *not* to change or omit dose.
 D. **Evaluation/outcome criteria**
   1. Changed facial affect.
   2. Improved: posture, ability to concentrate, sleep patterns.
   3. Assumption of self-care.

🔹 Anti-Parkinson Agents

I. Trihexyphenidyl HCl (*Artane*).
II. Benztropine mesylate (*Cogentin*).
   A. *Use*—counteract extrapyramidal reactions.
   ✉ B. **Assessment**
      1. *Artane*
         a. *Side effects*—dry mouth, blurred vision, dizziness, nausea, constipation, drowsiness, urinary hesitancy or retention, pupil dilation, headache, and weakness.
         b. *Precautions*—cautious use with cardiac, liver, or kidney disease or obstructive gastrointestinal-genitourinary disease. Do *not* give if glaucoma present.
      2. *Cogentin—side effects:* same as for *Artane*, plus:
         a. Effect on *body temperature* may result in life-threatening state.
         b. *Gastrointestinal distress.*
         c. *Inability to concentrate,* memory difficulties, and mild confusion (often mistaken for senility).
         d. May lead to toxic psychotic reactions.
         e. *Subjective sensations*—light or heavy feelings in legs, numbness and tingling of extremities, light-headedness or tightness of head, and giddiness.
   ✉ C. **Nursing care plan/implementation**
      1. Goal: *relieve GI distress* by giving *after* or *with* meals or at bedtime.
      2. Goal: *monitor adverse effects*
         a. Hypotension, tachycardia: check pulse, BP.
         b. Constipation and fecal impaction: add roughage to *diet.*
         c. Dry mouth: increase *fluid* intake; encourage frequent mouth rinsing.
         d. Blurred vision, dizziness: assist with ambulation; use side rail.
      3. *Health teaching.*
         a. *Avoid* driving, and limit activities requiring alertness.
         b. *Delayed* drug effect (2–3 d).
         c. Potential abuse due to hallucinogenic effects.
         d. *Avoid* alcohol and other CNS depressants.
   ✉ D. **Evaluation/outcome criteria**
      1. Less rigidity, drooling, and oculogyric crisis.
      2. Improved: gait, balance, posture.

Use of Restraints

I. **Principles**
   A. Use as a last resort in an emergency, only when other means have not been effective. "Freedom from unlawful restraint" is a basic human right protected by law (false imprisonment).

   B. Use only for a limited purpose of protecting the patient from injury, *not* for convenience of personnel.
   C. Can apply without an order, but must notify attending MD immediately.
   D. Consult with another staff member first.
   E. If possible, obtain the patient's consent.
   F. Document facts and reasons.
   G. Have coworkers witness the record.
✉ II. **Nursing care plan/implementation**
   A. Use soft material; restrain one limb at a time.
   B. For *safety* involve staff, if possible (one to direct, one for each of four limbs). Remove loose items.
   C. Approach patient from the side, *never* from the back.
☞ D. Check frequently to ensure that restraints do not impair *circulation* or cause pressure sores or other injury. Secure restraints to bed frame.
   E. Provide for hydration (drink), elimination, basic mouth care, and food.
   F. Have at least one staff member nearby, to reduce panic and feelings of abandonment.
   G. Test for readiness before releasing from seclusion room: give a directive (e.g., "Please sit on the bed") to see if patient has adequate self-control to listen and respond appropriately.
   H. Remove restraints (one at a time) at first opportunity.
   I. Document what was done and why.

💡 Study and Memory Aids

🔹 Prevent lithium toxicity

- Increase *fluids* (10–12 glasses)
- Adequate *salt* in daily diet
- Take *with* food or after meals (**p.c.**)
- Monitor blood lithium level (monthly, 8–12 hr after dose)
- *Avoid:* sodium bicarbonate (due to increased renal excretion) and ibuprofen (due to reduced renal clearance)
- *Report:* vomiting, diarrhea, diaphoresis

Indications for use of restraints

- Risk for injury to self or others
- Medication to control aggressive behavior not working
- Confusion that leads to injury related to wandering (e.g., in the streets)

🗝 Summary of Key Points

☞ Care of Patient Who Is to Have ECT

1. Check for or witness an informed consent.
2. *Preprocedure:* NPO, remove dentures, take vital signs; have patient empty bladder.
3. *During ECT:*
   - Patient may get oxygen (10 L/min × 2–3 min).
   - *Brevital* (methohexital sodium) is given to induce anesthesia.
   - *Succinylcholine chloride* is given to relax muscles and prevent active seizures.
   - Ambu bag with 100% oxygen is used for respirations during the electric impulse.
4. *After ECT:*
   - Take vital signs every 5 min until awake.
   - *Position:* side-lying after airway is out.
   - Reorient; to decrease confusion, same nurse is assigned pre- and postprocedure.
   - Observe for respiratory problems.

☞ Psychopharmacology

Antipsychotics (Neuroleptics)
- *Nursing implications:* watch for EPS and neuroleptic malignant syndrome; watch for hypotension, urinary retention, agranulocytosis (sore throat, fever). Give with *food/milk* to ↓ GI symptoms.
- *Teaching: avoid* sun, alcohol; use candy, gum, and ice chips to ↓ dry mouth; ↑ *fluids* to prevent constipation; caution in operating vehicles and machinery (due to visual disturbances).

Antidepressants
Teaching: Effect delayed 2–4 wk; *avoid* alcohol; take with food; rise slowly from sitting or lying position.

Monoamine-Oxidase Inhibitors (MAOIs)
- *Teaching:* delayed therapeutic effect (2–3 wk)
- *Tyramine-free diet* during treatment and for 2 wk after discontinuation (*avoid:* aged cheese, sour cream, raisins, caffeine, bananas, split peas, pizza, liver, pickled herring, soy sauce, licorice, beer, and red wine)
- Take early in day to avoid insomnia.

Antianxiety Agents
See Table 5.1.
Teaching: avoid alcohol, OTC, and sudden withdrawal; may be habit forming; suicide risk.

Antimanic Agents
- Lithium blood levels taken initially 2 times per wk until therapeutic level is reached (0.8–1.6 mEq/L), then every 2 mo.
- *Teaching:* ↑ *fluids* (3000 mL/d); regular meals with 3–6 g sodium daily; take with *food/milk*; delayed effect (1–3 wk); *avoid* strenuous exercise (due to sodium loss) and caffeine (due to diuretic effects).

Anti-Parkinson Agents
Teaching: avoid alcohol and other CNS depressants; delayed effect (2–3 d); ↑ *roughage* and *fluids* in diet; *avoid* activities requiring alertness; give p.c. or h.s.

☞ Care of a Patient in Restraints
- Need a team: coordinator and four or five staff members, for safety
- Remove all loose and potentially dangerous items from self and patient; staff should tie back own hair
- Restrain one limb at a time
- Secure restraints to bed frames
- Observe patient every 15 min
- Remove one restraint at a time at least every 2 hr; offer bathroom privileges every 2 hr; offer fluids and nutrition.
- Document: patient's behavior; reason for use of restraints; activities of daily living that are met during period of restraint (food, drink, safety, toilet)
- *Priority* concerns: safety and circulation

Glossary

agranulocytosis Decreased WBC (leukocytes) caused by reaction to drugs that affect bone marrow and impair the ability of the body's immune system to fight infections; potentially fatal if condition is not detected, and the drug not stopped, within 1–2 wk.

akathisia A reversible EPS reaction to antipsychotic drugs, causing restlessness (fidgeting, pacing); may be mistaken for anxiety or agitation. To treat, give anticholinergics or change to a different antipsychotic drug.

akinesia Absence, delay, or slowness in beginning and carrying through voluntary motor movements.

athetosis A condition in which there is a constant, repetitive succession of slow, writhing, involuntary movements of flexion, extension, pronation, and supination of fingers, hands, toes, feet.

dystonia Temporary reaction during *early* antipsychotic drug treatment that is characterized by spasms of head, neck, and back, with oculogyric effects (abnormal eye movements in which eyes roll to the back of the head). Relieved by injection of an anticholinergic drug.

electroconvulsive therapy (ECT), electroshock treatment (EST) A somatic therapy in which a grand mal seizure is produced by passing a controlled electric current of 70–130 V for 0.1–0.5 sec through electrodes placed at the temples. The patient is anesthetized and given a muscle relaxant. Best suited to treatment of depression.

neuroleptic malignant syndrome (NMS) A quick, potentially fatal reaction to antipsychotic medications that requires *immediate* treatment for symptoms (temperature up to 107°F, renal shutdown, unstable BP, dehydration). Other symptoms include muscle rigidity, ↑ CPK, confusion, and diaphoresis.

pseudo-parkinsonism (also known as parkinsonian symptoms, parkinson-like symptoms) A reaction to antipsychotic drugs that is characterized by *reversible* motor and muscular symptoms, e.g., rigid appearance to muscles in face, trunk, and limbs; shuffling gait; tremors; drooling. To treat, change to different antipsychotic drug or give anticholinergic drug.

psychotropic drug A drug with mind-altering effects.

somatic therapy Use of physical measures to treat mental/emotional conditions (ECT, restraints).

tardive dyskinesia (TD) Severe and potentially *irreversible* reaction to *long-term* use of high dose of antipsychotic drugs occurring when drug dosage is *decreased or discontinued*. No treatment; prevent by periodic screening for TD.

Questions

1. What behavior would the nurse expect to see in a patient following ECT (electroconvulsive therapy)?
   1. Loss of short-term memory.
   2. Hyperalertness.
   3. Hyperkinesis.
   4. Suspiciousness about the food.
2. What should the nurse do first after a patient has had electroconvulsive therapy?
   1. Check vital signs.
   2. Give pain medication.
   3. Put the patient in restraints.
   4. Stay with the patient to reassure and orient.
3. What is a nursing priority during ECT?
   1. Monitoring BP and TPR.
   2. Controlling spasmodic movements.
   3. Maintaining airway.
   4. Applying electric charges.
4. Electroconvulsive therapy is ordered as a treatment for a patient who is depressed. What is the most important point for the nurse to consider in planning immediate posttreatment care?
   1. The patient will not be as depressed as before, and therefore will be at higher risk for suicide.
   2. The patient needs to be left alone to sleep.

3. The patient may look bewildered, be confused, and experience memory loss.
   4. The patient will be hungry after being NPO, and will need nourishment on awakening.
5. The nursing assessment of a patient who is on Thorazine reveals muscular tremors, agitation, restlessness, continuous movement, and finger tapping. What would be an appropriate nursing evaluation of these specific side effects?
   1. Dystonia.
   2. Akathisia.
   3. Extrapyramidal symptoms (EPS).
   4. Pseudo-parkinsonism.
6. A patient is placed on Cogentin after developing side effects from Thorazine. What signs would the nurse look for as indicators of improvement as a result of being on Cogentin?
   1. Skin will be less photosensitive.
   2. Visual problems will improve.
   3. Extrapyramidal symptoms will lessen.
   4. Blood pressure will be normotensive.
7. What antidote would the nurse have ready for a patient on Thorazine?
   1. Haldol.
   2. Artane.
   3. Elavil.
   4. Prolixin.
8. The nurse would be most concerned about side effects of chlorpromazine (Thorazine) when a patient is:
   1. Watching a movie.
   2. Going to a picnic.
   3. Going shopping in the mall.
   4. Attending a concert.
9. What should the nurse give a patient who is on Thorazine and experiencing side effects?
   1. Antiemetic medication.
   2. Antidiarrheal medication.
   3. Hard candy or gum.
   4. Aspirin.
10. A patient has been ordered benztropine (*Cogentin*) 2 mg bid to decrease extrapyramidal symptoms. For which possible side effect must the nurse evaluate this patient?
    1. Pupil constriction. (dilation
    2. Urinary frequency.
    3. Hypertension.
    4. Constipation.
11. A patient taking Navane has several prn medications ordered. Which would be the most appropriate drug to give if this patient develops neck spasms and protruding tongue?
    1. Diphenhydramine (Benadryl) 10 mg IM q4h prn.
    2. Chlorpromazine (Thorazine) 25 mg IM q4h prn.
    3. Temazepam (Restoril) 15 mg PO q4h prn.
    4. Lorazepam (Ativan) 2 mg PO q4h prn.
12. Twenty-four hours after the initial dose of thiothixene (Navane), a patient has neck spasms, dysphagia, and tongue protrusion. The nurse accurately evaluates these symptoms as:
    1. Parkinsonian.
    2. Dystonia.

   3. Akathisia.
   4. Tardive dyskinesia.

13. A patient has been ordered 5 mg of thiothixene (Navane) qid. The nurse recalls that the major action of this medication is to: *(antipsychotic)*
   ✓1. Reduce distorted thoughts and perceptions.
   2. Increase appetite.
   3. Promote sleep.
   4. Relieve depression.

14. A patient who has been on Elavil for 3 days complains of not feeling better. How should the nurse respond?
   1. Suggest the patient report it to the MD.
   2. Suggest the patient stop taking the medication.
   ✓3. Encourage the patient to continue taking the medication.
   4. Record the patient's response to the medication.

15. The nurse would teach the patient to report which serious side effect of amitriptyline hydrochloride (Elavil) to the MD?
   1. Diarrhea.
   2. Dizziness.
   3. Insomnia.
   ✓4. Urinary retention.

16. A patient who has been on haloperidol (Haldol) 10 mg HS for 3 weeks tells the nurse, "I just can't sit still any more!" The nurse assesses that the patient is experiencing:
   1. Akinesia.
   ✓2. Akathisia.
   3. Parkinsonism.
   4. Torticollis.

17. As part of home care for a patient on Haldol (haloperidol), for what common side effect should the nurse assess?
   ✓1. Extrapyramidal symptoms (EPS).
   2. Hypoglycemia.
   3. High blood pressure.
   4. Involuntary movements.

18. What is a possible consequence of sudden withdrawal from Valium?
   1. Drowsiness.
   2. Ataxia.
   3. Confusion.
   ✓4. Seizures.

19. A patient is going home on an MAO inhibitor. What is the most important health teaching that the nurse needs to provide?
   1. The importance of monitoring for signs of hypotension.
   ✓2. Information about dietary restrictions.
   3. Information about activity restrictions.
   4. The importance of staying on the medication regimen.

20. While a patient is on tranylcypromine sulfate (Parnate), which food should be avoided?
   ✓1. Aged cheeses.
   2. Green vegetables.
   3. Nuts.
   4. Whole wheat.

21. What should the primary care nurse do when a patient's serum lithium is 0.5 mEq/L?
   1. Withhold the next lithium dose.
   ✓2. Give the next lithium dose.
   3. Ask the MD to check the patient.
   4. Determine the patient's compliance with the prescribed medication regimen.

22. The nurse observes that a patient on lithium has a coarse hand tremor, slurred speech, and ataxia. Vital signs indicate a decrease in blood pressure and irregular pulse. At this time the nurse would:
   1. Give the next dose of lithium to raise the blood level of the drug.
   2. Assure the patient that these are common side effects of lithium, and not reason for concern.
   ✓3. Withhold the next dose of lithium and request a lithium blood level.
   4. Give the next dose of lithium along with trihexyphenidyl hydrochloride (Artane) 5 mg PO, prn, to decrease the tremors.

23. Discharge teaching for a patient with a bipolar disorder includes explaining how lithium interacts with diet. The nurse would instruct this patient to:
   1. Maintain a table-salt–free diet, to reduce edema.
   2. Maintain a reduced table-salt diet, since lithium is a salt.
   3. Maintain a regular table-salt diet, to reduce lithium toxicity.
   4. Not worry about table salt, because it does not affect lithium levels.

24. When a patient is taking lithium, the nurse must evaluate for the possibility of toxicity. Initial signs are:
   ✓1. Polyuria, diarrhea, nausea, and vomiting.
   2. Motor weakness, headache, and edema.
   3. Lethargy, drowsiness, and slurred speech.
   4. Convulsions, delirium, and stupor.

25. A patient with bipolar disorder, manic phase is prescribed 600 mg bid of lithium. The nurse recalls that the therapeutic blood level, with an expected alteration in the patient's mood, will be reached in:
   1. 4–6 hours.
   2. 4–6 days.
   ✓3. 1–3 weeks.
   4. 1–2 months.

26. The patient is given disulfiram (Antabuse) to discourage drinking when discharged. In health teaching, the nurse would instruct the patient that it is safe to use:
   1. Mouthwash.
   2. Cough elixirs.
   3. Aftershave lotion.
   ✓4. Antacids.

27. After applying mechanical restraints to a patient who is delirious and combative, the nurse should:
   ✓1. Check extremities for circulation.
   2. Secure the restraints to the bed rails.
   3. Check and chart the patient's mental status q2h.
   4. Offer a bedpan or urinal once per shift.

Answers/Rationale

1. **(1)** This is the *desired* result; the therapeutic aim is to erase memories that may be perpetuating depression.

Hyperalertness (**No. 2**) and hyperkinesis (**No. 3**) are incorrect because the opposite occurs. Following ECT, the person is *drowsy* and *lethargic*, and is likely to be sleeping. (*Safety* will therefore be a primary goal; put the side rails up, as the patient will be confused and disoriented as to time and place.) Paranoid behavior (**No. 4**) is irrelevant, as it is not an expected result of ECT. **EV, 2, PsI**

2. **(1)** The nurse needs to take vital signs every 15 minutes for the first 45 minutes after ECT, to watch for *bradycardia*. Pain medications (**No. 2**) are not indicated after ECT. It is *not* necessary to put the patient in restraints (**No. 3**) *after* ECT. No. 4 is a good intervention, but *not right after* ECT, as the patient will, in all likelihood, sleep for the first 15 minutes. **IMP, 1, PhI**

💡 *Test-taking tip:* A priority answer focuses on *assessment* (vital signs, **No. 1**) and physiologic integrity.

3. **(3)** Seizures will be induced as part of the procedure; therefore maintaining an airway, as always, is the *priority*. Monitoring vital signs (**No. 1**) is the *next* priority. It is important to watch for bradycardia, especially *after* the procedure. Controlling spasms (**No. 2**) is unnecessary because a muscle relaxant (Brevital) is given *before* ECT, to control jerking movements caused by ECT. The electric charges (**No. 4**) are applied by the *MD*, not the nurse. **IMP, 1, PhI**

💡 *Test-taking tip:* Remember, the priority is always **ABC**: **A**irway, **B**reathing, **C**irculation.

4. **(3)** The patient will be in a confused state after treatment and will require side rails, as a safety measure, and the reassuring presence of a nurse. Suicide (**No. 1**) and hunger (**No. 4**) are *not* immediate posttreatment concerns. No. 2 is incorrect because the patient *needs someone present* to help with orientation, as the patient is likely to wake up somewhat disoriented. **AN, 7, SECE**

💡 *Test-taking tip:* Concern with safety is a priority answer ("most important"). Also note key word: "immediate."

5. **(2)** The *specific* behaviors are descriptive of akathisia, a *specific* side effect of Thorazine. Dystonia (**No. 1**) is wrong because it is characterized by *specific* muscular spasms, tongue protrusion, and oculogyric crisis. Extrapyramidal symptoms (**No. 3**) is wrong because it refers to a *general* category of side effects; akathisia is *one specific type* of EPS, as are dystonia (**No. 1**) and pseudo-parkinsonism (**No. 4**). Pseudo-parkinsonism (**No. 4**) is wrong because the characteristic specific be-

Key to Codes

Nursing process: AS = Assessment; **AN** = Analysis; **PL** = Planning; **IMP** = Implementation; **EV** = Evaluation. (See Appendix E for explanation of nursing process steps.)

Category of human function: 1 = Protective; **2** = Sensory-Perceptual; **3** = Comfort, Rest, Activity, and Mobility; **4** = Nutrition; **5** = Growth and Development; **6** = Fluid-Gas Transport; **7** = Psychosocial-Cultural; **8** = Elimination. (See Appendix G for explanation.)

Client need: SECE = Safe, Effective Care Environment; **PhI** = Physiologic Integrity; **PsI** = Psychosocial Integrity; **HPM** = Health Promotion/Maintenance. (See Appendix H for explanation.)

haviors include: a shuffling gait, drooling, pill-rolling motion, and blank facies. **EV, 3, PsI**

💡 *Test-taking tip:* Look at the question stem to determine whether it calls for a *specific* or general answer. In this question, the *specific* behaviors described call for a *specific* category of side effects (akathisia), *not* the *general* EPS category.

6. **(3)** The patient is improving, and the Cogentin has been effective, when extrapyramidal symptoms lessen. Photosensitivity (**No. 1**) *will* still be a problem, and it is *not* an extrapyramidal symptom. Visual problems (**No. 2**) will *not* improve. The patient will *not* be normotensive (**No. 4**), but *hypotensive*. What are some common extrapyramidal symptoms to remember? The first is *akathisia*, which is a shaking, tremulous feeling; the person will tell the nurse that he or she feels like there is a bowl of Jell-O inside of the body and everything is sort of shaking and quivering. Second is *dystonia*: the eyes roll to the back of the head, into an oculogyric crisis. There is a spasm between the neck and shoulder blades (sternocleidomastoid muscles), and there is a terrible feeling that this is a bizarre happening (although it is not life-threatening). The third main symptom is a *Parkinson-like syndrome* (also called Parkinsonian, pseudo-parkinsonism): a fine tremor, drooling, eyes and face in a sort of a blank stare, a pill-rolling motion, and a shuffling gait. **EV, 3, PsI**

💡 *Test-taking tip:* Focus on the key word: *improvement*.

7. **(2)** Although the term "antidote" is awkward in referring to these drugs, it can be read, "drug that counteracts side effects"; Artane and Cogentin are given to counteract the side effects of Thorazine. Haldol (**No. 1**) and Prolixin (**No. 4**) are not used to counteract phenothiazine side effects because Haldol *is like* a phenothiazine and Prolixin *is* a phenothiazine (it is the *long*-acting one). Elavil (**No. 3**) is a tricyclic drug that is used to treat depression. **IMP, 1, SECE**

💡 *Test-taking tip:* Don't get "hung up" if a question is phrased awkwardly as an exam question. Translate it in your mind (as above: "*antidote . . . that means it counteracts the side effects*").

8. **(2)** Due to photosensitivity, there is danger of sunburn with use of Thorazine; a picnic is the only activity listed here that usually takes place outdoors. A movie (**No. 1**), shopping (**No. 3**), and a concert (**No. 4**) would all usually take place *indoors*, with little risk of sunburn. **AN, 1, PhI**

💡 *Test-taking tip:* Look at the option that is different from the others. In this case, three options are typically indoor activities, but one option is typically an *outdoor* activity. When in doubt and you need to guess, choose the option that is different.

9. **(3)** Dry mouth (cholinergic effect) is a side effect of Thorazine; candy and gum provide an *anti*cholinergic effect. (Other side effects related to phenothiazines such as Thorazine are akathisia, pseudo-parkinsonism,

and dystonia.) **Nos. 1 and 2** are incorrect because neither nausea nor diarrhea is a typical side effect. Aspirin **(No. 4)** is not relevant when a patient is on Thorazine. **IMP, 7, PsI**

💡 *Test-taking tip:* Which option is not like the others? Three **(Nos. 1, 2, and 4)** are *medications,* but one **(No. 3)** is *not* a medication.

10. **(4)** Constipation is a side effect of Cogentin. Cogentin also causes pupil *dilation* (not constriction, **No. 1**), urinary *retention* (not frequency, **No. 2**), and *hypo*tension (not hypertension, **No. 3**). **EV, 8, PsI**

11. **(1)** Only Benadryl would reduce all the extrapyramidal symptoms. Thorazine **(No. 2)** would *increase* the symptoms. Restoril **(No. 3)** is used to promote *sleep.* Ativan **(No. 4)** reduces anxiety and agitation, not neck spasms and tongue protrusion. **IMP, 3, PsI**

12. **(2)** Acute dystonic reaction is characterized by limb and neck spasms, rigidity of back muscles, oculogyric crisis, speech and swallowing difficulties, and tongue protrusion. It occurs within the first few hours, extending through the first few weeks after starting Navane. Parkinsonian symptoms **(No. 1)** are characterized by fine motor tremors; akathisia **(No. 3)** is characterized by motor restlessness. Tardive dyskinesia **(No. 4)** would occur only after *long-term* use (at least 3 mo). **EV, 3, PsI**

13. **(1)** Thiothixene (Navane) is an antipsychotic medication. It reduces thought disorders and altered perceptions. **Nos. 2, 3, and 4** are not major actions of this medication. **PL, 2, PsI**

14. **(3)** It may take 2–4 weeks before a patient experiences a change, so the nurse should explain this and encourage the patient to continue taking the Elavil. **Nos. 1 and 2** both imply that there is something wrong if no noticeable effect is seen in 2–3 days, whereas a *lag* in time *is typical.* **No. 4** is not a good choice because "recording the patient's response" applies to *all* situations, *not specifically* to this one. **IMP, 7, PsI**

💡 *Test-taking tip:* Look at contradictory options; in this case, **No. 2** is *stop* the med, and **No. 3** is *continue* the med. If you need to guess, narrow your choices to these two; then, recalling a point of theory (e.g., time lag) will help with the final choice **(No. 3).**

15. **(4)** Urinary retention is a serious, autonomic nervous system (ANS) side effect of Elavil. Diarrhea **(No. 1)** is incorrect because the opposite, constipation, occurs. Dizziness **(No. 2)** and insomnia **(No. 3)** are *not* known to occur as common side effects of Elavil. *To remember ANS side effects* of tricyclics (e.g., Elavil), think of what would help if a lion was chasing you, so that you could make a quick getaway: you would need to hold on to your bodily fluids (urine, feces, saliva), leading to urine retention, constipation, and dry mouth. Another important ANS side effect is ECG changes (flattened T waves and arrhythmias). Remember also that it takes 2–4 weeks before desired results are seen. **PL, 8, HPM**

💡 *Test-taking tip:* Look for the *most serious* side effect.

16. **(2)** Akathisia refers to the continuous motor restlessness, fidgeting, and pacing that occur with use of neuroleptics (antipsychotics). Anticholinergics (Artane, Cogentin) can be used to treat extrapyramidal side effects like this. Akinesia **(No. 1)** is the *opposite* of movement and restlessness; it means fatigue and muscular weakness. Parkinsonism **(No. 3),** or more specifically, pseudo-parkinsonism, involves pill-rolling motion, drooling, fine tremors, and a shuffling gait. The question does not indicate that the patient is experiencing these side effects. Torticollis **(No. 4)** involves neck spasms—acute dystonia. This is not what the patient is experiencing in this question. **AN, 3, PsI**

💡 *Test-taking tip:* When you need to make an "educated guess," look at two opposites (here, **No. 1,** *lack* of movement, and **No. 2,** *restless* movement).

17. **(1)** It is important for the nurse to assess for extrapyramidal symptoms, including involuntary movements (akathisia), dystonia, and pseudo-parkinsonism. Because it *includes* akathisia **(No. 4),** this option is the more inclusive response. Hypoglycemia **(No. 2)** is *not* relevant to assess as a side effect of Haldol. *Hypotension, not hypertension* **(No. 3)** is a side effect that is important to monitor. Involuntary movements **(No. 4)** are covered by **No. 1,** the more inclusive answer. **AS, 7, PsI**

💡 *Test-taking tip:* Choose the "telescope" answer, the one that includes another option and is therefore more comprehensive.

18. **(4)** This option is the best answer by process of elimination. The person withdrawing from Valium does have seizures, which are serious. Look at the key words: "possible consequence," i.e., potentially serious problem. Of the options here, seizures seem to be the most potentially serious problem. Drowsiness **(No. 1)**, ataxia **(No. 2)**, and confusion **(No. 3)** are side effects when *on* Valium, not when withdrawing from it. **AS, 2, PsI**

💡 *Test-taking tips*

- Exam takers often miss questions like this because of missing the *key word;* in this case, missing "withdrawal," and focusing on side effects instead. Be sure to look for the key word in the stem of a question.
- When you are unsure as to the best answer, you won't get clues from reading and rereading the options, but rather from the *question stem;* therefore, reread the stem.

19. **(2)** It is most important to *avoid* foods containing tyramine (which is a pressor amine), which can potentiate the CNS stimulant effects of the MAOIs, and may result in stroke and death. The long list of food items to avoid includes caffeine products, wine (especially red), cheese, and herring. (The nurse must also teach the importance of not taking any over-the-counter antihistamine medications, like Sudafed, for the same reason.) **No. 1** is incorrect because the danger to watch for is a *hyper*tensive crisis, *not hypotension.* Activity **(No. 3)** has no relation to MAOIs. Staying on the regimen **(No.**

4), while important, is not *specific* to MAOIs; it applies to most drugs. **IMP, 7, HPM**

20. **(1)** Parnate (like Niamid, Nardil, and Marplan) is an MAO inhibitor. Monoamine-oxidase inhibitors interact with tyramine-containing foods (such as fermented or pickled foods). Toxicity can result in hypertensive crisis. Other common foods to avoid are: herring, wine (especially red), pickles, beer, salami, chocolates, cola and any caffeine product, avocado, bananas, raisins, licorice, yogurt, liver, sour cream, soy sauce, and meat tenderizers. Green vegetables (**No. 2**), nuts (**No. 3**), and whole wheat (**No. 4**) are not contraindicated because they do *not* contain tyramine. **PL, 4, PsI**

21. **(2)** The therapeutic range is 0.8–1.6 mEq/L; 0.5 mEq/L is below the therapeutic level, so the nurse needs to *give* the next dose. Withholding the drug (**No. 1**) is incorrect because it is the opposite of the correct response. The drug would be withheld if serum lithium was over 2.0 mEq/L. **Nos. 3 and 4** would *follow* giving the next dose in the sequence of actions when the serum lithium level is below therapeutic level. **IMP, 1, SECE**

💡 *Test-taking tip:* When in doubt, focus on two options that are diametrically opposed (here, **No. 1** is "don't give" and **No. 2** is "give").

22. **(3)** Coarse hand tremors, slurred speech, and ataxia are major symptoms of lithium toxicity; the next dose should be withheld to decrease the lithium, and the blood level should be checked. Giving the lithium (**Nos. 1 and 4**) would increase the toxicity; also, Artane (**No. 4**) is given for extrapyramidal reactions, not lithium toxicity. **No. 2** is incorrect because these symptoms *are* serious side effects and require intervention. **EV, 3, PsI**

💡 *Test-taking tip:* When two options contradict each other, and you don't know which to pick, you may want to make an educated guess, choosing the one that is *different*. In this case, **Nos. 1, 2, and 4** all focus on *giving* the drug. **No. 3** is the one that is different ("withhold").

23. **(3)** To cross the neuron membrane, the lithium needs to be transported with sodium, so a normal amount of salt should be included in the diet. By limiting the salt,

Nos. 1 and 2 would limit the utilization of the lithium. **No. 4** is incorrect because salt *does* play an important role in lithium management. **IMP, 4, HPM**

24. **(1)** These symptoms of lithium toxicity may occur at lithium levels of 1.6–2.0 mEq/L. The symptoms in **Nos. 2 and 3** are not the *initial* signs; they tend to occur at levels above 2.0 mEq/L. The symptoms in **No. 4** occur even later, at levels above 2.5 mEq/L. **EV, 1, 7**

25. **(3)** It takes 1 to 3 weeks to reach the therapeutic blood level and begin seeing results. The time periods in **Nos. 1 and 2** are too short. The time period in **No. 4** is too long. **EV, 7, PSI**

26. **(4)** When a patient on Antabuse uses alcohol, the patient vomits; antacids do *not* contain alcohol and are therefore safe to use. Mouthwash (**No. 1**) and cough elixirs (**No. 2**) often contain alcohol as an ingredient, and may therefore induce vomiting. Most aftershaves (**No. 3**) also contain alcohol. It is better not to have it on hand, as some alcohol-dependent individuals will even drink aftershave lotion when no other source of alcohol is available. When Antabuse and alcohol are paired and the patient vomits, the patient learns to associate intake of alcohol with the noxious result of vomiting. This is called aversive conditioning, or aversion therapy. See also *aversion therapy* in Chap. 1. **IMP, 1, PsI**

💡 *Test-taking tip:* Choose the one that is not like the others (**Nos. 1, 2, and 3** contain alcohol, only **No. 4** does not).

27. **(1)** Safety and physiologic integrity (e.g., hydration, elimination) are the important concerns, so checking for circulation is the priority. Restraints should be secured to the bed frames, never the bed *rails* (**No. 2**). **No. 3** is incorrect because checking and charting status every 2 hours implies that there is no one with the patient in the meantime. **No. 4** is definitely incorrect. A shift may be 8 hours or more! Basic needs like elimination need to be taken care of more often than once every 8–12 hours! **IMP, 1, SECE**

💡 *Test-taking tip:* A *priority* answer is called for, even if not explicitly worded in the question stem. Safety and circulation are commonly the priority concerns.

Psychiatric Emergencies

Chapter Outline

- General Characteristics
- Categories of Psychiatric Emergencies
  - Acute Nonpsychotic Reactions
  - Delirium
    Acute Alcohol Intoxication
    Hallucinogenic Drug Intoxication
    Acute Delirium
  - Acute Psychotic Reactions
    Acute Schizophrenic Reaction
    Manic Reaction
  - Disease States That May Produce Psychotic Symptoms
  - Homicidal or Assaultive Reaction
  - Suicidal Ideation
- Crisis Intervention
- Study and Memory Aids
- Glossary
- Summary of Key Points
- Questions
- Answers/Rationale

A psychiatric emergency* is the sudden onset (days or weeks, not years) of unusual (for that individual), disordered (without pattern or purpose), or socially inappropriate behavior caused by emotional or physiologic situation. For example: suicidal feelings or attempts, overdose, acute psychotic reaction, acute alcohol withdrawal, acute anxiety.

General Characteristics

▶ I. **Assessment:** the presence of great distress without reasonable explanation; *extreme* behavior in comparison with antecedent event.
  A. *Fear*—related to a particular person, activity, or place.
  B. *Anxiety*—fearful feeling without any obvious reason, not specifically related to a particular person, activity, or place (e.g., adolescent turmoil).
  C. *Depression*—continual pessimism, easily moved to tears, hopelessness, and isolation (e.g., student despondency around exam time, middle-aged crisis, elderly hopelessness).
  D. *Mania*—unrealistic optimism.
  E. *Anger*—many events seen as deliberate insults.
  F. *Confusion*—diminished awareness of who and where one is; memory loss.
  G. *Loss of reality contact*—hallucinations or delusion (as in acute psychosis).

H. *Withdrawal*—neglect or giving away of belongings and neglect of appearance; loss of interest in activities; apathy.
▶ II. **Analysis/nursing diagnosis**—*Ineffective individual coping* related to degree of seriousness:
  A. *Life-threatening emergencies*—violence toward self or others (e.g., suicide, homicide).
  B. *Serious emergencies*—confused and unable to care for or protect self from dangerous situations (as in substance abuse).
  C. *Potentially serious emergencies*—anxious and in pain; disorganized behavior; can become worse or better (as in grief reaction and rape).
▶ III. **General nursing care plan/implementation**
  A. *Remove* from stressful situation and persons.
  B. Engage in *dialogue* at a nonthreatening distance, to offer help.
  C. Use *calm, slow, deliberate* approach to relieve stress and disorganization.
  D. *Explain* what will be done about the problem and the likely outcome.
  E. *Avoid* using force, threat, or counterthreat.
  F. Use *confident, firm, reasonable* approach.
  G. Encourage client to relate.
  H. Elicit *details*.
  I. Encourage *ventilation* of feelings without interruption.
  J. Accept distortions of reality *without arguing*.
  K. Give form and *structure* to the conversation.
  L. Contact significant others to gain information and to be with client, including previous therapist.

*Adapted from Aguilera D, Messick J. *Crisis Intervention: Therapy for Psychological Emergencies*. St. Louis: Mosby, 1986.

M. Treat emergency as *temporary* and *readily resolved.*

N. Check every half hour if cannot remain with client.

Categories of Psychiatric Emergencies

Acute Nonpsychotic Reactions

Acute anxiety attack or panic reaction is the most common acute nonpsychotic reaction (for symptoms, see Anxiety and Anxiety Disorders, pp. 2–3 and Chap. 9). *Hyperventilation syndrome* may occur.

I. Assessment includes differentiating hyperventilation that is anxiety connected *from* asthma, angina, and heart disease.

II. Nursing care plan/implementation in *hyperventilation syndrome*—Goal: prevent paresthesia, tetanic contractions, disturbance in awareness; reassure client that vital organs are not impaired.

A. Have patient increase carbon dioxide in lungs by rebreathing from paper bag.

B. Minimize secondary gains; *avoid* reinforcing behavior.

C. *Health teaching:* demonstrate how to slow down breathing rate.

III. Evaluation/outcome criteria: respirations slowed down; no evidence of effect of hyperventilation.

Delirium

Delirium refers to conditions produced by changes in the cerebral chemistry or tissue by metabolic toxins, direct trauma to the brain, drug effects, and/or withdrawal. Different from dementia (see pp 148–150).

I. Acute alcohol intoxication (see also **Alcohol Abuse and Dependence,** pp 162–165).

A. Assessment: signs of head or other injury (past and recent), emotional lability, memory defects, loss of judgment, disorientation.

B. Nursing care plan/implementation
1. Observe, monitor *vital signs* (autonomic nervous system effects).
2. *Prevent aspiration* of vomitus by positioning.
3. *Decrease* environmental stimuli:
    a. Place in quiet area of emergency room.
    b. Speak and handle calmly.
4. Give medication (diazepam [Valium]) to control agitation.

C. Evaluation/outcome criteria: oriented to time, place, person; appears calmer.

II. Hallucinogenic drug intoxication—Common agents include lysergic acid diethylamide (LSD), mescaline, amphetamines, cocaine, scopolamine, and belladonna.

A. Assessment
1. Perceptual and cognitive distortions (e.g., feels heart stop beating).
2. Anxiety (apprehension → panic).

3. Subjective feelings (omnipotence → worthlessness).
4. Interrelationship of dose, potency, setting, expectations, and experiences of user.
5. Eyes: *red*—marijuana; *dilated*—LSD, mescaline, belladonna; *constricted*—heroin and derivatives.

B. Nursing care plan/implementation
1. "Talk down."
    a. Establish *verbal* contact, attempt to have client verbally express what is being experienced.
    b. *Environment*—few people, normal lights, calm, supportive.
    c. Allay fears.
    d. Encourage to keep eyes *open.*
    e. Have client focus on *inanimate* objects in room as a bridge to reality contact.
    f. Use simple, *concrete, repetitive* statements.
    g. *Repetitively* orient to time, place, and temporary nature.
    h. Do *not* moralize, challenge beliefs, or probe into life-style.
    i. Emphasize confidentiality.
2. *Medication*—Administer a minor tranquilizer such as diazepam (*Valium*) or *Librium*:
    a. Allay anxiety.
    b. Reduce aggressive behavior.
    c. Reduce suicidal potential; check client every 5–15 min.
    d. Avoid anticholinergic crisis (precipitated by use of *phenothiazines, belladonna,* and *scopolamine* ingestion) with 2–4 mg IM or PO of *physostigmine salicylate.*
3. *Hospitalization:* if hallucinations, delusions last more than 12–18 hr; if client has been injecting amphetamines for extended time; if client is paranoid and depressed.

C. Evaluation/outcome criteria: less frightened; oriented to time, place, person.

III. Acute delirium—seen in postoperative electrolyte imbalance, systemic infections, renal and hepatic failure, oversedation, metastatic cancer. Different from dementia (see pp. 148–150).

A. Assessment
1. Disorientation regarding time, especially at night.
2. Hallucinations, delusions, illusions.
3. Alterations in mood.
4. Increased emotional lability.
5. Agitation.
6. Lack of cooperation.
7. Withdrawal.
8. Sleep pattern reversal.
9. Alterations in food intake.

B. Nursing care plan/implementation
1. Identify and remove *toxic* substance.
2. Reality orientation—well-lit room; constant attendance to inform *repetitively* of place and time and to *protect* from injury to self and others.

3. Simplify environment.

👁 4. *Avoid* excessive medication and restraints; use low-dose *phenothiazines;* do **not** give barbiturates or sedatives (these increase agitation, confusion, disorientation).

✉ **C. Evaluation/outcome criteria:** oriented to time, place, person; cooperative; less agitated.

Acute Psychotic Reactions

Acute psychotic reactions are disorders of mood or thinking characterized by hallucinations, delusions, excessive euphoria (mania), or depression.

I. Acute schizophrenic reaction (see also **Schizophrenic Disorders,** pp. 127–130).

✉ **A. Assessment**

1. History of previous hospitalization, no illicit drug ingestion; use of major tranquilizers and recent withdrawal from them or alcohol.

2. Auditory hallucinations and delusions.

3. Violent, assaultive, suicidal behavior directed by auditory hallucinations.

4. Assault, withdrawal, and panic related to paranoid delusions of persecution; fear of harm.

5. Disturbance in mental status (associative thought disorder).

✉ **B. Nursing care plan/implementation** (see also **Hallucinations,** pp. 128–130).

1. Hospitalization.

2. Safe environment, away from others.

👁 3. Medication—phenothiazines are given to ↓ psychotic symptoms.

4. *Avoid* physical restraints or touch when fears and delusions of sexual attack exist.

5. Allow client to *diffuse* anger and intensity of panic through talk.

6. Use simple, *concrete* terms; *avoid* figures of speech or content subject to multiple interpretations.

7. Do *not* agree with reality distortions; point out that client's thoughts are difficult to understand but you are willing to listen.

✉ **C. Evaluation/outcome criteria:** doesn't hear frightening voices; less fearful and combative behavior.

II. Manic reaction (see also **Bipolar Disorders,** pp. 139–141).

✉ **A. Assessment**

1. History of depression requiring antidepressants.

2. *Thought disorder* (flight of ideas, delusions of grandeur).

3. *Affect* (elated, irritable, irrational anger).

4. *Speech* (loud, pressured).

5. *Behavior* (rapid, erratic, chaotic).

✉ **B. Nursing care plan/implementation**

1. Hospitalization to protect from injury to self and others.

👁 2. Medication: *lithium carbonate* is given to ↓ manic symptoms.

3. Same as for acute schizophrenic reaction, *ex-*

cept do not encourage talk, as need to decrease stimulation.

4. Provide food and fluids that can be consumed while on-the-go.

✉ **C. Evaluation/outcome criteria:** speech and activity slowed down; thoughts less disordered.

Disease States That May Produce Psychotic Symptoms

This list is not intended to be comprehensive. It is provided simply as a reminder that "psychiatric" symptoms may be the result of physical illness. Assess every "psychotic" patient carefully!

I. Toxic and Deficiency States

  A. Drug-induced psychoses, especially from

    1. Digitalis

    2. Steroids

    3. Disulfiram

    4. Amphetamines

    5. LSD, PCP, and other psychedelics

  B. Alcoholic hallucinosis

  C. Wernicke's encephalopathy

  D. Korsakoff's psychosis

  E. Poisoning with bromide or other heavy metals

  F. Pellagra and other vitamin deficiencies

  G. Uremia

  H. Liver failure

II. Infections

  A. Syphilis

  B. Toxoplasmosis

  C. Viral encephalitis

  D. Brain abscess

III. Neurologic Disease

  A. Seizure disorders (especially temporal lobe seizures)

  B. Primary and metastatic tumors of the brain

  C. Presenile and senile dementias

  D. Postencephalitic states (e.g., after measles encephalitis)

IV. Cardiovascular Disorders

  A. Low cardiac output (e.g., in heart failure)

  B. Hypertensive encephalopathy

V. Endocrine Disorders

  A. Thyrotoxicosis

  B. Myxedema

  C. Adrenal hyperfunction (Cushing's syndrome)

VI. Metabolic Disorders

  A. Electrolyte imbalances (e.g., after severe diarrhea)

  B. Hypoglycemia

  C. Diabetic ketoacidosis

Source: Caroline N. *Emergency Care in the Streets* (5th ed). Boston: Little, Brown, 1995. P 902.

Homicidal or Assaultive Reaction

Homicidal or assaultive reaction is seen in acutely drug-intoxicated, delirious, paranoid, acutely excited manic, or acute anxiety-panic conditions.

✉ **I. Assessment**—history of obvious antisocial behavior, paranoid psychosis, previous violence, sexual conflict, rivalry, substance abuse, recent moodiness, and withdrawal.

✉ **II. Nursing care plan/implementation**

☞ **A.** Physically restrain if client has a weapon; use group of trained people to help. See Chap. 5, restraints, p. 70.

  B. Allow person to "save face" in giving up weapon.

  C. *Separate* from intended victims.

  D. Approach: calm, unhurried; *one person* to offer support and reassurance; use clear, unambiguous statements.

  E. Immediate and rapid admission procedures.

  F. Observe for *suicidal* behavior that may follow homicidal attempt.

✉ **III. Evaluation/outcome criteria:** client regains impulse control.

Suicidal Ideation

Suicidal ideation is seen in anxiety attacks, substance intoxication, toxic delirium, schizophrenic auditory hallucinations, and depressive reactions.

  I. Concepts and principles related to suicide

  A. *Based on social theory:* Suicidal tendency is a result of collective social forces rather than isolated individual motives (Durkheim's *Le Suicide*).

   1. Common factor: increased *alienation* between person and social group; psychological isolation, called "anomie," when links between groups are weakened.

   2. "Egoistic" suicide: results from lack of integration of individual with others.

   3. "Altruistic" suicide: results from insufficient individualization.

   4. *Implication:* increase group cohesiveness and mutual interdependence, making group more coherent and consistent in fulfilling needs of each member.

  B. *Based on symbolic interaction theory*

   1. Person evaluates self according to *others' assessment*.

   2. Thus, suicide stems from *social rejection* and disrupted social relations.

   3. Perceived failure in relationships with others may be inaccurate but seen as real by the individual.

   4. *Implication:* need to recognize difference in perception of alienation between own viewpoint and others'.

  C. *Based on psychoanalytic theory*

   1. Suicide stems mainly from the individual, with external events only as precipitants.

   2. There is a strong life urge in people.

   3. *Universal death instinct* is always present (Freud).

   4. Person may be balancing life wishes and death wishes. When self-preservation instincts are diminished, death instincts may find direct outlet via suicide.

  5. When *love instinct* is frustrated, *hate* impulse takes over (Menninger).

   a. Desire to kill → desire to be killed → desire to kill oneself.

   b. Suicide may be an act of extreme *hostility, manipulation,* and *revenge* to elicit guilt and remorse in significant others.

   c. Suicide may also be act of *self-punishment* to handle own guilt or to control fate.

  6. *Implication:* support person's life wishes.

  D. *Based on synthesis of social and psychoanalytic theories:*

   1. Suicide is seen as *running away* from an intolerable situation in order to interrupt it rather than *running to* something more desirable.

   2. Process *defined in operational terms* involves:

   a. Despair over inability to cope.

   b. Inability to feel hope or adequacy.

   c. Frustration with others when others cannot fill needs.

   d. Rage and aggression experienced toward significant other is turned inward.

   e. Psychic blow acts as precipitant.

   f. Life seen as harder to cope with, with no chance of improvement in life situation.

   g. *Implication:* persons who experience suicidal impulses can gain a certain amount of control over these impulses through the support they gain from meaningful relationships with others.

  E. *Based on crisis theory (Dublin):* concept of emotional disequilibrium:

   1. Everyone at some point in life is in a crisis, with temporary inability to solve problems or to master the crisis.

   2. Usual coping mechanisms do not function.

   3. Person unable to relate to others.

   4. Person searches consciously and unconsciously for useful coping techniques, with suicide as one of various solutions.

   5. With inadequate communication of needs and isolation, suicide is possible.

   6. *Implication:* assist person to get in touch with previous coping mechanisms.

  F. *Based on the view that suicide is an individual's personal reaction and decision, a final response to own situation:*

   1. *Process* of anger turned inward → self-inflicted, destructive action.

   2. *Definition* of concept in *operational steps:*

   a. Frustration of individual needs → anger.

   b. Anger turned inward → feelings of guilt, despair, depression, incompetence, hopelessness, and exhaustion.

   c. Stress felt and perceived as unbearable and overwhelming.

   d. Attempt to communicate hopelessness and defeat to others.

   e. Others do not provide hope.

   f. Sudden change in behavior, as noted when depression appears to lift, may indicate *danger,* as person has more energy to act on suicidal thoughts and feelings.

g. Decision to end life → plan of action → self-induced, self-destructive behavior.

3. May be *pseudo-suicide* attempts, where there is no actual or realistic desire to achieve finality of death. Intentions or causes may be:

a. "Cry for help," where nonlethal attempt notifies others of deeper intentions.

b. Desire to *manipulate* others.

c. Need for *attention and pity.*

d. *Self-punishment.*

e. Symbol of *utter frustration.*

f. Wish to *punish* others.

g. *Misuse* of alcohol and other drugs.

4. Other reasons for self-destruction, where the individual *gives own life* rather than takes it, include:

a. Strong parental love that can overcome fear and instinct of self-preservation to save child's life.

b. "Sacrificial death" during war, such as kamikaze pilots in World War II.

c. Submission to death for religious beliefs (martyrdom).

5. *Implication:* preventive interventions are needed to reduce anger, frustration, hopelessness, need for attention, pity, and manipulation.

II. Assessment of suicide

A. *Assessment of risk regarding statistical probability of suicide—composite picture:* over-45-year-old male, unemployed, divorced, living alone, depressed (weight loss, somatic delusions, sleep disturbance, preoccupied with suicide), history of substance abuse and suicide within family.

B. *Ten factors* to predict potential suicide and assess risk:

1. *Age, sex, and race*—teenage, older age; more women make attempts; more men complete suicide act. Highest risk: older women rather than young boys; older men rather than young girls. Suicide occurs in all races and socioeconomic groups.

2. *Recent stress*—family problems: death, divorce, separation, alienation; financial pressures; loss of job; loss of status; failing grades.

3. *Clues to suicide:* suicidal thoughts are usually time-limited and do not last forever. Early assessment of behavioral and verbal clues is important.°

a. *Verbal clues—Direct:* "I am going to shoot myself." *Indirect:* "It's more than I can bear." *Coded:* "This is the last time you'll ever see me." "I want you to have my coin collection."

b. *Behavioral clues—Direct:* trial run with pills or razor, for example. *Indirect:* sudden lifting of depression, buying a casket, giving away cherished belongings, putting affairs in order, writing a will.

c. *Syndromes—Dependent-dissatisfied:* emotionally dependent but dislikes dependent state, irritable, helpless. *Depressed:* detachment from life; feels life is a burden; hopelessness, futility. *Disoriented:* delusions or hallucinations, confusion, delirium tremens, dementia. *Willful-defiant:* active need to direct and control environment and life situation, with low frustration tolerance and rigid set, rage, shame.

4. *Suicidal plan*—the more details about method, timing, and place, the higher the risk.

5. *Previous suicidal behavior*—history of prior attempt increases risk. Eight out of ten suicide attempts give verbal and behavioral warnings as listed above.

6. *Medical status*—chronic ailments, terminal illness, and pain increase suicidal risk.

7. *Communication*—the more noncommunicative (i.e., nonverbal) and apathetic, the greater potential for suicide, *unless* extreme *psychomotor* retardation is present.

8. *Style of life*—high risks include substance abusers, those with sexual-identity conflicts, unstable relationships (personal and job-related). Suicidal tendencies are not inherited but learned from family and other interpersonal relationships.

9. *Alcohol*—can reinforce helpless and hopeless feelings; may be lethal if used with barbiturates; can decrease inhibitions, result in impulsive behavior.

10. *Resources*—the fewer the resources, the higher the suicide potential. Examples of resources: family, friends, colleagues, religion, pets, meaningful recreational outlets, satisfying employment.

C. Assess *needs* commonly communicated by individuals who are suicidal:

1. To trust.

2. To be accepted.

3. To bolster self-esteem.

4. To "fit in" with groups.

5. To experience success and interrupt the failure syndrome.

6. To expand capacity for pleasure.

7. To increase autonomy and sense of self-mastery.

8. To work out an acceptable sexual identity.

III. Analysis/nursing diagnosis—*Risk for self-directed violence* related to:

A. Feelings of alienation.

B. Feelings of rejection.

C. Feelings of hopelessness, despair.

D. Feelings of frustration and rage.

IV. Nursing care plan/implementation

A. Long-term goals

1. Increase client's self-reliance.

2. Help client achieve more realistic and positive

°Adapted from the *American Journal of Nursing* 65(5):112–115, 1965.

feelings of self-esteem, self-respect, acceptance by others, and sense of belonging.

3. Help client experience success, interrupt failure pattern, and expand views about pleasure.

B. Short-term goals

☞ 1. Medical: assist as necessary with *gastric lavage;* provide *respiratory* and *vascular* support; assist in repair of inflicted *wounds;* administer ordered medications (e.g., tricyclics for depression)

2. Provide protection from self-destruction until client is able to assume this responsibility.

3. *Allow outward and constructive* expression of hostile and aggressive feelings.

4. Provide for physical needs.

C. Suicide precautions to institute under emergency conditions:

1. One-to-one supervision at *all* times for maximum precautions; check whereabouts every 15 min, if on basic suicide precautions.

2. Prior to instituting these measures, explain to client what you will be doing and why; MD must also explain; document this explanation.

3. Do not allow client to leave the unit for tests, procedures.

4. Look through client's belongings *with* the client and remove any potentially harmful objects, e.g., pills, matches, belts, razors, glass, tweezers.

5. Allow visitors and phone calls, but maintain one-to-one supervision during visits.

6. Check that visitors do not leave potentially harmful objects in the client's room.

7. Serve meals in an isolation meal tray that contains no glass or metal silverware.

8. Do not discontinue these measures without an order.

D. General approaches

1. *Observe* closely at all times to assess suicide potential.

2. Be *available.*
   a. Demonstrate concern for client as a person.
   b. Be sensitive, warm, and consistent.
   c. Listen with empathy.
   d. *Avoid* imposing your own feelings of reality on client.
   e. *Avoid* extremes in your own mood when with client (especially exaggerated cheerfulness).

3. *Focus directly* on client's self-destructive ideas.
   a. Reduce alienation and immobilization by discussing this "taboo" topic.
   b. Acknowledge suicidal threats with calmness and without reproach—do not ignore or minimize threat.
   c. *Find out details* about suicide plan and reduce environmental hazards.
   d. Help client *verbalize* aggressive, hostile, and hopeless feelings.
   e. *Explore death fantasies*—try to take "romance" out of death.

4. Acknowledge that suicide is one of several options.

5. *Make a contract* with the client, and structure a plan of alternatives for coping when next confronted with the need to commit suicide (e.g., the client could call someone, express feeling of anger outwardly, or ask for help).

6. Point out client's *self-responsibility* for suicidal act.
   a. *Avoid* manipulation by client who says, "You are responsible for stopping me from killing myself."
   b. Emphasize protection against self-destruction *rather than* punishment.

7. *Support* the part of the client that wants to live.
   a. Focus on *ambivalence.*
   b. Emphasize meaningful past relationships and events.
   c. Look for reasons left for wanting to live. Elicit what is meaningful to the client at the moment.
   d. Point out effect of client's death on others.

8. *Remove sources of stress.*
   a. Decrease uncomfortable feelings of *alienation* by initiating one-to-one interactions.
   b. Make all *decisions* when client is in severe depression.
   c. Progressively let client make simple decisions: what to eat, what to watch on TV, etc.

9. *Provide hope.*
   a. Let client know that problems can be solved with help.
   b. Bring in new resources for help.
   c. Talk about likely changes in client's life.
   d. Review past effective coping behaviors.

10. *Provide with opportunity to be useful.* Reduce self-centeredness and brooding by planning diversional activities within the client's capabilities.

11. *Involve as many people as possible.*
    a. Gradually bring in others, e.g., other therapists, friends, staff, clergy, family, coworkers.
    b. Prevent staff "burn-out," found when only one nurse is working with suicidal client.

12. *Health teaching:* teach client and staff principles of crisis intervention and resolution. Teach new coping skills. Discuss effects of antidepressants, if ordered (e.g., tricyclics).

▶ **V. Evaluation/outcome criteria:** physical condition is stabilized; able to verbalize feelings rather than acting them out.

Crisis Intervention

Crisis intervention is a type of brief psychiatric treatment in which individuals and/or their families are helped in their efforts to forestall the process of mental decompensation in reaction to severe emotional stress by direct and immediate supportive approaches.

I. Definition of crisis—sudden event in one's life that disturbs homeostasis, during which usual coping mechanisms cannot resolve the problem. Types of crisis:

 A. *Maturational* (internal): see Erik Erikson's eight stages of developmental crises anticipated in the development of the infant, child, adolescent, and adult (Chap. 1).

 B. *Situational* (external): occurs at any time; e.g., loss of job, loss of income, death of significant person, illness, hospitalization, rape.

 C. *Adventitious* (external): sudden, uncommon, results in multiple losses and significant changes (e.g., destruction related to tornado, earthquake).

II. Concepts and principles related to crisis intervention:

 A. Crises are turning points where changes in behavior patterns and life-styles can occur; individuals in crisis are most amenable to altering old and unsuccessful coping mechanisms and are most likely to learn new and more functional behaviors.

 B. Social milieu and its structure are contributing factors in both the development of psychiatric symptoms and eventual recovery from them.

 C. If crisis is handled effectively, the person's mental stability will be maintained; individual may return to a precrisis state or better.

 D. If crisis is not handled effectively, individual may progress to a worse state with exacerbations of earlier conflicts; future crises may not be handled well.

 E. There are a number of universal developmental crisis periods (maturational crises) in every individual's life.

 F. Each person tries to maintain equilibrium through use of adaptive behaviors.

 G. When individuals face a problem they cannot solve, tension, anxiety, narrowed perception, and disorganized functioning occur.

 H. *Immediate relief* of symptoms (e.g., anxiety) produced by crisis is more urgent than *exploring* their cause.

III. Characteristics of crisis intervention:

 A. Acute, sudden onset related to a stressful precipitating event of which individual is aware but which immobilizes previous coping abilities.

 B. Responsive to brief therapy with focus on immediate problem.

 C. Focus shifted from the psyche in the individual to the *individual in the environment;* deemphasis on intrapsychic aspects.

 D. Crisis period is *time-limited* (usually up to 6 wk).

IV. Assess the crisis:

 1. Identify stressful *precipitating* events: duration, problems created, and degree of significance.

 2. Assess *suicidal and homicidal risk.*

 3. Assess amount of *disruption* in individual's life and effect on significant others.

 4. Assess *current coping skills,* strengths, and general level of functioning.

V. Nursing care plan/implementation in crises:

 A. **General goals**

 1. *Avoid* hospitalization if possible.

 2. Return to precrisis level and preserve ability to function.

 3. Assist in problem solving, with *here-and-now* focus.

 B. **Plan** the intervention:

 1. Consider *past coping* mechanisms.

 2. Propose *alternatives* and untried coping methods.

 C. **Implementation**

 1. Help client relate the crisis event to current feelings.

 2. Encourage expression of all feelings related to disruption.

 3. Explore past coping skills and *reinforce adaptive* ones.

 4. Use all means available in *social network* to take care of client's *immediate needs* (e.g., significant others, law enforcement agencies, housing, welfare, employment, medical, school).

 5. Set limits.

 6. *Health teaching:* provide anticipatory guidance; teach additional problem-solving approaches.

VI. Evaluation/outcome criteria

 A. Client returns to precrisis level of functioning.

 B. Client learns new, more effective coping skills.

 C. Client can describe realistic plans for future in terms of own perception of progress, support system, and coping mechanisms.

💡 Study and Memory Aids

Crisis intervention—four points of theory:

Crisis intervention theory emerged from research on the grieving process.

The first step in crisis intervention is to get the patient's perception of the event.

To clarify what happened, help the client to place the events in chronologic sequence.

Goal: Mobilize patient's support system.

Glossary

Suicide

suicide The act of taking one's own life voluntarily and intentionally.

Summary of Key Points

General Characteristics of a Psychiatric Emergency

Presence of extreme fear, anxiety, depression, mania, anger, confusion, withdrawal. Treat as potentially life-threatening.

Care of Patient with Acute Nonpsychotic Reactions (e.g., Anxiety Attack, Panic Reaction)

Assess and treat hyperventilation symptoms.

Care of a Patient with Delirium

Focus on physical and environmental aspects of care in *alcohol-related* condition.

Focus on "talking down" and environmental aspects of care in *hallucinogenic drug* intoxication.

Focus on removing toxic substances and providing reality orientation when *acute delirium* is due to electrolyte imbalances, infections, and metastatic cancer.

Care of a Patient with Acute Schizophrenic Reaction

1. Build trust with consistency and short, frequent contacts.
2. Verbalize the observable: "You seem frightened," or "I heard you speaking to someone."
3. Provide safe environment away from others; give antipsychotic medications.
4. Give your perception: "I don't hear voices."

Care of a Patient in Manic Reaction

Same as for *acute schizophrenic reaction* except:
Avoid stimulation; minimize talking.
Medication: *Lithium carbonate.*

Care of a Patient Who is Homicidal or Assaultive

1. Assess for clues of impending loss of self-control (e.g., agitation). The priority is prevention of violence.
2. Continue to speak quietly and firmly; inform the patient that violence is not acceptable.
3. Take patient out of immediate area, to a quiet room.

4. Call for extra help.
5. Consider prn medications and physical restraints.

Care of a Patient Who is Suicidal

1. *Assess for suicide risk factors:* age (under 19, older than 45); higher in men; history of previous suicide attempt; substance abuse; lack of social support (unmarried/no significant relationship); chronic or painful illness; organized *suicide plan;* recent crisis (stress, loss); identity crisis.
2. *Assessment of suicide clues*
   • Depression and sudden recovery
   • Mania
   • Auditory hallucinations
   • Sleep deprivation
   • Direct verbal comments
   • Cancelling plans
   • Giving away belongings
   • Putting affairs in order (will, funeral plans)
   • Social withdrawal
3. *Suicide precautions:* remove harmful objects (e.g., no phone cords, extension and equipment cords; no curtain cords; no belts; no matches or cigarettes; no razors); lock windows; have only break-proof glass and mirrors; use plastic flatware.
4. **Care of patient who is suicidal**
   • Keep patient always in view, especially when patient goes to bathroom.
   • Ensure complete swallowing of medications.
   • Assess: mood, body posture, eye contact, and response to *direct* questions such as "Do you feel like hurting yourself?" "Do you have a plan?"
   • Give simple, clear directions.
   • Provide activities that do *not* require thinking or competition (e.g., folding papers, sticking labels on papers).
   • Increase suicide precautions when patient's behavior *appears* better (e.g., better groomed).

Crisis Intervention

Characteristics: brief; focus on here-and-now, immediate needs, and adaptive behaviors; relief of symptoms more important than exploring causes.

---

suicide attempt A deliberate action by the individual that will result in death, if carried out.

suicide gesture A suicide attempt that is aimed at being discovered, used for the purpose of controlling others' behavior.

suicide threat A verbal or nonverbal warning of plans to attempt suicide; may be a direct, indirect, or coded warning.

Crisis Intervention

adventitious crisis Unexpected, uncommon, accidental crisis that results in many losses and significant changes (e.g., destruction caused by a hurricane).

anticipatory guidance Suggestions and information given to a patient, to help the patient in future situations.

crisis A sudden change in an individual's life situation, in which usual coping methods fail or are inadequate; a disturbance in psychological equilibrium caused by a stressful event that is seen as a threat. It may be a developmental crisis and a turning point in one's life.

crisis intervention Short-term, directive, therapeutic approach, with the goal of problem solving of the here-and-now concerns in order to restore physiologic equilibrium.

maturational crisis An event that occurs during and is associated with a particular developmental period or stage (e.g., death of a parent), that disturbs an individual's equilibrium.

situational crisis A specific, *external* event that upsets an individual's psychological equilibrium (e.g., a crisis that results when caught cheating on an exam).

Questions

1. A woman comes to the emergency department with ripped clothing, periorbital edema, ecchymoses all over her body, and a misshapen, bloody nose. She is crying but reluctant to talk about what happened, saying only that she fell down her basement stairs. Which nursing action would be most appropriate when the nurse is alone with this patient?
   1. Ask her if someone hurt her.
   2. Collect physical evidence of possible sexual abuse.
   3. Point out the discrepancy between her explanation and her appearance and the extent of her injuries.
   4. Suggest that she seek shelter away from home.
2. A patient is seen in the emergency department and is diagnosed with major depression. The patient has had symptoms of a month's duration that include difficulty in concentration, apathy, rumination, a 12-pound weight loss, anorexia, and insatiable desire for sleep. What need should be a priority nursing concern?
   1. Self-care.
   2. Nutrition.
   3. Sleep.
   4. Interaction.
3. A patient is seen in the emergency department with symptoms of acute onset of delirium: confusion, limited attention span, fearfulness, impulsive actions (e.g., undressing in the lobby), and agitated, restless activity. Which would be the most relevant physical indicator in determining the cause of the delirium?
   1. Respirations.
   2. Pulse.
   3. Changes in activity level.
   4. Changes in accuracy of perceptions.
4. What observable characteristic(s), seen in a patient who presents in the emergency department, would help the nurse distinguish delirium from dementia?
   1. Inappropriate social behavior and loss of memory.
   2. Progressive loss of intellectual functioning.
   3. Sudden disorientation that is usually reversible.
   4. Symptoms that mimic depression.
5. A patient is found wandering on the streets, without shoes, looking disheveled and mumbling incoherently. In the emergency department, the patient crouches in a fetal position, with the face covered by the arms, look-

ing frightened. How should the nurse approach this patient?
   1. Sit 2–3 feet away from the patient and say, "Hello, I'm a nurse here. You look frightened," and wait for a response.
   2. Allow the patient to remain alone to watch what is going on for an hour or so, until the patient is more comfortable.
   3. Sit quietly next to the patient, touch the patient's hand, saying "I'm your nurse," and wait for a response.
   4. Enthusiastically approach the patient, saying, "Hi! I'm your nurse. You'll like it here. Everyone is warm and friendly. Let's go meet the other patients."
6. A patient is brought in for evaluation after hitting a cab driver. It is determined that the patient has a history of violence and assaultive behavior with a lack of remorse. The most appropriate short-term goal in fostering change in behavior would be that this patient will:
   1. Discuss the reasons for the acts of violence.
   2. Not strike out at anyone when upset.
   3. Discuss feelings of anger.
   4. Ask for medication when feeling out of control.
7. The nurse would assess that a teenage patient is less of a suicide risk when the patient:
   1. Says, "I cooked for myself last night and didn't cry about my ex-boyfriend."
   2. Says, "I feel better about myself and started an exercise program."
   3. Gives away her stereo and sits alone in her room.
   4. Says, "My parents don't believe I'm sick, but they'll find out soon!"
8. A patient threatens suicide as an attention-seeking mechanism, but does not talk about a plan. The nurse should view this behavior as:
   1. Anger turned inward.
   2. Manipulation.
   3. Ambivalence.
   4. Hopelessness.
9. A patient states, "I have nothing to live for." How should the nurse respond?
   1. Ask directly about the patient's suicide plans.
   2. Keep watching the patient.
   3. Say nothing and wait for the patient to go on.
   4. Focus the patient's thinking on the positive aspects of life.
10. During emergency hospitalization for depression, the nurse should reassess the patient's risk for a suicide attempt when:
    1. The patient's family does not visit.
    2. The patient's energy level returns.
    3. The patient is withdrawn and stays in bed.
    4. The patient has difficulty sleeping.
11. After being treated in the ICU for a deliberate overdose of *Elavil*, the patient is transferred to the medical floor for further observation. For what clues of highest suicide risk must the nurse watch?
    1. Continued expression of feelings of rejection and hopelessness.
    2. Specific plans for suicide and hallucinatory behavior (olfactory and visual).

3. Availability of sharp objects and delusions of grandeur.
4. Sudden improvement in appearance, with autism.

12. Recently, a patient took an intentional overdose of antidepressant medication. Based on the dynamics of suicide, which nursing intervention would be most therapeutic?
    1. Avoiding talking about the suicide attempt.
    2. Encouraging verbalization of feelings of hopelessness and helplessness.
    3. Providing time alone for self-reflection.
    4. Urging participation in group activity to decrease isolation.

13. When a patient overdoses by taking a full bottle of *Tofranil* (imipramine hydrochloride), for what toxic effect is it most important that the nurse monitor?
    1. Hypertensive crisis.
    2. Confusion and visual hallucination.
    3. Hypothermia.
    4. Arrhythmias.

14. What information is most important for the nurse to assess when a patient is in crisis?
    1. How the patient perceives the problem.
    2. Suicide risk.
    3. Availability of supportive resources.
    4. Usual coping behaviors.

15. What factor will determine the outcome of crisis intervention with a patient who was driving the car at the time of a crash in which family members were seriously hurt?
    1. The severity of the injuries.
    2. The number of family members injured.
    3. The patient's reaction to the crisis situation.
    4. The effectiveness of the crisis intervention.

16. A crisis caller spends 5 minutes telling the nurse that he "can't make it" and that his "life is over." The nurse's best response would be:
    1. "Are you thinking of killing yourself?"
    2. "Do you have a mental illness?"
    3. "Do you realize you may change your mind?"
    4. Say nothing; wait and listen.

Answers/Rationale

1. **(1)** This provides an opportunity for relief of symptoms (reluctance to talk, denial) to help the woman to discuss what happened. A private room may help her to bring up the topic of spousal abuse. Gathering evidence of possible rape (**No. 2**) is not a nursing action, but rather

is done by the M.D. with the nurse's assistance. Pointing out the discrepancy (**No. 3**) is too confrontational at this time. Suggesting shelter (**No. 4**) is premature at this time. **IMP, 1, PsI**

2. **(2)** A 12-pound weight loss in 1 month is significant when the person is also anorexic and thus apt to lose even more weight. Self-care needs (**No. 1**) are not a primary concern because this patient has *physiologic* needs, which are paramount. Sleep disturbance (**No. 3**) usually is resolved when the patient is started on antidepressant medications. The need for interaction (**No. 4**) is a *later* focus. **AN, 4, PhI**

💡 *Test-taking tip:* Remember Maslow's hierarchy of needs in "priority" questions; in this question, it can be used to narrow the choices down to food (**No. 2**) and sleep (**No. 3**).

3. **(2)** Delirium is often evaluated by the accompanying autonomic signs. Blood pressure and pulse are very important when the delirium is related to substance withdrawal or metabolic abnormalities. Respirations (**No. 1**) are not as good an indicator of the autonomic changes that usually accompany delirium. Although changes in activity level (**No. 3**) and perceptions (**No. 4**) do occur in delirium, they do not improve in a *predictable* enough way to provide a reliable measure of the progression of delirium (as the delirium resolves). **AS, 1, PhI**

4. **(3)** Abrupt confusion with return to previous level of awareness and self-care ability is most characteristic of *delirium*. The behaviors in **No. 1** and **No. 2** are characteristic of *dementia* rather than delirium. **No. 4** is incorrect because this applies to *both* dementia and delirium. **AS, 7, PsI**

5. **(1)** It is important not to violate the patient's personal space by moving too close, too fast, before assessing a new patient's behavior. Leaving the patient alone (**No. 2**) is inappropriate; an intervention is needed. Proximity and physical contact (**No. 3**) could easily frighten a patient who fears closeness and could cause a violent outburst. Touch may be misinterpreted by a frightened person. The approach in **No. 4** may overload the patient, contains false reassurances, and focuses on socialization with others, which is not what is needed for a new, frightened patient with psychotic behaviors. **IMP, 7, PsI**

6. **(3)** Discussion of feelings of anger will provide an opportunity for the nurse to help the patient to find an appropriate expression of anger. Discussion of reasons (**No. 1**) will usually evoke defensive rationalization and displacement, without attempts at self-control. Not assaulting others (**No. 2**) is a *long-term* goal and does not deal with *learning* how to handle angry feelings appropriately. Asking for medication (**No. 4**), as a short-term goal, will not help the patient *deal* with angry feelings. **EV, 1, SECE**

7. **(2)** This focuses on improving her self-concept (which is an antithesis of suicidal behavior). Also, working on a *long-range* goal and plan of action (like exercise) is more likely to be indicative of improvement, and therefore less of a suicide risk. **No. 1** is positive, but may be short-lived. On *one* recent (but *past*) occasion, she did

---

Key to Codes

Nursing process: AS = Assessment; **AN** = Analysis; **PL** = Planning; **IMP** = Implementation; **EV** = Evaluation. (See Appendix E for explanation of nursing process steps.)

Category of human function: 1 = Protective; **2** = Sensory-Perceptual; **3** = Comfort, Rest, Activity, and Mobility; **4** = Nutrition; **5** = Growth and Development; **6** = Fluid-Gas Transport; **7** = Psychosocial-Cultural; **8** = Elimination.

Client need: SECE = Safe, Effective Care Environment; **PhI** = Physiologic Integrity; **PsI** = Psychosocial Integrity; **HPM** = Health Promotion/Maintenance.

something for herself (cooked dinner) and did not despair (i.e., cry about her ex-boyfriend). Giving away something of value (**No. 3**) and a hostile expression (a "they'll be sorry" type of response, **No. 4**) are signs of *higher* risk of suicidal behavior. **AN, 7, PsI**

8. **(2)** All threats of suicide need to be taken seriously; however, if a person verbalizes a plan, it is a more serious threat than repeated verbalized threats used to get attention. This latter behavior needs to be confronted, as attention seeking is a form of manipulation when it is designed to move others into action, to elicit a response from others. Anger turned inward (**No. 1**) usually refers to *depression*. Ambivalence (**No. 3**) is exhibited by a voice for and steps toward "life" and a voice for "death"—a decision not yet made. There are insufficient data to indicate that the lack of a verbalized plan stems from hopelessness (**No. 4**). **AN, 7, PsI**

9. **(1)** This is an *active* verbal intervention, with the purpose of increasing suicide prevention; the nurse needs to find out what the person is considering. The patient is offering an opening in the ambivalence about "life vs. death." Watching (**No. 2**) and saying nothing (**No. 3**) are *passive* interventions. **No. 4** is a much *later* intervention. **PL, 7, PsI**

💡 *Test-taking tip:* Which option is not like the others? Two of the immediate interventions are passive (**Nos. 2 and 3**); one is *direct* (**No. 1**).

10. **(2)** Suicide precautions should be increased when the patient shows signs of *increased energy;* with more physical energy, the patient is more likely to put suicidal thoughts and plans into action. **No. 1** *may* be a factor in *some* cases, if the patient appears angry, dejected, and rejected when the family doesn't visit; however, there are no descriptive data in the question to establish a pattern of depressive reaction leading to suicidal behavior related to lack of family visits. When the patient has *no* energy (**No. 3**) it is the *opposite* of the correct option (**No. 2**), and is therefore incorrect. Insomnia (**No. 4**) is *not* a relevant factor in determining high risk for suicide. **AN, 7, PsI**

💡 *Test-taking tip:* When you need to make an "educated guess," consider selecting one of two contradictory options (see **Nos. 2 and 3**).

11. **(1)** By process of elimination, feelings of rejection and hopelessness are the most significant clues to suicide. All other options are only *partially* correct: plans (**No. 2**), availability of tools for self-destruction (**No. 3**), and a sudden improvement in appearance (**No. 4**) are all important clues. However, each also contains elements of *psychotic* behavior that are *not* indicative of high risk of suicide: olfactory and visual hallucinations (**No. 2**), delusions of grandeur (**No. 3**), and autistic behavior (**No. 4**). **No. 2** is incorrect because *auditory* hallucinations (*not* olfactory and visual) can accompany a suicide attempt. **No. 3** is incorrect because delusions of perse-

cution (*not* grandeur) may be part of a high suicide risk profile. **No. 4** is incorrect because a person with *depression* (*not* autism) is a high risk for suicide when there is a sudden change in appearance. **AS, 7, PsI**

💡 *Test-taking tip:* Choose the option in which there are *no* incorrect aspects; eliminate options that are *partially* correct.

12. **(2)** Verbalization will facilitate recognition of sources of hopelessness and provide an opportunity to talk through more adaptive coping strategies. **No. 1** is incorrect because it is a *myth* that talking about suicide will cause suicidal behavior. **No. 3** is incorrect because the nurse needs to be with this patient, to observe, and to communicate empathy and support. **No. 4** can be ruled out because this patient first needs a one-to-one relationship. **IMP, 7, PsI**

13. **(4)** With tricyclic antidepressant (TCA) overdose, there is a high risk for serious cardiac problems, including arrhythmias, tachycardia, and myocardial infarction. [*Note:* In addition, the nurse should monitor for respiratory failure.] The risk is for postural *hypo*tension, not hypertension (**No. 1**). While hallucinations (**No. 2**) may occur as an early sign, this is a side effect, not a serious *toxic* effect (like arrhythmias). Confusion is also an early sign of overdose, not a toxic effect. *Hyper*thermia is a toxic effect, not hypothermia (**No. 3**). **AS, 6, PhI**

14. **(2)** Assessment of suicide risk is important in ensuring *physical* safety, as a priority. The patient's perception of the problem (**No. 1**), the availability of supportive resources (**No. 3**), and the patient's coping mechanisms (**No. 4**) are all important, but are not as high in priority as physiologic integrity, namely safety. **AS, 7, PsI**

💡 *Test-taking tip:* Three options (**Nos. 1, 3, and 4**) focus on higher levels of Maslow's hierarchy of needs. Choose the option (**No. 2**) that is the *first*, basic level on *Maslow's hierarchy,* the need for safety.

15. **(3)** How any one crisis is resolved depends on the patient's coping mechanisms and response to crisis in the past. **Nos. 1 and 2** are not the determinant factors in ultimate resolution of this crisis. **No. 4** does not answer the question, which asks for a *factor* in the outcome; the outcome itself ("effectiveness," as determined by the outcome criteria) is not a factor. **EV, 7, PsI**

16. **(1)** This is an *active*, direct verbal intervention with the purpose of preventing suicide. The nurse needs to find out what the person is considering and to ask directly about suicide plans. The client is offering an opening in the ambivalence between life vs. death. **No. 2** is a "conversation stopper." What will the patient say to someone who abruptly asks about a mental illness? ("Huh?") **No. 3** focuses on a later time ("tomorrow") and therefore is not the best response. The nurse needs to focus on what action the patient may take *now*. **No. 4** is a *passive* intervention, and therefore the opposite of the correct response (**No. 1**), a direct, active intervention. **IMP, 7, PsI**

Common Disruptive or Problematic Behaviors

Chapter Outline

- Anger
- Combative-Aggressive Behavior
- Confusion/Disorientation
- Demanding Behavior
- Denial of Illness
- Dependence
- Hopelessness
- Hostility

- Manipulation
- Noncompliance and Uncooperative Behavior
- Violent Behavior
- Study and Memory Aids
- Glossary
- Summary of Key Points
- Questions
- Answers/Rationale

Anger

I. **Definition:** feelings of resentment in response to anxiety when threat is perceived; need to discharge tension of anger.

▷ II. **Assessment**

A. **Degree and frequency** of anger: Scope of anger ranges on a continuum from everyday *mild annoyance* → *frustration* from interference with goal accomplishment → *assertiveness* (behavior used to deal with anger effectively) → *anger* related to helplessness and powerlessness that may interfere with functioning → *rage and fury,* when coping means are depleted or not developed.

B. **Mode of expression** of anger

1. *Covert, passive* expression of anger
   a. Being overly nice.
   b. Body language: little or no eye contact, arms close to body, soft voice, little gesturing.
   c. Sarcasm through humor.
   d. *Sublimation* through art and music.
   e. *Projection* onto others.
   f. *Denying* and pushing anger out of awareness.
   g. *Psychosomatic* illness in response to internalized anger (e.g., headache).
2. *Overt, active* expression of anger
   a. Physical activity to work off excess physical energy associated with biologic response (e.g., hitting punching bag, taking a walk).
   b. *Aggression.*
   c. Assertiveness.

C. **Physiologic behaviors**—result of secretion of epinephrine and sympathetic nervous system stimulation preparing for "fight" or "flight."

1. *Cardiovascular* response: increased BP and pulse, increased free fatty acid in blood.
2. *Gastrointestinal* response: increased nausea, salivation, decreased peristalsis.
3. *Genitourinary* response: urinary frequency.
4. *Neuromuscular* response: increased alertness, increased muscle tension and deep tendon reflexes, ECG changes.

D. **Positive functions** of anger

1. Energizes behavior.
2. Protects positive image.
3. Provides ego defense during high anxiety.
4. Gives greater control over situation.
5. Alerts to need for coping.
6. A sign of a healthy relationship.

▷ III. **Analysis/nursing diagnosis**—*Defensive coping* related to source of stress (stressors):

A. *Biologic stressors*

1. Instinctual drives (Lorenz, on aggressive instincts, and Freud).
2. *Endocrine imbalances.*
3. Seizures.
4. Tumors.
5. *Hunger.*
6. *Fatigue.*

B. *Psychological stressors*

1. Inability to resolve frustration that leads to aggression.
2. Real or imagined threatened loss of self-esteem.
3. Conflict.
4. Lack of control.

5. Anger as a learned expression and a reinforced response.
6. Prolonged stress.
7. An attempt to protect self.
8. Desire for retaliation.
9. A normal part of grief process.

C. *Sociocultural stressors*
1. Lack of early training in self-discipline and social skills.
2. Crowding, personal space intrusion.
3. *Role-modeling* of abusive behavior by significant others and by media personalities.

◙ **IV. Nursing care plan/implementation—Long-term goal:** constructive use of angry energy to accomplish tasks and motivate growth.

A. *Prevent* and *control* violence.
1. Approach unhurriedly.
2. Provide atmosphere of acceptance; listen attentively, refrain from arguing and criticizing.
3. Encourage expression of feelings.
4. Offer feedback of client's expressed feelings.
5. Encourage mutual problem solving.
6. Encourage realistic perception of others and situation and respect for the rights of others.

B. *Limit-setting*
1. Clearly state *expectations* and *consequences* of acts.
2. Enforce consequences.
3. Encourage client to assume responsibility for behavior.
4. Explore reasons and meaning of negative behavior.

C. Promote *self-awareness* and *problem-solving* abilities. Encourage and assist client to:
1. Accept self as a person with a right to experience angry feelings.
2. Explore reasons for anger.
3. Describe situations where anger was experienced.
4. Discuss appropriate alternatives for expressing anger (including assertiveness training).
5. Decide on one feasible solution.
6. Act on solution.
7. Evaluate effectiveness.

D. *Health teaching*
1. Explore other ways to express feelings, and provide activities that allow appropriate expression of anger.
2. Recommend that behavior limits be set (by the family).
3. Explain how to set behavioral limits.
4. Advise against causing defensive patterns in others.

◙ **V. Evaluation/outcome criteria**
A. Demonstrates insight (awareness of factors that precipitate anger; identifies disturbing topics, events, and inappropriate use of coping mechanisms).
B. Uses appropriate coping mechanisms.
C. Reaches out for emotional support before stress level becomes excessive.

D. Evidence of increased reality perception and problem-solving ability.

Combative-Aggressive Behavior

I. Definition: *acting out* feelings of frustration, anger, anxiety, etc. through *physical or verbal* behavior.

◙ **II. Assessment**—Recognize *precombative* behavior:
A. Demanding, fist clenching.
B. Boisterous, loud.
C. Vulgar, profane.
D. Limited attention span.
E. Sarcastic, taunting, verbal threats.
F. Restless, agitated, elated.
G. Frowning.

◙**III. Analysis/nursing diagnosis**—*Risk for violence* related to:
A. Frustration as response to *breakdown of self-control* coping mechanisms.
B. Acting out as customary response to anger (*defensive coping*).
C. Confusion (*sensory-perceptual alterations*).
D. Physical restraints, such as when postoperative patient discovers wrist restraints.
E. Fear of intimacy; intrusion on emotional and physical space (*altered thought processes*).
F. Feelings of helplessness, inadequacy (*situational or chronic low self-esteem*).

◙ **IV. Nursing care plan/implementation**
A. **Long-term goal:** channel aggression—help person express feelings rather than act them out.
B. **Immediate goal:** *prevent injury to self and others.*
1. Calmly call for assistance; do *not* try to handle *alone*.
2. Approach cautiously. Keep client within *eye contact*, observing client's personal space.
3. *Protect* against self-injury and injury to others; be aware of your position in relation to the weapon, door, escape route.
4. *Minimize* stimuli, to control the environment—clear the area, close doors, turn off TV so person can hear you.
5. *Divert* attention from the act; engage in talk and lead away from others.
6. Assess *triggering* cause.
7. Identify immediate problem.
8. Focus on *remedy for immediate* problem.
9. Choose one calm, quieting individual to interact with person; nonauthoritarian, nonthreatening.
10. Maintain *verbal contact* to keep communication open; offer empathetic ear, but be firm and consistent in setting *limits* on dangerous behavior.
11. Negotiate, but don't make false promises or argue.
☞**12.** Restraints may be necessary as a *last* resort.

13. Place person in quiet room so he or she can calm down.

C. Health teaching

1. Explain how to obtain release from stress and how to rechannel emotional energy into acceptable activity.
2. Advise against causing defensive responses in others.
3. Explain what is justifiable aggression.
4. Emphasize importance of how to recognize tension in self.
5. Explain why self-control is important.
6. Explain to family, staff, how to set behavioral limits.
7. Explain causes of maladaptive coping related to anger.
8. Teach how to use problem-solving method.

V. Evaluation/outcome criteria

A. Is aware of causes of anger; can recognize the feeling of anger and utilize alternative methods of expressing anger.
B. Expression of anger is appropriate, congruent with the situation.
C. Replaces aggression and acting-out with assertiveness.

Confusion/Disorientation

I. Definition: loss of reality orientation as to person, time, place, events, ideas.

II. Assessment—Note unusual behavior:

A. Picking, stroking movements in the air or on clothing and linens.
B. Frequent crying or laughing.
C. Alternating periods of confusion and lucidity (e.g., confused at night, when alone in the dark).
D. Fluctuating mood, actions, rationality (argumentative, combative, withdrawn).
E. Increasingly restless, fearful, leading to insomnia, nightmares.
F. Acts bewildered; has trouble identifying familiar people.
G. Preoccupied; irritable when interrupted.
H. Unresponsive to questions; problem with concentration and setting realistic priorities.
I. Sensitive to noise and light.
J. Has unrealistic perception of time, place, and situation.
K. Nurse no longer seen as supportive but as threatening.

III. Analysis/nursing diagnosis—*Altered thought processes and sensory-perceptual alterations* related to:

A. *Physical and physiologic disturbances*
1. Metabolic (uremia, diabetes, hepatic dysfunction), fluid, and electrolyte imbalances.
2. Cardiac arrhythmias, heart failure.
3. Anemia, massive blood loss with low hemoglobin.
4. Organic brain disease.
5. Nutritional deficiency.

6. Pain.
7. Sleep disturbance.
8. Drugs (antidepressants, tranquilizers, sedatives, antihypertensives, diuretics, alcohol, phencyclidine hydrochloride [PCP], street drugs).

B. *Unfamiliar environment*—unfamiliar routine and people; procedures that threaten body image; *noisy* equipment.
C. *Loss of sensory acuity* from partial or incomplete reception of orienting stimuli or information.
D. *Disability in screening out* irrelevant and excessive sensory input.
E. *Memory impairment.*

IV. Nursing care plan/implementation

A. Check *physical signs;* e.g., vital signs, neurologic status, fluid and electrolyte balance, and blood urea nitrogen.
B. Be calm; make contact to *reorient to reality:*
1. *Avoid* startling if person is alone, in the dark, sedated.
2. Make sure person can *see, hear, and talk* to you—turn off TV; turn on light, put on client's glasses, hearing aids, dentures.
3. Call by name, clearly and distinctly.
4. Approach cautiously, close to *eye* level.
5. Keep your *hands visible;* e.g., on bed.

C. Take care of *immediate problem;* e.g., disconnected IV tube or catheter.
1. Give instructions slowly and distinctly; *avoid* threatening tone and comments.
2. *Stay* with person until reoriented.
3. Put *side rails* up.

D. Use *conversation* to *reduce* confusion:
1. Use *simple, concrete phrases;* language the person can understand; *repeat* as needed.
2. *Avoid* shouting, arguing, false promises, use of medical abbreviations (e.g., NPO).
3. Give *more time to concentrate* on what you said.
4. Focus on *reality-oriented* topics or objects in the environment.

E. Establish a *reality-oriented relationship* (to prevent confusion).
1. Introduce self by name.
2. Jointly establish routines to prevent confusion from unpredictable changes and variations. Determine client's usual routine; attempt to incorporate this to lessen disruption in lifestyle.
3. Explain what to expect in understandable words—where client is and why, what will happen, noises and activities client will hear and see, people client will meet, tests and procedures client will have.
4. Find out what meaning hospitalization has to client; reduce anxiety related to feelings of apprehension and helplessness.
5. Spend as much time as possible with client.

F. *Maintain orientation by providing nonthreatening environment.*

1. Assign to room *near nurse's station*.
2. Surround with *familiar* objects from home (e.g., photos).
3. Provide *clock, calendar, and radio*.
4. Have flexible visiting hours.
5. Open curtain for *natural light*.
6. Keep glasses, dentures, hearing aids nearby.
7. Check client often, especially at night.
8. *Avoid* using intercom to answer calls.
9. *Avoid* low-pitched conversation.

G. *Take care of other needs.*
  1. Promote sleep according to usual habits and patterns in order to *prevent sleep deprivation*.
  2. *Avoid sedatives,* which may lead to or increase confusion.
  3. Promote independent functions, self-help activities, to *maintain dignity*.
  4. Encourage *nutritional* adequacy; incorporate familiar foods, ethnic preferences.
  5. Maintain *routine; avoid* being late with meals, medication, or procedures.
  6. Have *realistic expectations*.
  7. *Discover hidden fears.*
    a. Do not assume confused behavior is unrelated to reality.
    b. Look for clues to meaning from client's background, occupation.
  8. *Provide support to family.*
    a. Encourage expression of feelings; *avoid* being judgmental.
    b. Check what worked in previous situations.

H. *Health teaching:* explain possible causes of confusion. Reassure that it is common. Teach family, friends how to react to confused behavior.

V. Evaluation/outcome criteria
A. Less restlessness, fearfulness, mood lability.
B. More frequent periods of lucidity; oriented to time, place, and person; responds to questions.

Demanding Behavior

I. Definition: a strong and persistent struggle to obtain satisfaction of self-oriented needs (such as control, self-esteem) or relief from anxiety.

II. Assessment
A. Attention-seeking behavior.
B. Multiple requests.
C. Frequency of questions.
D. Lack of reasonableness; irrationality of request.

III. Analysis/nursing diagnosis. *Defensive coping* and *impaired social interaction* related to:
A. Feelings of *helplessness* and *hopelessness*.
B. Feelings of *powerlessness* and *fear*.
C. A way of coping with anxiety.

IV. Nursing care plan/implementation
A. *Control* own irritation; assess reasons for own annoyance.
B. *Confront* with behavior; discuss reasons for behavior.

C. *Anticipate* and meet client's needs; set time to discuss requests.
D. *Ignore* negative attention seeking and *reinforce appropriate* requests for attention.
E. Make plans with *entire staff* to set *limits*.
F. Set up *contractual* arrangement for brief, frequent, regular, uninterrupted attention.
G. *Health teaching:* teach appropriate methods for gaining attention.

V. Evaluation/outcome criteria: fewer requests for attention; assumes more responsibility for self-care.

Denial of Illness

I. Definition: an attempt or refusal to acknowledge some anxiety-provoking aspect of oneself or external reality. Denial may be an acceptable first phase of coping as an attempt to allow time for adaptation.

II. Assessment
A. Observe for *coping mechanisms* such as dissociation, repression, selective inattention, suppression, displacement of concern to another person.
B. Note behaviors that may indicate *denial of diagnosis:*
  1. Failure to follow treatment plan.
  2. Missed appointment.
  3. Refusal of medication.
  4. Inappropriate cheerfulness.
  5. Ignoring symptoms.
  6. Use of flippant humor.
  7. Use of second or third person in reference to illness.
  8. Flight into wellness, overactivity.
C. Note *body language*—use of earliest and most primitive defense by closing eyes, turning head away to separate from what is unpleasant and anxiety provoking.
D. Note *range* of denial: *explicit* verbal denial of obvious facts, disowning → *ignoring* aspects → *minimizing* by understatement.
E. Be aware of situations such as long-term physical disability that make people more prone to denial of anger. *Denial of illness protects the ego from overwhelming anxiety.*

III. Analysis/nursing diagnosis—*Ineffective denial* related to:
A. Untenable wishes, needs, ideas, deeds, or reality factors.
B. Inability: to adapt to full realization of painful experience or to accept changes in body image or role perception.
C. Intense stress and anxiety.

IV. Nursing care plan/implementation
A. **Long-term goal:** understand needs met by denial.
B. **Short-term goal:** *avoid* reinforcing denial patterns.
  1. Recognize behavioral cues of denial of some reality aspect; be aware of level of awareness and degree to which reality is excluded.
  2. Determine if denial interferes with treatment.
  3. Support moves toward greater reality orientation.

4. Determine person's stress tolerance.

5. Supportively help person discuss events leading to, and feelings about, hospitalization.

C. *Health teaching*

1. Explain that emotional response is appropriate and common.

2. Explain to family and staff that emotional adjustment to painful reality is done at own pace.

✠ **V. Evaluation/outcome criteria:** indicates desire to discuss painful experience.

Dependence

I. Definition: reliance on other people to meet basic needs, usually for love and affection, security and protection, and support and guidance; *acceptable in early phases* of coping.

✠ **II. Assessment**

A. Excessive need for advice and answers to problems.

B. Lack of confidence in own decision-making ability and lack of confidence in self-sufficiency.

C. Clinging, too-trusting behavior.

D. Gestures, facial expressions, body posture, recurrent themes conveying "I'm helpless."

✠ **III. Analysis/nursing diagnosis**

A. Chronic *low self-esteem* related to inability to meet basic needs or role expectations.

B. *Helplessness* and *hopelessness* related to inadvertent reinforcement by staff's expectations.

C. *Powerlessness* related to holding a belief that one's own actions cannot affect life situations.

✠ **IV. Nursing care plan/implementation**

A. **Long-term goal:** increase self-esteem, confidence in own abilities.

B. **Short-term goals:** provide activities that promote independence.

1. *Limit-setting*—clear, firm, consistent; acknowledge when demands are made; accept client but refuse to respond to demands.

2. *Break cycle* of: nurse avoids client when he or she is clinging and demanding → client's anxiety increases → demands for attention increase → frustration and avoidance on nurse's part increase.

3. *Give attention before* demand exists.

☞ 4. Use *behavior modification* approaches—

a. *Reward* appropriate behavior (such as making decisions, helping others, caring for own needs) with attention and praise.

b. Give *no response* to attention seeking, dependent, infantile behavior; goal is to increase incidence of mature behavior as client realizes little gratification from dependent behavior.

5. *Avoid secondary gains* of being cared for, which impede progress toward above goals.

6. Assist in developing *ability to control panic* by responding less to client's high anxiety level.

7. Help client develop ways to seek gratification other than excessive turning to others.

8. *Resist* urge to act like a parent when client becomes helpless, demanding, and attention seeking.

9. *Promote decision making* by not giving advice.

10. *Encourage accountability* for own feelings, thoughts, and behaviors.

a. Help identify feelings through nonverbal cues, thoughts, recurrent themes.

b. Convey expectations that client does have opinions and feelings to share.

c. Role model how to express feelings.

11. *Reinforce self-esteem* and ability to work out problems independently. (Consistently ask: "How to you feel about . . ." "What do you think?")

12. *Health teaching*

a. Teach family ways of interacting to enforce less dependency.

b. Teach problem-solving skills, assertiveness.

✠ **V. Evaluation/outcome criteria**

A. Performs self-care.

B. Asks less for approval and praise.

C. Seeks less attention, proximity, physical contact.

Hopelessness

I. Definition: a subjective state in which an individual sees no alternatives or personal choices available and cannot mobilize energy on own behalf.

✠ **II. Assessment**

A. Decreased verbalization.

B. Lack of initiative.

C. Decreased response to stimuli (e.g., avoids eye contact).

D. Decreased affect.

E. Decreased appetite.

F. Lack of involvement in care (passivity).

G. Increased sleep.

H. Expression of verbal cues such as: "I can't," "I don't care."

✠ **III. Analysis/nursing diagnosis**

A. *Hopelessness* related to failing or deteriorating physiologic condition.

B. *Low self-esteem* related to abandonment.

C. *Ineffective individual coping* related to long-term stress.

D. *Powerlessness* related to loss of spiritual belief.

✠ **IV. Nursing care plan/implementation**

A. Increase social support system to decrease feelings of abandonment.

B. Explore alternative coping behaviors.

C. Explore with patient factors that contribute to feelings of hopelessness.

D. Assess and document risk for suicide; institute precautions.

E. Provide opportunities for patient to initiate interactions and activities.

F. Involve family/significant other in treatment plan.

G. Provide positive reinforcement for behaviors that demonstrate initiative (e.g., eye contact, self-disclosure, self-care, increased appetite, reduction in amount of sleep time).

V. Evaluation/outcome criteria
  A. Identifies personal strengths.
  B. Initiates behaviors that may reduce feelings of hopelessness.

Hostility

I. Definition: a feeling of *intense* anger or an attitude of antagonism or animosity, with the *destructive* component of intent to inflict harm and pain to another or to self; may involve *hate, anger, rage, aggression, regression.*

II. Operational definition
  A. Past experience of frustration; loss of self-esteem; unmet needs for status, prestige, or love.
  B. Present expectations of self and others not met.
  C. Feelings of humiliation, inadequacy, emotional pain, and conflict.
  D. Anxiety experienced and converted into hostility, which can be:
    1. Repressed, with result of becoming withdrawn.
    2. Disowned to the point of overreaction and extreme compliance.
    3. Overtly exhibited: verbal, nonverbal.

III. Concepts and principles
  A. Aggression and violence are two *outward* expressions of hostility.
  B. Hostility is often unconscious, automatic response.
  C. Hostile wishes and impulses may be underlying motives for many actions.
  D. Perceptions may be *distorted* by hostile outlook.
  E. Continuum: extreme politeness → *externalization* as murderous rage or homicide → *internalization* as depression or suicide.
  F. Hostility seen as a defense *against* depression as well as a *cause* of it.
  G. Hostility may be repressed, dissociated, or expressed covertly or overtly.
  H. *Normal* hostility may come from justifiable fear of *real* danger; *irrational* hostility stems from *anxiety.*
  I. *Developmental roots* of hostility
    1. *Infants* look away, push away, physically move away from threat; give defiant look. Role modeling by parents.
    2. *Three-year-olds* replace overt hostility with protective shyness, retreat, and withdrawal. Feel weak, inadequate in face of powerful person against whom cannot openly ventilate hostility.
    3. Frustrated or unmet needs for status, prestige, or power serve as a basis for *adult* hostility.

IV. Assessment
  A. Fault finding, scapegoating, sarcasm, derision.
  B. Arguing, swearing, abusiveness, verbal threatening.
  C. Deceptive sweetness, joking at others' expense, gossiping.

D. Physical abusiveness, violence, murder, vindictiveness.

V. Analysis/nursing diagnosis
  A. Causes
    1. *Anxiety* related to a learned means of dealing with an interpersonal threat.
    2. *Risk for violence* related to a reaction to *loss of self-esteem* and *powerlessness.*
    3. *Defensive coping* related to intense frustration, insecurity, and/or apprehension.
    4. *Impaired social interaction* related to low anxiety tolerance.
  B. Situations with high potential for hostility
    1. *Enforced illness* and *hospitalization* cause anxiety, which may be expressed as hostility.
    2. Dependency feelings related to acceptance of illness may result in hostility as a coping mechanism.
    3. Certain illnesses or physical disabilities may be conducive to hostility:
      a. *Preoperative cancer* client may displace hostility onto staff and family.
      b. Postoperatively, if diagnosis is *terminal,* the family may displace hostility onto nurse.
      c. Anger, hostility is a *stage of dying* the person may experience.
      d. *Amputee* may focus frustration on others due to dependency and jealousy.
      e. Patients on *hemodialysis* are prone to helplessness, which may be displaced as hostility.

VI. Nursing care plan/implementation
  A. Long-term goal: help alter response to fear, inadequacy, frustration, threat.
  B. Short-term goals: express and explore feelings of hostility without injury to self or others.
    1. Remain calm, nonthreatening; endure verbal abuse in impartial manner, within limits; speak quietly.
    2. *Protect from self-harm,* acting out.
    3. Discourage hostile behavior while showing acceptance of client.
    4. Offer support to *express* feelings of frustration, anger, and fear *constructively, safely,* and *appropriately.*
    5. Explore hostile feelings *without* fear of retaliation, disapproval.
    6. *Avoid* arguing, advice giving, reacting with hostility, punitiveness, fault finding.
    7. *Avoid* joking and teasing, which can be misinterpreted.
    8. *Avoid* words like *anger, hostility;* use client's words (*upset, irritated*).
    9. Do not minimize problem or give client reassurance or hasty, general conclusions.
    10. *Do not stop verbal* expression of anger unless detrimental.
    11. Respond *matter-of-factly* to attention-seeking behavior, not defensively.
    12. *Avoid* physical contact; allow client to set pace in "closeness."

13. Look for clues to antecedent events and focus *directly* on those areas; *do not evade* or ignore.
14. Constantly focus on *here and now* and affective component of message rather than on content.
15. Reconstruct what happened and why, discuss client's reactions; seek observations, *not* inferences.
16. Learn how client would like to be treated.
17. Look for ways to help client relate better without defensiveness, *when ready*.
18. Plan to channel feelings into *motor* outlets (occupational and recreational therapy, physical activity, games, debates).
19. Explain procedures beforehand; approach frequently.
20. Withdraw attention, *set limits*, when acting out.
   C. **Health teaching:** teach acceptable motor outlets for tension.
VII. **Evaluation/outcome criteria:** identifies sources of threat and experiences success in dealing with threat.

Manipulation

I. **Definition:** process of playing upon and using others by unfair, insidious means to serve own purpose without regard for others' needs; may take many forms; occurs consciously, unconsciously to some extent, in all interpersonal relations.
II. **Operational definition** (Figure 7.1)
   A. Conflicting needs, goals exist between client and other person (e.g., nurse).
   B. Other person perceives need as unacceptable, unreasonable.
   C. Other person refuses to accept client's need.
   D. Client's tension increases, and he begins to relate to others as objects.
   E. Client increases attempts to influence others to fulfill his need.
      1. Appears unaware of others' needs.
      2. Exhibits excessive dependency, helplessness, demands.
      3. Sets others at odds (especially staff).
      4. *Rationalizes*, gives logical reasons.
      5. Uses deception, false promises, insincerity.
      6. Questions and *defies nurse's authority* and competence.
   F. Nurse feels powerless and angry at having been used.
III. **Assessment**
   A. Acts out sexually, physically.
   B. Dawdles, always last minute.
   C. Uses insincere flattery; expects special favors, privileges.
   D. Exploits generosity and fears of others.
   E. Feels no guilt.
   F. Plays one staff member against another.
   G. *Tests limits.*
   H. Finds weaknesses in others.

I. Makes excessive, unreasonable, unnecessary *demands* for staff time.
J. *Pretends* to be helpless, lonely, distraught, tearful.
K. Can't distinguish between truth and falsehood.
L. *Plays on sympathy* or *guilt.*
M. Offers many excuses, lacks insight.
N. Pursues unpleasant issues without genuine regard for or feelings of individuals involved.
O. *Intimidates*, derogates, threatens, bargains, cajoles, violates rules to obtain reactions or privileges.
P. Betrays information.
Q. Uses communication as a medium for manipulation, as verbal, nonverbal means to get others to cooperate, to behave in certain way, to get something from another for own use.
R. May be coercive, illogical, or skillfully deceptive.
S. *Unable to learn from experience;* i.e., repeats unacceptable behaviors despite negative consequences.
IV. **Analysis/nursing diagnosis**—*Impaired adjustment* related to:
   A. Mistrust and contemptuous view of others' motivations.
   B. Life experience of rejection, deception.
   C. Low anxiety tolerance.
   D. Inability to cope with tension.
   E. Unmet dependency needs.
   F. Need to avoid anxiety when cannot obtain gratification.
   G. Need to obtain something that is forbidden, or need for *instant gratification.*
   H. Attempt to put something over on another when no real advantage exists.
   I. *Intolerance of intimacy*, maneuvering effectively to keep others at a safe distance in order to dilute the relationship by withdrawing and frustrating others or distracting attention away from self.
   J. Attempt to demand attention, approval, disapproval.
V. **Nursing care plan/implementation**
   A. **Long-term goal:** define relationship as a mutual experience in *learning and trust* rather than a struggle for *power and control.*
   B. **Short-term goal:** increase awareness of self and others; increase self-control; learn to accept limitations.
   C. Promote use of "three C's": *cooperation, compromise, collaboration,* rather than exploitation or deception.
   D. *Decrease level and extent of manipulation.*
      1. Set *firm, realistic goals,* with clear, consistent expectations and limits.
      2. *Confront* client regarding exploitation attempts; examine, discuss behavior.
      3. Give *positive reinforcement* with concrete reinforcers for nonmanipulation, to lessen need for exploitative, deceptive, and self-destructive behaviors.
      4. *Ignore* "wooden-leg" behavior (feigning illness to evoke sympathy).
      5. *Allow verbal* anger; don't be intimidated; *avoid*

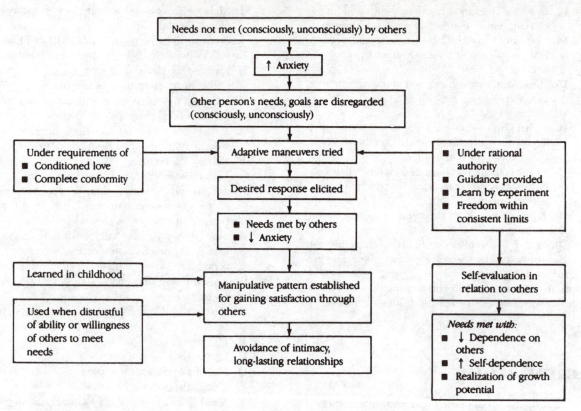

FIGURE 7.1   OPERATIONALIZATION OF THE BEHAVIORAL CONCEPT OF MANIPULATION

giving desired response to obvious attempts to irritate.

6. Set *consistent, firm, enforceable limits* on *destructive*, aggressive behavior that impinges on others' health, rights, and interests, and on excessive dependency; *give reasons* when you can't meet requests.

7. Keep staff informed of rules and reasons; obtain staff *consensus*.

8. Enforce *direct* communication; encourage openness about *real* needs, feelings.

9. Do *not* accept gifts, favors, flattery, or other guises of manipulation.

E. Increase responsibility for *self-control* of actions.

1. Decide who (client, nurse) is responsible for what.

2. Provide opportunities for *success* to increase self-esteem, experiencing acceptance by others.

3. Evaluate actions, *not* verbal behavior; point out the difference between talk and action.

4. Support efforts to be responsible.

5. Assist client to increase emotional repertoire; explore *alternative* ways of relating interpersonally.

6. *Avoid submission* to control based on fear of punishment, retaliation, loss of affection.

F. Facilitate awareness of, and *responsibility* for, manipulative behavior and its *effects on others*.

1. Reflect back client's behavior.

2. Discourage distortion and misuse of information.

3. *Increase tolerance* for differences.

4. Promote *delayed gratification* through behavior modification.

5. Insist on clear, consistent staff communication.

G. *Avoid:*

1. Labeling client as a "problem."

2. Hostile, negative attitude.

3. Making a public issue of client's behavior.

4. Being excessively rigid or permissive, inconsistent or ambiguous, argumentative or accusatory.

H. *Health teaching:* act as a role model; demonstrate how to deal with mistakes, human imperfections, by admitting mistakes in nonshameful, nonvirtuous ways.

▶ VI. **Evaluation/outcome criteria:** accepts limits; able to compromise, cooperate rather than deceive and exploit; acts responsibly; self-dependent.

Noncompliance and Uncooperative Behavior

I. **Definition:** consistently failing to meet the requirements of the prescribed treatment regimen; e.g., refusing to adhere to dietary restrictions or take required medications.

II. Assessment
  A. Refuses to participate in routine or planned activities.
  B. Refuses medication.
  C. Violates rules, ignores limits, and abuses privileges; acts out anger and frustration.

III. Analysis/nursing diagnosis—*Noncompliance* related to:
  A. *Psychological factors:* lack of knowledge; attitudes, beliefs, and values; denial of illness; rigid, defensive personality type; anxiety level (very high or very low); can't accept limits or dependency (rebellious counterdependency).
  B. *Environmental factors:* finances; transportation; lack of support system.
  C. *Health care agent–client relationship:* client feels discounted and like an "object"; sees staff as uncaring, authoritative, controlling.
  D. *Health care regimen:* too complicated; not enough benefit from following regimen; results in social stigma or social isolation; unpleasant side effects.

IV. Nursing care plan/implementation
  A. *General goal:* reduce need to act out by nonadherence.
    1. Take *preventive* action—be alert to signs of noncompliance, such as intent to leave against medical advice.
    2. *Explore* feelings and reasons for lack of cooperation.
    3. Assess and *allay fears* in client in reassuring manner.
    4. Provide *adequate* information about, and reasons for, rules and procedures.
    5. *Avoid* threats or physical restraints; maintain calm composure.
    6. Demonstrate *tact and firmness* when confronting violations.
    7. Offer *alternatives.*
    8. Firmly insist on cooperation in selected important activities but not all activities.
  B. *Health teaching:* increase knowledge base regarding health-related problem, procedures, or treatments, consequences.

V. Evaluation/outcome criteria: follows prescribed regimen.

Violent Behavior

I. Characteristics of violence
  A. Destructive, overt expression of aggression that involves physical harm to people and/or property.
  B. Differs from aggression in intensity; intense uncontrolled, sudden, and excessive furor.
  C. Tends to escalate.
  D. Is addictive due to adrenaline rush accompanying expression of violence, with a sense of ecstasy and accomplishment brought about by change.
  E. Involves continuity (habit), reciprocal behaviors, and repetitive acts, with intent to harm others.

II. Four theories of aggression

  A. Aggression is an *instinctive* behavior (based on theories of Freud, Lorenz).
    1. It is innate, inevitable; it has survival value; aggression constantly seeks release.
    2. *Controlled by:* catharsis.
  B. Aggression is an *elicited drive* (based on Dollard's theories).
    1. External factors (e.g., accumulated frustration, pain and loss of face) arouse a strong drive to harm others.
    2. *Controlled by:* removing or decreasing external sources of frustration, or displacement and sublimation through sports.
  C. Aggression is *learned social behavior* (based on Bandura's theory).
    1. Although potential exists for aggressive acts, aggression is not inevitable. It is learned by imitating role models and by experiencing rewards following aggression.
    2. *Controlled by:* demonstrating nonviolent solutions to problems and not rewarding aggressive behaviors.
  D. Aggression is based on an *interaction of biology and cultures* (based on Wilson's theory).
    1. Violence develops out of biologic potential for aggression interacting with certain environmental conditions.
    2. *Controlled by:* altering environmental conditions.

III. Assessment
  A. *Sequence of antecedent events,* with combination of factors that lead to violent behavior:
    1. **Anger:** a strong emotional response to provocation; has autonomic nervous system (ANS) and CNS components; is short-lived; if not expressed, may result in hostility, fear, suppression of anger with motor or sensory symptoms; may be *displaced* onto someone else or repressed.
    2. **Hostility:** long-lasting antagonism toward one or many; is usually anger that is hidden, unexpressed; anger may come through as fantasies of revenge; can easily result in aggression, but may not necessarily involve overt physical acts of violence.
    3. **Shame:** when feeling humiliated, rage may be an immediate response ("shame-rage," or "humiliation-fury"), which is often repressed. Repressed shame and rage from the past can be triggered by current feelings of shame, resulting in an overwhelming, out-of-proportion rage reaction (i.e., violent outbursts).
    4. **Low self-esteem** and **powerlessness:** aggression may be an attempt to compensate for, defend, or promote self-image. Aggressive acts may represent opportunities to restore a sense of power by producing pain in others.
  B. Assess **risk factors** (potential) for violence:
    1. Signs of *frustration* and anger noted in body language, (e.g., clenched fists, rigid posture); argumentative, demanding, threatening.

2. Signs of *pain or hurt:* tears, melancholy.

3. Signs of increasing *anxiety:* continuous complaints, repetitive questions; misperceived messages from others; pacing.

4. Signs of *low self-esteem:* easily slighted and quick to take offense; overreactive; feelings of loss of control.

5. Situations where the patient may have felt *insignificant or humiliated:* feeling ignored due to long wait to be seen; lack of information; ignored requests; sarcastic remarks by personnel taken as criticism.

6. *Physical factors:* steroids, premenstrual syndrome (PMS), substance abuse or withdrawal, toxic reactions to medications, delirium.

7. *Emotional/mental conditions:* Paranoid or overly suspicious behavior; lack of basic trust; *depression* with feelings of inferiority, inadequacy, and pessimism; feelings of betrayal, rejection, or injury by others.

8. *History of violence,* as either the perpetrator (gang or criminal activity), or the victim of domestic violence or child abuse.

C. Rationalizations offered as *reasons* for violent acts (with sample statements):

1. *Projecting blame:* "He asked for it."

2. *Comparison:* "I only hit her with the belt; others beat her with a pipe."

3. *Minimizing injury:* "He only has a black eye, rather than a broken nose."

4. *Dehumanizing:* "The child is retarded and useless anyway."

5. *Relabeling:* "It was just in fun."

6. *Moral justification:* "He murdered my daughter . . . an eye for an eye."

7. *Conformity:* "All the others were raping her—I went along with the gang."

✉ IV. Analysis/nursing diagnosis

A. *Ineffective individual coping.*

B. *Fear.*

C. *Hopelessness.*

D. *Powerlessness.*

E. *Self-esteem disturbance.*

F. *High risk for trauma.*

✉ V. Nursing care plan/implementation

A. Identify risk for violent behavior to prevent violence (see **Assessment,** p. 97).

B. Diffuse the momentum of present anger.

C. Address underlying hurt and pain of betrayal, injury, and rejection.

D. Use empathy and reflection to help the patient to verbalize the anger and pain.

E. Explore frustrations related to the situation.

F. Convey acceptance and understanding of the feelings (but *not* the behavior), to help the patient regain self-control.

G. Assess staff behavior, to *avoid* demeaning comments and ignoring the patient.

✉ VI. Evaluation/outcome criteria

A. Demonstrates use of reason rather than out-of-control rage.

B. Seeks and utilizes constructive problem solving in order to see options and take alternative actions.

C. Addresses underlying feelings of frustration, pain, and injury; shame, humiliation, and powerlessness; consequences of violence (e.g., injuries, property damage) are minimized.

💡 Study and Memory Aids

Care of a patient who is combative—"OUT of CONTROL"

Out of range (maintain distance from patient)
Unhurried approach
T ranquil environment and attitude
  (of)
Consistent firmness
Overt aggression needs to be prevented
Neutral attitude
Tools (sharp objects) of "combat" removed
Restraints are *last* resort
Outbursts need to be controlled and channeled
Limit-setting

Manipulative behavior: therapeutic interventions

1. Limit-setting
2. Consistency
3. *Avoid:* arguments, power struggles; keep a matter-of-fact tone.
4. Use contracts (behavior modification)
5. Group, not 1:1 sessions

Manipulation—promote "3 C's"

Cooperation
Compromise
Collaboration

Glossary

aggression   An action aimed at destruction; overt or suppressed hostility, either innate or resulting from continued frustration.

anger   A strong *feeling* of displeasure in response to anxiety related to a real or imagined threat, injustice, injury, frustration, or exasperation.

confusion   A series of behaviors that include disorientation, memory loss, and difficulties with self-care related to cognitive impairment.

demanding   Strong, persistent struggle to obtain satisfac-

☞ Summary of Key Points

Care of a Patient Who Exhibits Anger, Combative-Aggressive Behavior, Hostility, or Violent Behavior

Nursing implications:
- Increase awareness of anger (precipitating factors).
- Set limits on acting-out; establish acceptable hierarchy of behaviors.
- Reinforce self-control.
- Control of violent behavior through *prevention, self-protection,* and *intervention.*
- Teach/model assertiveness.

Care of a Patient Who Exhibits Confusion or Disorientation

Nursing implications:
- Provide environmental safety.
- Focus on reality orientation; provide clock, calendar, radio, natural light.
- Rule out physiologic factors (i.e., check vital signs, fluid, electrolytes, and BUN; assess for sleep deprivation).
- *Avoid* sedatives.

Care of a Patient Who Exhibits Demanding Behavior

Nursing implications:
- Anticipate needs and respond to *requests,* rather than to attention-seeking demands.
- Provide a range of acceptable choices.

Care of a Patient Who Exhibits Denial of Illness

Nursing implications:
- Accept initial denial related to painful reality; give patient time for emotional adjustment at own pace; understand needs being met by denial.
- Support and encourage attempts to discuss some aspect of reality.

Care of a Patient Who Exhibits Dependence

Nursing implications:
- Promote interactions at "adult-to-adult" level.
- Reinforce *independent* behavior.

Care of a Patient Who Exhibits Hopelessness

Nursing implications:
- Assess suicide risk.
- Consider etiologic factors (e.g., progression of illness despite compliance with therapy, fear about illness or its outcome, long-term stressors, abandonment, isolation, chronic low self-esteem).
- Reduce isolation.
- Encourage active role in care and treatment, to help patient feel more *in control.*
- Convey *hope* by reflecting on positive aspects and patient's progress; help recall of previous successes; set an attainable goal for the future.

Care of a Patient Who Exhibits Manipulation

Nursing implications:
- Be consistent.
- Set limits.
- Use behavior modification approach.
- Use peer *group* method of treatment.

Care of a Patient Who Exhibits Noncompliance and Uncooperative Behavior

Nursing implications:
- Determine and intervene with *psychological* factors (e.g., lack of knowledge, high anxiety level, rebelliousness, denial of illness) and *environmental* factors (e.g., finances, transportation, lack of support system) that contribute to uncooperative behavior.
- Offer alternatives; prioritize which aspect(s) of prescribed treatment regimen is most important.

---

tion of self-oriented needs (e.g., control, self-esteem) or relief from anxiety.

denial   A defense mechanism that is demonstrated by avoidance of disagreeable reality by the mind's refusal to acknowledge at a conscious level the existence of some anxiety-provoking aspect of oneself or external reality (e.g., experience, idea, or memory). May or may not be adaptive.

dependence   Reliance on others to meet one's basic needs (e.g., for love, affection, security, protection, support, and guidance).

hostility   A *feeling* of intense anger, or an attitude of antagonism or animosity, with the destructive component of in-

tent to inflict harm and pain to another or to self; may involve hate, rage, aggression, regression.

manipulation   Meeting one's goals at the *expense* of another, by influencing and controlling the behavior of others.

noncompliance   Failure to perform prescribed activities.

projection   The attribution of one's feelings, impulses, thoughts, and wishes onto others or onto the environment.

rationalization   Offering a socially acceptable or logical explanation to justify feelings or behavior.

repression   An unconscious mechanism used to avoid painful experiences, unacceptable thoughts and impulses, and disagreeable memories by "forgetting."

sublimation   The transformation of psychic energy associated with unacceptable sexual or aggressive behaviors into socially acceptable outlets.

Questions

1. When a patient demonstrates self-awareness of anger, what would be the next appropriate nursing action?
   1. Let the patient know that it is all right to be angry.
   2. Let the patient know anger is unnecessary.
   3. Help the patient express anger in acceptable ways.
   4. Encourage the patient to take up sports or other physical activity to discharge tension associated with anger.

2. What is the rationale behind encouraging physical exercise for a person who has a tendency to become easily angered?
   1. To keep anger from escalating into physical aggression, with intent to cause harm to a person or object.
   2. To provide a constructive outlet for angry feelings.
   3. To maintain a stable blood pressure.
   4. To prevent violent behavior.

3. How would the nurse evaluate the outcome of nursing interventions with a patient who has a history of uncontrolled anger, when the patient says, "I am really upset and angry"?
   1. This statement is indicative of suppression of anger.
   2. This is an indication of a positive outcome.
   3. The patient is being manipulative toward the nurse.
   4. This statement is aimed at getting the nurse's attention.

4. What is the best nursing intervention for a patient who manifests anxiety by combative, aggressive behavior and angry outbursts?
   1. Avoiding confrontation about the outbursts.
   2. Allowing this expression of anger.
   3. Offering choices to the patient.
   4. Providing structure and limits.

5. A 75-year-old patient in a nursing home exhibits confusion and has severe memory loss. At 7:30 A.M., the patient tells the nurse that he is going to work and starts for the front door. What should the nurse do?
   1. Tell the patient that today is a holiday, so he does not have to go to work.
   2. Remind the patient that he retired years ago.
   3. Ask the patient if he would like to go for a walk with a staff member.
   4. Let the patient know that it is time for breakfast and take him to the dining room where it is being served.

6. A patient who is demanding has had many different nurses. The primary nurse is responsible for:
   1. Assigning the same staff nurse as yesterday.
   2. Asking a new staff nurse to care for the patient.
   3. Asking the staff about the patient's needs and assigning an appropriate staff person.
   4. Assigning the most experienced staff person.

7. A patient with insomnia comes to the nurses' station shouting and demanding something to help her sleep. The nurse's first action should be to:

   1. Set limits on her shouting before allowing her to go on.
   2. Ask her about her sleeping problem.
   3. Give her a choice of what can be done.
   4. Give her the prn sleeping med.

8. A middle-aged man states that he does not remember ever seeing his wife take an alcoholic drink and that he has never seen his wife drunk or tipsy. Given the fact that his wife has admitted to drinking several alcoholic drinks each day, what coping mechanism should the nurse identify that the man is using?
   1. Projection.
   2. Denial.
   3. Repression.
   4. Sublimation.

9. A nursing diagnosis of ineffective individual coping is established when a patient exhibits dependent behavior. What related behavior is the nurse most likely to observe in this patient?
   1. Avoidance of group activities.
   2. Resentment of suggestions.
   3. Fears of separation.
   4. Scorn and criticism of others.

10. A patient in the terminal stages of AIDS is despondent upon hearing that a close friend, who also had AIDS, has just died. The patient begins to cry and says to the nurse, "What's the use of hanging on when there is no hope? I'll die soon too." What is the best response by the nurse?
    1. "A cure for AIDS is bound to be discovered soon; don't give up yet."
    2. "No one knows how long you'll have to live. Make the most of the time you have left."
    3. "Let's talk about pleasant memories."
    4. "Would you like to talk?"

11. Which need is being expressed by manipulative behavior?
    1. Affection.
    2. Control.
    3. Appreciation.
    4. Superiority.

12. A woman's refusal to see a physician about a lump in her breast can be interpreted by the nurse as:
    1. Rationalization.
    2. Projection.
    3. Sublimation.
    4. Denial.

13. What is the most important short-term nursing goal with a patient whose behavior is manipulative?
    1. Peer group therapy for confrontation.
    2. Limit-setting.
    3. Establishing rules.
    4. Providing feedback regarding the effect of this behavior on others.

14. When a patient is manipulative, which step is most significant in reaching the long-term goal of change in behavior?
    1. Confront patient and set limits.
    2. Confront patient and impose sanctions.
    3. Encourage awareness of the manipulative behavior.
    4. Encourage expression of feelings.

15. A patient with psychotic behavior was admitted to the psychiatric unit because he would not comply with the medication regimen. What would be the initial approach by the nurse in dealing with this problem of noncompliance?
    1. Explain to the patient the importance of regular use of the medication.
    2. Ask a member of the family to ensure that the medication is taken.
    3. Ask the patient for the reason(s) why he does not take the medication.
    4. Suggest that the doctor order a more palatable form of medication.

Answers/Rationale

1. **(1)** Guilt is often associated with feelings of anger. As the next step in the therapeutic nursing process, it is important for the patient to accept anger as an understandable reaction to frustration, pain, fear, and a sense of powerlessness. **(No. 2)** is the opposite of the correct response. Helping the patient express anger in acceptable ways **(No. 3)**, for example, through sports **(No. 4)**, *follows* as the *next* step, after acknowledging that anger is understandable. **PL, 7, PsI**

   Test-taking tip: When in doubt, look for two *contradictory* options (here, **Nos. 1 and 2**). Then choose the option that states an action **(No. 1)** that must *come before* subsequent actions **(Nos. 3 and 4)**.

2. **(2)** Physical exercise can channel angry feelings into socially acceptable channels. Although **Nos. 1 and 4** are appropriate, they are both desired *results* of channeling the feelings. There are no data here about the patient's blood pressure **(No. 3)**; people who have a tendency to become easily angered may or may not have a problem with blood pressure. **PL, 3, PsI**

   Test-taking tip: When two options are very similar (such as **Nos. 1 and 4**), look for another.

3. **(2)** It is a sign of progress when the patient can *verbalize* anger rather than acting it out. This may be indicative of suppression of an angry *act*, but it is not an example of suppression of angry *feelings* **(No. 1)**. There is nothing here to indicate that this patient is using manipulation **(No. 3)** to demand attention **(No. 4)**, or to take control of the nurse through a threat of impending violent behavior. **EV, 7, PsI**

Key to Codes

Nursing process: AS = Assessment; **AN** = Analysis; **PL** = Planning; **IMP** = Implementation; **EV** = Evaluation. (See Appendix E for explanation of nursing process steps.)

Category of human function: 1 = Protective; **2** = Sensory-perceptual; **3** = Comfort, Rest, Activity, and Mobility; **4** = Nutrition; **5** = Growth and Development; **6** = Fluid-Gas Transport; **7** = Psychosocial-Cultural; **8** = Elimination.

Client need: SECE = Safe, Effective Care Environment; **PhI** = Physiologic Integrity; **PsI** = Psychosocial Integrity; **HPM** = Health Promotion/Maintenance.

4. **(4)** Providing guidelines for appropriate behavior helps to reduce acting-out. Ignoring excessive angry outbursts **(No. 1)** will not control them; the opposite is needed for change in behavior to occur. Expressing anger through combative, aggressive behavior is considered excessive, and *cannot* be allowed **(No. 2)**. The patient must be guided into acceptable expression of anger. Providing choices **(No. 3)** is unrealistic at this stage; by the time anxiety takes the form of combative behavior, the patient's anger is out of control. **PL, 7, SECE**

   Test-taking tip: Focus on the two options that are opposites; in this case, offering *choices* **(No. 3)** and providing *structure* **(No. 4)**. Narrow down the options to the one in which safety is the issue—the need to reduce acting-out by providing rules, limits, and guidelines for acceptable behavior, i.e., structure. (Because safety is the priority, *allowing* the behavior—**Nos. 1 and 2**—can be eliminated.)

5. **(4)** Of the four options, this is the best attempt at reality orientation when a patient is confused. **No. 1** serves to *reinforce* the confusion and disorientation. **No. 2** may increase the patient's anxiety by reminding him of his memory loss. **No. 3** is not *bad*, but it does not deal with the need to provide reality orientation. **IMP, 2, SECE**

6. **(3)** The theory about demanding behavior calls for understanding the difference between a *demand* and a *need*. It is important to learn about and meet underlying needs that are not being met when a patient is exhibiting demanding behaviors, and then to assign the staff person who is likely to be *most effective*. The *same* staff person **(No. 1)**, a *new* staff person **(No. 2)**, or the *most experienced* staff person **(No. 4)** may not be the *most effective*. **PL, 1, SECE**

7. **(3)** Giving choices helps give a demanding patient an appropriate method of self-control. A person who engages in attention-seeking behaviors, makes many requests, and seems unreasonable and irrational is a person who feels *helpless, fearful, powerless;* this person is struggling to obtain satisfaction of self-oriented needs (such as control, self-esteem) or relief from anxiety. Nursing measures include anticipating and meeting the patient's needs, and reinforcing appropriate requests for attention (in this case, help with insomnia). The patient exhibiting demanding behavior needs control over his or her environment, *not* to first *be controlled* **(No. 1)**. **No. 2** is not good because asking about the sleeping problem may result in more shouting; the patient wants the nurse to *do* something, *not* talk about a sleep problem. **No. 4** can be eliminated because "pushing a pill" is not the best *initial* nursing action. **PL, 7, PsI**

8. **(2)** Denial is the failure to acknowledge the existence of an affect, experience, idea, or memory. The person blocks from conscious awareness that which is painful, anxiety provoking, or threatening. The man may perceive that his behavior contributes to his wife's use of alcohol and may use denial to avoid facing feelings of guilt. Projection **(No. 1)** is the attribution of one's feelings, impulses, thoughts, and wishes onto others or onto the environment. Repression **(No. 3)** is an unconscious

mechanism used to avoid painful experiences, unacceptable thoughts and impulses, and disagreeable memories by "forgetting." Sublimation (**No. 4**) is the transformation of psychic energy associated with unacceptable sexual or aggressive behaviors into socially acceptable outlets. **AN, 7, PsI**

9. (3) The individual who is dependent on others is clingy and fears being rejected. The individual is preoccupied with fears of being left alone to care for him- or herself. The *opposite* of the other options is true: individuals who are dependent *need* to be with others and to avoid *solitary* activities (**No. 1**); they constantly *seek* advice from others (**No. 2**); and they are *reluctant* to disagree or argue with others (**No. 4**) because of fear of being rejected. **AS, 7, PsI**

10. (4) Although this response calls for a yes or no answer, it is the best option of the four. It is an attempt to provide an opportunity for the patient to express feelings of hopelessness and sadness related to the loss of a friend and a sense of loss related to the patient's own condition. Listening to the patient who is dying is important. **Nos. 1, 2, and 3** are trite, nonfeeling responses, which discourage the patient from expressing feelings. **IMP, 7, PsI**

11. (2) Control needs are dominant in patients with manipulative behavior. Much time and effort is spent in attempting to gain and maintain control over others. Neither the need for affection (**No. 1**) nor for appreciation (**No. 3**) is the cornerstone need in a manipulative personality. The need for feeling safe in a relationship is instead met by maneuvers to maintain distance. Who can get close to another person who is aloof, controlling, and uses people for his or her own gain? An attitude of superiority (**No. 4**) is used to maintain control of others, through intimidation; however, it is only one aspect of the central theme of control. **AN, 7, PsI**

Test-taking tip: First look at patterns: There are two "positive" options, **No. 1** (affection) and **No. 3** (appreciation). Eliminate these, as they do not go with a "negative" behavior (manipulation). Then, look for a *telescope* answer —one that includes the other. Here, **No. 2** (control) is more inclusive because it takes in **No. 4** (superiority).

12. (4) Denial is defined as the avoidance of disagreeable realities by ignoring or refusing to recognize them; *avoidance* implies refusing to take action. Rationalization (**No. 1**) involves offering a socially acceptable or logical explanation to justify feelings or behavior. In rationalization, one does not need to take action; one merely offers an explanation. Projection (**No. 2**) in-

volves attributing one's feelings, thoughts, or impulses to others. Sublimation (**No. 3**) is the channeling of a socially unacceptable behavior into substitute or outlet. **AN, 2, PsI**

13. (2) Limit-setting is the most important initial intervention; it calls for rules (**No. 3**) that need to be consistently reinforced at all times, by all staff. [*Note:* The *combined* approach of "confrontation, feedback, and control," through rules, peer group pressure, and corrective feedback is needed in working with patients whose behavior is manipulative.] A *peer* group (**No. 1**) is not a *nursing* action. Rules (**No. 3**) are *part* of limit-setting. Providing feedback (**No. 4**) is not enough; limits need to be placed on behaviors that have negative effects. **PL, 7, PsI**

Test-taking tip: Look for key words; in this case, "nursing" goal. Also, when two options seem correct, select the one that incorporates the other; in this case, *rules* (**No. 3**) are part of *limits* (**No. 2**); limit-setting requires rules.

14. (3) As part of the long-term goal (for change to occur), patients with manipulative modes of interaction must increase their limited self-awareness; they need to learn what effect their behavior has on others. Limits (**No. 1**) and sanctions (**No. 2**) are short-term goals, which serve to provide external controls for this maladaptive behavior rather than facilitating change (the long-term goal). Feelings (**No. 4**) are not the focus in dealing with manipulation. **PL, 7, PsI**

Test-taking tip: The best answer must meet the conditions of the question stem; here, the question asks about meeting the *long-term* goal (thus **Nos. 1 and 2,** short-term goals, can be eliminated).

15. (3) It is important to assess the reasons for noncompliance before action can be taken. Two common reasons for noncompliance include lack of understanding about how to *take* the medication and lack of resources to *get* the medication. Explaining the importance of regular use (**No. 1**) is premature. The nurse must first determine if the problem is one of knowledge deficit. Before enlisting the assistance of family (**No. 2**), the nurse must know if the reason for noncompliance is one that will be aided by family participation. (If the problem of noncompliance is due to denial of illness, it may cause a family conflict.) There is not enough information here to suggest that changing the form of medication (**No. 4**) will result in compliance. **IMP, 7, PsI**

Test-taking tip: When in doubt, look first for the option that calls for assessment (**No. 3:** "Ask why . . .").

Sleep Pattern Disturbances and Eating Disorders

Chapter Outline

- Sleep Pattern Disturbances
  - Types of Sleep
  - Sleep Deprivation (Dyssomnias)
  - Other Sleep-Related Conditions/Disturbances
- Eating Disorders
  - Anorexia Nervosa
    - Definition
    - Concepts and principles
    - Assessment
    - Analysis/nursing diagnosis
    - Nursing care plan/implementation
    - Evaluation/outcome criteria
  - Bulimia Nervosa
    - Definition
    - Concepts and principles
    - Assessment
    - Analysis/nursing diagnosis
    - Nursing care plan/implementation
    - Evaluation/outcome criteria
- Summary of Key Points
- Study and Memory Aids
- Glossary
- Questions
- Answers/Rationale

Sleep Pattern Disturbances

Types of Sleep

I. *Rapid eye movement (REM) sleep:* colorful, dramatic, emotional, implausible dreams.

II. *Non–REM sleep—stages*
- A. Stage 1: lasts 30 sec to 7 min—falls asleep, drowsy; easily awakened; fleeting thoughts.
- B. Stage 2: more relaxed; no eye movements, clearly asleep but readily awakens; 45% of total sleep time spent in this stage.
- C. Stage 3: (Delta sleep) deep muscle relaxation; ↓ TPR (temperature, pulse, respirations).
- D. Stage 4: (Delta sleep) very relaxed; rarely moves.

III. *Sleep cycle*—common progression of sleep stages:
- A. Stages 1, 2, 3, 4, 3, 2, REM, 2, 3, 4, etc.
- B. *Delta* sleep most common during first third of night, with *REM* sleep periods increasing in duration during night from 1–2 min at start to 20–30 min by early morning.
- C. REM sleep varies.
  - 1. Adolescents spend 30% of total sleep time in REM sleep.
  - 2. Adults spend 15% of total sleep time in REM sleep.

Sleep Deprivation (Dyssomnias)

I. **Assessment**
- A. *Non–REM sleep loss:* physical fatigue due to less time spent in normal deep sleep.
- B. *REM sleep loss:* psychological effects—irritability, confusion, anxiety, short-term memory loss, paranoia, hallucinations.
- C. *Desynchronized sleep:* occurs when sleep shifts more than 2 hr from normal sleep period. Irritability, anoxia, decreased stress tolerance.
- D. Obtain sleep history.
  - 1. Normal sleep pattern: amount and quality of sleep.
  - 2. Bedtime rituals.
- E. Current specific problem.
  - 1. Symptoms.
  - 2. Alleviating factors.
- F. Recent physical illnesses.
- G. Current/recent emotional stressors.
- H. Current medications and possible effects on sleep (Table 8.1).

II. **Analysis/nursing diagnosis**—*Sleep pattern disturbance* may be related to:
- A. Interrupted sleep cycles before 90-min sleep cycle is completed.
- B. Unfamiliar sleeping environment.
- C. Alterations in normal sleep/activity cycles (e.g., jet lag).

103

Table 8.1   MEDICATIONS THAT MAY AFFECT SLEEP

Drug/Drug Class	Assessment: Effect
Alcohol	Disruption of REM sleep Rapid onset of sleep Frequent awakening (intermittent insomnia) Difficulty returning to sleep (terminal insomnia)
Antidepressants and **stimulants**	Suppression of REM sleep
Beta-adrenergic blockers	Nightmares Frequent awakening
Caffeine	Prevention of sleep (initial insomnia) Frequent awakening
Digoxin	Nightmares
Diuretics	Nocturia
Hypnotics	Interference with deep sleep *Temporary* increase (1 wk) in length of sleep "Hangover" during day: drowsiness, lethargy, confusion Older adults: sleep apnea
Narcotics (e.g., *Demerol, Morphine*)	Suppression of REM Increased awakening and drowsiness If discontinued abruptly: cardiac dysrhythmias
Valium	Decrease in Stages 2 and 4, and REM

D. Preexisting sleep deficits prior to hospital admission.

E. Medications (e.g., alcohol withdrawal or abrupt discontinuation of hypnotic or antidepressant medications).

F. Pain.

III. Nursing care plan/implementation

A. Obtain sleep history as part of nursing assessment. Determine: normal sleep hours, bedtime rituals, factors that promote or interrupt sleep.

B. Duplicate normal bedtime rituals when possible.

C. Make *environment* conducive to sleep: lighting, noise, temperature.

   1. Close door, dim lights, turn off unneeded machinery.

   2. Encourage staff to muffle conversation at night.

D. Encourage *daytime* exercise periods.

E. Allow *uninterrupted periods of 90 min of sleep.* Group nighttime treatments and observations that require touching the client.

F. *Minimize* use of hypnotic medications.

   1. Substitute backrubs, warm milk, relaxation exercises.

   2. Encourage physician to consider prescribing hypnotics that minimize sleep disruption (e.g.,

chloral hydrate and *flurazepam hydrochloride* [*Dalmane*]).

   3. *Taper* off hypnotics rather than abruptly discontinuing.

G. Observe client while asleep.

   1. Evaluate quality of sleep.

   2. It may be sleep apnea if client is extremely restless and snoring heavily.

H. *Health teaching: avoid* caffeine and hyperstimulation at bedtime; teach how to promote sleep-inducing environment, relaxation techniques.

IV. Evaluation/outcome criteria: verbalizes satisfaction with amount, quality of sleep.

Other Sleep-Related Conditions/Disturbances

These include bruxism, enuresis, insomnia, narcolepsy, sleep apnea, somnambulation. (See **Glossary** at end of chapter).

Eating Disorders

Definition: *Anorexia nervosa* is a mental disorder, usually seen in adolescent women, characterized by refusal to attain or maintain minimum normal body weight for age and height, intense fear of being fat, and body image disturbance. Patients are often underweight (15% or more *under* ideal body weight) and emaciated. It can result in death due to irreversible metabolic processes.

Bulimia nervosa is another type of eating disorder, also encountered among older women and younger men as well. It is characterized by at least two binge-eating episodes of large quantities of high-calorie food over a couple of hours followed by disparaging self-criticism and depression. Self-induced vomiting is commonly associated since it decreases physical pain of abdominal distention, may reduce postbinge anguish, and may provide a method of self-control. Bulimic episodes may occur as part of anorexia nervosa, but these clients rarely become emaciated, and not all have a body image disturbance.

Anorexia Nervosa

I. **Concepts and principles** related to anorexia nervosa:
A. *Not* due to lack of appetite (only in late stages) or problem with appetite center in hypothalamus; rather a need to demonstrate control.
B. Normal stomach hunger is *repressed, denied, depersonalized;* no conscious awareness of hunger sensation.

II. **Assessment** of anorexia nervosa:
A. *Body image disturbance*—delusional, obsessive (e.g., doesn't see self as thin and is bewildered by others' concern). Denies probability of illness or death as a result of starvation.
B. Usually obsessively *preoccupied* with food, yet dreads gaining too much weight. *Ambivalence:* avoids food, hoards food. Restrictive *diet;* eliminates high-calorie foods.
C. Feels ineffectual, with low sex drive. *Repudiation of sexuality.*
D. *Pregnancy* fears, including misconceptions of oral impregnation through food.
E. *Self-punitive* behavior leading to starvation, suicidal attempts (especially following forced weight gain).
F. *Physical signs and symptoms*
1. Weight loss (20% of previous "normal" body weight).
2. *Amenorrhea* (absence of three or more menstrual cycles) and secondary sex organ atrophy (or significant delayed psychosexual development in adolescents).
3. *Hyperactivity;* compulsiveness.
4. Constipation—marked.
5. *Hypotension, bradycardia, hypothermia.*
6. *Hyperkeratosis* of skin; dry hair (may fall out).
7. Blood: leukopenia, anemia, hypoglycemia, hypoproteinemia, hypercholesterolemia, hypokalemia.

III. **Analysis/nursing diagnosis**
A. *Risk for self-inflicted injury* related to starvation from refusal to eat or ambivalence about food or strive for control and "perfection."
B. *Risk for altered physical regulation processes:*
amenorrhea related to starvation; hypotension, bradycardia.
C. *Altered nutrition, less than body requirements,* related to attempts to vomit food after eating and refusal to eat, related to need to demonstrate control.
D. *Altered eating:* excessive dieting
E. *Compulsive behaviors* (e.g., excessive exercising) related to need to maintain control of self, represented by losing weight.
F. *Body image disturbance* related to anxiety over assuming an adult role and concern with sexual identity.

IV. **Nursing care plan/implementation**
Long-term goals
A. Improve self-esteem, self-image, self-concept through cognitive therapy and assertiveness training.
B. Promote awareness of fears about sexuality and intimacy; help with transition from adolescence to intimacy.
C. Break through maladaptive denial.
D. Encourage participation in family therapy.
Immediate goal
A. Help reestablish connections between body sensations (hunger) and responses (eating). Use *stimulus-response conditioning* methods to set up *eating* regimen (see **Behavior Modification;** pp. 56–57).
B. *Monitor physiologic signs and symptoms* (amenorrhea, constipation, hypoproteinemia, hypoglycemia, anemia, secondary sexual organ atrophy, hypothermia, hypotension, leg cramps and other signs of hypokalemia, including weight loss).
1. *Weigh* regularly, at same time and with same amount of clothing.
2. Make sure water drinking is *avoided* before weighing.
3. Give one-to-one supervision during and 2 h after mealtimes to *prevent* attempts to vomit food.
C. *Health teaching*
1. Explain normal sexual growth and development to improve knowledge deficit.
2. Use behavior modification to reestablish awareness of hunger sensation and to relate it to the clock and regular meal times.
3. Teach parents skills in communication related to adolescent's control needs, conflicts between dependence/independence needs of adolescent around decision making.

V. **Evaluation/outcome criteria**
A. Attains and maintains signs of physical improvement (e.g., minimal normal weight for age and height; menstrual cycles resume; skin turgor and muscle tone reveal improved nutritional state).
B. Eats regular meal (standard nutritional diet).
C. No incidence of self-induced vomiting, bulimia, or compulsive physical activity (e.g., absence of preoccupation with strenuous exercise and food preparation, while eating little or nothing).
D. Acts on increased internal emotional awareness

and recognition of body sensation of hunger (i.e., talks about being hungry and feeling hunger pangs).

E. Relates increased sense of effectiveness (i.e., being "in control") with less need to control food intake.

F. Normal fluid and electrolyte levels.

Bulimia Nervosa

Definition: A type of eating disorder similar to *anorexia nervosa.* It is characterized by recurrent binge eating episodes coupled with methods to prevent weight gain (see also definition on p. 105). **Differences** from *anorexia nervosa* are outlined below.

I. Concepts and principles

A. Bulimic episodes may occur as *part* of anorexia nervosa, but *not all* anorexics are bulimic.

B. *Different* characteristics from anorexia:

1. Young *men* and *older* women *also* have bulimia.

2. Many do *not* have body image disturbance.

3. *Rarely* become emaciated.

4. Frequent *weight fluctuations.*

5. Maintain *awareness* (rather than denial) of abnormal eating pattern.

6. Fear of *not* being able to *voluntarily stop* eating.

7. History of *depression,* which generally occurs a year before the onset of bulimic symptoms.

▷◁ II. Assessment

A. *Binge eating:* at least two episodes per week (for 3 mo) of consuming large quantities of high-calorie foods in a frenzy over a couple of hours; eating is often done secretively; may experience feelings of dissociation, followed by disparaging self-criticism, guilt, and *depression* as person deals with postbinge remorse or despair.

B. *Purge cycles* through use of diuretics, laxatives, enemas, and self-induced vomiting, as compensatory techniques used to decrease physical pain of abdominal distention; may reduce postbinge anguish; may provide a method of self-control. Results:

1. Dental erosion (poor teeth enamel) and many decayed teeth as a result of acidic gastric secretions from frequent vomiting episodes.

2. Dehydration.

3. Irreversible perimolysis on lingual surfaces of incisors due to frequent contact with gastric secretions from emesis and sugary foods.

4. Sore throats.

5. *Lab* values: hypokalemia; low serum phosphate (from massive laxative abuse); low serum chloride; metabolic acidosis (renal effect of chronic vomiting).

C. *Cardiac*

1. Myocardial contractility problems.

2. Cardiac dysrhythmias or cardiac arrest due to hypokalemia.

D. *Muscle:* weakness and contractility problems due to hypokalemia.

E. *G.I.:* acute gastric dilation and stomach rupture; esophageal or rectal bleeding; stomach ulcers.

F. *Thyroid:* delayed thyroid-stimulating hormone (TSH) response to thyroid-releasing hormone (TRH).

▷◁ III. Analysis/nursing diagnosis

A. *Altered eating* related to binge-purge behaviors.

B. *Defensive coping* (i.e., purging) related to self-criticism for binge eating.

C. *Diarrhea* related to laxative abuse and frequent dietary changes.

D. *Altered nutrition:* more than body requirements related to psychological impairment (bulimia).

▷◁ IV. Nursing care plan/implementation

Long-term goals

A. Help patient to gain control in areas *other than* dieting, fasting, and binging, by promoting feelings of self-control through *independent* decision making in managing own daily activities, work, leisure time, social functions.

B. Encourage expression of angry and negative feelings to reduce depression related to self contempt (anger turned inward).

C. Determine possible sources of irrational beliefs; give permission to be less than "perfect" and still be a worthwhile person.

D. Focus on strengths and capabilities to build self-esteem and discourage guilt and self-criticism.

E. Lessen obsession with food, weight, and physical appearance.

Short-term goals

A. Help to regain self-control of binge-purge behaviors through 1:1 *observation* by staff for *2 hr after meals* in order to monitor eating-related behaviors.

B. Minimize compulsive purging by encouraging participation in social activities that discourage secret binge-purge episodes and increase healthy social interactions. *Limit weighing to once* a week.

C. *Diet:* Fluids and high-fiber foods to prevent constipation and resulting temptation to use enemas and laxatives.

D. *Avoid* discussion of foods as focal point of family visits.

E. Facilitate a behavior modification program that provides a structured eating situation.

▷◁ V. Evaluation/outcome criteria

A. Ceases binge-purge episodes; absence of use of laxatives or diuretics, in order to lose weight.

B. Stops dieting or fasting in order to prevent weight gain.

C. No longer need to weigh self daily.

D. Maintains normal weight for age and height.

E. Demonstrates internal locus of control, rather than control of life through binge-purge episodes.

F. Demonstrates normal social eating patterns without attempts to conceal food or eat in isolation.

G. Eats nutritionally balanced meals, rather than soft, sweet high-calorie foods (e.g., ice cream, pastries).

☞ Summary of Key Points

Care of a Patient with a Sleep Pattern Disturbance (Dyssomnia)

1. Be aware of medications that may affect sleep.
2. Make environment conducive for uninterrupted 90-min sleep cycles.
3. There are other sleep-related disturbances: bruxism, enuresis, narcolepsy, sleep apnea, somnambulation.

Care of a Patient with an Eating Disorder

1. *Identify eating disorder:* use of laxatives and cathartics; poor tooth enamel and many decayed teeth, red fingers and hands; preoccupation with appearance.
2. *Commonality* between anorexia and bulimia is a feeling of loss of control and low self-esteem.
3. *Differences* between anorexia and bulimia
   - *Anorexia nervosa:* intense fear of becoming fat; weight is 20% less than original body weight. No known physical illness; *body image disturbance.*
   - *Bulimia nervosa:* cycle of binge-purge. Depression follows binge; fear of not being able to stop eating voluntarily; awareness of abnormal eating pattern.
4. Goals
   - *Treatment of choice:* behavior modification program, with rewards when weight is gained; firm, consistent approach.
   - Limited exercise (based on weight lost or gained).
   - 1:1 observation until control over behavior is regained (i.e., no longer: refuses to eat, overexercises, or binge-purges).
5. *Interventions*
   - Encourage expression of *feelings* (especially angry and negative feelings).
   - Encourage *independent decision making* to promote feelings of control.
   - *Weigh* daily (use same scales immediately on rising and after first void—as a short-term goal).
   - Offer *positive reinforcement* for improvements in eating behaviors.
   - *Do not* discuss food or eating after a plan is developed by patient and dietitian.

☼ Study and Memory Aids

Anorexia nervosa: clinical features— "A²NOREX²I²C²"

Adolescent female, **A**menorrhea
Nutritional deficits
Obsession: with need to lose weight, with fear of becoming fat
Refusal to eat → 10% mortality
Electrolyte abnormality (hypokalemia)
e**X**cessive e**X**ercise
Induced vomiting; **I**ntelligence above average
Cardiac arrhythmias related to hypokalemia resulting from starvation and possible **C**athartic and diuretic abuse

Source: Modified from Rogers PT. *The Medical Student's Guide to Top Board Scores.* Boston: Little, Brown, 1995. P 78.

anorexia nervosa   A mental disorder that is characterized by eating disorder and body image disturbance, in which an individual who is not obese has a self-perception of obesity and an intense, pathologic fear of being fat; characterized by *denial* of current low body weight, refusal to eat, or excessive dieting and emaciation. No loss of appetite occurs until the late stages of the disease.

binge eating   Rapid consumption of large amounts of food in a short period of time with feeling of lack of control during binge episode.

bulimia nervosa   An eating disorder that is characterized by recurrent cycles of abnormal, uncontrolled *binge* eating of large quantities of food followed by compensatory *purging* (through vomiting, use of laxatives, enema, and diuretics), fasting, and overexercising. The individual suffers from persistent overconcern with body shape and weight, but *lacks* the body image distortion and degree of weight loss experienced by individual with anorexia nervosa.

cachexia   Physical condition with appearance of wasting and emaciation related to medical condition and malnutrition.

depersonalization   An alteration in the perception of self in which one's usual sense of reality is temporarily changed or lost.

Glossary

Eating Disorders

amenorrhea   After menarche, female misses at least three consecutive menstrual periods; before menarche, menstrual cycle is delayed.

Sleep Pattern Disturbances

bruxism   Grinding or clenching teeth while asleep. Believed to be related to repressed aggression, emotional tension, anger, fear, and frustration.

dyssomnia   Any disorder of sleep.

enuresis   Involuntary bed-wetting after the age at which urinary control is normally attained.

insomnia　Chronic difficulty with sleeping.
　initial insomnia　Difficulty falling asleep.
　intermittent insomnia　Difficulty remaining asleep.
　terminal insomnia　Difficulty going back to sleep.
narcolepsy　Uncontrollable desire for sleep; brief and recurrent episodes of falling asleep without warning.
sleep apnea　Cessation of breathing during sleep.
sleep deprivation　Decrease in length and quality of sleeping time.
sleep disorder　A chronic disturbance of sleep patterns (amount, quality, or timing of sleep; nightmares).
somnambulation (also called **somnambulism**)　Sleepwalking, usually occurring in the first third of the night and lasting a few minutes to a half hour.

Questions

1. A patient with anorexia nervosa exhibits a body image disturbance when she looks into a mirror and exclaims that she sees a person who is obese. The nurse will be most correct in identifying this behavior as which psychodynamic defense mechanism?
   1. Depersonalization.
   2. Disassociation.
   3. Denial.
   4. Displacement.
2. During the initial hospitalization period of a 15-year-old with anorexia, the nurse should:
   1. Assess how the patient feels about herself.
   2. Determine what causes the eating disorder.
   3. Allow the patient to set her own limits for how much she wants to eat.
   4. Offer small portions to encourage eating.
3. A patient who has a diagnosis of anorexia nervosa stands up in the dining room and says, "I don't want to stay here and eat." The nurse's most therapeutic response would be to say:
   1. "You may go to your room," and allow her to leave.
   2. "You need to eat," and explain why, offering nutritional reasons.
   3. "You need to stay with the group," and set limits.
   4. "If you do not eat, you will have to stay here longer," and restate the therapeutic regimen.
4. With which problem should the nurse be concerned when planning care for an adolescent patient who is being treated for anorexia nervosa?
   1. Lack of self-esteem.
   2. Lack of self-control.
   3. Low intelligence.
   4. An attitude of superiority.
5. What is the most common family issue that the nurse needs to be aware of in working with an adolescent girl with anorexia nervosa?
   1. Lack of self-control.
   2. Control of others.
   3. Confusion of sexual identity.
   4. Dependency.
6. What is the most significant finding that the nursing assessment is likely to reveal in a patient with bulimia who engages in frequent purging?
   1. Amenorrhea.

2. Bradycardia.
3. Dehydration.
4. Cachexia.
7. In working with a patient with bulimia, the nurse must be aware of what serious problem that affects electrolyte balance and causes cardiac irregularities?
   1. Hypocalcemia.
   2. Hypokalemia.
   3. Hyperkalemia.
   4. Hypernatremia.
8. A patient with bulimia is on the hospital unit. What would be the most indicative sign that she is improving?
   1. She no longer continuously talks about her weight.
   2. She no longer continuously talks about food.
   3. She no longer weighs herself daily.
   4. She no longer limits her food intake.
9. Which intervention should the nurse perform first to help a patient with insomnia?
   1. Provide active exercise during the day.
   2. Administer hypnotic medication at bedtime.
   3. Encourage daily naps.
   4. Provide a warm cup of cocoa at bedtime.

Answers/Rationale

1. **(1)** The patient feels that she is separate from her body and feelings. Disassociation (**No. 2**) refers to Sullivan's theory of "not-me," splitting off an aspect of self that is painful from conscious awareness (e.g., multiple personalities). There are no data here to indicate that this patient is exhibiting a dissociative disorder. Denial (**No. 3**) is a defense mechanism by which a person refuses to acknowledge an aspect of reality (e.g., drinking wine when told of impending liver failure). In displacement (**No. 4**), feelings about a person or object are directed toward another person or object that is less threatening. **AN, 7, PsI**
2. **(4)** The basis for primary nursing intervention in anorexia is reality- and success-orientation in achieving *physiologic* integrity (i.e., eating behaviors). **No. 1** is *not* the priority during *initial* hospitalization. Self-image, self-concept, and self-esteem are at the *upper* levels of Maslow's categories of human needs and are long-term goals; *physiologic* integrity (eating) is *primary*. **No. 2** is not important in the *initial* hospitalization period. Intellectual *understanding* of cause does *not* necessarily lead to a change in anorexic behavior. **No. 3** is incorrect because the major problem is that the patient *doesn't* eat; limits need to be placed *for* her, not set *by* her. **PL, 4, PsI**

Key to Codes

Nursing process: AS = Assessment; **AN** = Analysis; **PL** = Planning; **IMP** = Implementation; **EV** = Evaluation. (See Appendix E for explanation of nursing process steps.)

Category of human function: 1 = Protective; **2** = Sensory-Perceptual; **3** = Comfort, Rest, Activity, and Mobility; **4** = Nutrition; **5** = Growth and Development; **6** = Fluid-Gas Transport; **7** = Psychosocial-Cultural; **8** = Elimination.

Client need: SECE = Safe, Effective Care Environment; **PhI** = Physiologic Integrity; **PsI** = Psychosocial Integrity; **HPM** = Health Promotion/Maintenance.

3. **(3)** This option focuses on limit-setting and the use of stimulus-response conditioning (i.e., behavior modification) methods to set up an eating regimen. Behavior modification is used to reestablish awareness of hunger sensation and to relate it to the clock and regular mealtimes (lunchtime, dinnertime, etc.). Even if the patient won't eat, it is important to be in setting with others who *are* eating. **No. 1** is the opposite of the correct response. **No. 2** is not helpful; it provides cognitive input, when intellectual understanding is not the problem. **No. 4** can be eliminated because it sounds and *is* threatening. **IMP, 7, PsI**

💡 *Test-taking tip:* When you need to make an "educated guess," look for and focus on two options that are opposite; in this case, **No. 1** ("go") and **No. 3** ("stay").

4. **(1)** The patient with anorexia nervosa usually does not have a positive self-image. This low self-esteem serves as a barrier to taking charge of the patient's own life. *Lack of self-control* (**No. 2**) is not the problem; the patient uses *too much* control over own eating-related behaviors (e.g., controlling hunger by not eating and by exercising beyond reasonable limits). Neither low intelligence (**No. 3**) nor an attitude of superiority (**No. 4**) is a factor related to anorexia. **AS, 7, PsI**

5. **(2)** A central family issue that needs to be addressed is the adolescent girl's control of other family members (often the father), as expressed by eating-related behaviors. **No. 1** is incorrect because the question asks for a *family* issue, not a *self*-oriented issue; also, the problem in anorexia nervosa is *too much* self-control (in controlling own eating-related behavior). A problem is *concern* with (fear of) maturity and responsibilities connected with sexual development, *not* confusion of sexual identity (**No. 3**). Dependency (**No. 4**) is *not a central family* issue with anorexia nervosa, but rather the *adolescent's* own conflicting dependence/independence needs. **AN, 7, PsI**

6. **(3)** The pattern of binge eating and purging (used as compensatory behavior to prevent weight gain) leads to dehydration, through the use of self-induced vomiting, diuretics, and laxatives. Amenorrhea (**No. 1**), bradycardia (**No. 2**), and cachexia (**No. 4**)—a "wasting-away" condition—are more common in *anorexia* than in *bulimia*. **AN, 4, PhI**

7. **(2)** Due to frequent vomiting in the typical "eat-and-purge" behavior, with consequent loss of potassium, the major nursing concern is hypokalemia. The serious problem is *not* related to a loss and/or deficiency of calcium (**No. 1**). The problem is *loss* of potassium through vomiting, rather than an excess, hyperkalemia (**No. 3**). Excessive sodium (**No. 4**) is not the electrolyte imbalance problem. The concern is with cardiac irregularities that are associated with loss of potassium. **EV, 6, PhI**

8. **(3)** Eating *disturbance* is often accompanied by frequent weighing, as if to validate a need to take *action* to purge excess poundage, to maintain control of self as represented by losing weight. **Nos. 1 and 2** can be eliminated. It's not *talking* about the preoccupation with food and dread of gaining weight that is the problem, but what the person *does* about the concern, i.e., the compulsive activity (e.g., self-induced vomiting, avoiding eating, taking laxatives, hyperactivity) that is undertaken. *Talking* about weight and food, and disturbed eating patterns are behaviors that frequently *persist* in bulimia; when the person can stop daily weighing, *that* is most indicative of improvement. **No. 4** is not correct because bulimic behavior can be one of binging, and at other times, not eating (anorexic behavior). **EV, 7, HPM**

💡 *Test-taking tip:* Look at patterns: Which option is not like the others? When you need to make an "educated guess," consider choosing the one option that is different. In this case, there are two *talks* (**Nos. 1 and 2**) and an *action* (weighing, **No. 3**). Go with the one that is different, in this case, **No. 3**.

9. **(1)** Exercise at least 2 hours prior to bedtime helps induce sleep. Providing hypnotic medication (**No. 2**) would be a later intervention, not first. Naps (**No. 3**) will *decrease* the quality of nighttime sleep. **No. 4** is incorrect because cocoa contains caffeine, which is a stimulant. **IMP, 3, SECE**

Anxiety and Related Disorders

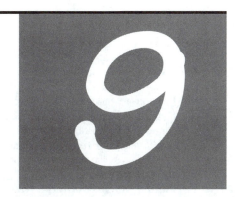

Anxiety Disorders

General Introduction

I. **Definition:** Anxiety disorders are emotional illnesses characterized by *fear* and *autonomic nervous system* (*ANS*) *symptoms* (e.g., palpitations, tachycardia, dizziness, tremor); and avoidance behavior.

An *anxiety disorder* is a mild to moderately severe functional disorder of personality in which *repressed* instinctual impulses (related to sexuality, aggression, or dependence) may be in conflict with the ego, superego, or sociocultural environment.

II. **General concepts and principles** related to anxiety disorders:
- **A.** Behavior may be an attempt to "bind" anxiety: to *fix* it in some particular area (*hypochondriasis*) or to *displace* it from the rest of personality (*phobic, conversion,* and *dissociative* disorders—amnesia, fugue, multiple personalities; *obsessive-compulsive* disorders).
- **B.** *Purpose of symptoms*
    1. To intensify *repression* as a defense.
    2. To exhibit some repressed content in *symbolic* form.

III. **General assessment** of anxiety disorders:
- **A.** Uses behavior to *avoid* tense situations.
- **B.** Frightened, suggestible.
- **C.** Prone to *minor* physical complaints (e.g., fatigue, headaches, indigestion) and reluctance to admit recovery from physical illnesses.
- **D.** Attitude of martyrdom.
- **E.** Often feels helpless, insecure, inferior, inadequate.
- **F.** Uses *repression, displacement,* and *symbolism* as key coping mechanisms.

Generalized Anxiety Disorder

I. **Definition:** Chronic excessive unrealistic worry and anxiety over 2 or more situations in the person's life.

II. **Assessment**
- **A.** Persistent, diffuse, free-floating, painful anxiety for at least 6 mo.
- **B.** Motor tension, autonomic hyperactivity.
- **C.** Hyperattentiveness expressed through vigilance and scanning.

III. **Analysis/nursing diagnosis**
- **A.** *Anxiety: excessive worry* related to threat to security.
- **B.** *Altered attention* related to overwhelming anxiety.
- **C.** *Fear* related to sudden object loss.
- **D.** *Guilt* related to inability to meet role expectations.
- **E.** *Risk for alteration in self-concept* related to feelings of inadequacy.
- **F.** *Altered role performance* related to inadequate support system.
- **G.** *Impaired social interaction* related to use of avoidance in tense situations.
- **H.** *Distractibility* related to pervasive anxiety.
- **I.** *Hopelessness* related to feelings of inadequacy.

IV. **Nursing care plan/implementation**
- **A.** Fulfill needs as promptly as possible.
- **B.** Listen attentively.

C. Stay with client.
D. *Avoid* decision making and competitive situations, but provide physical activities.
E. Promote rest; decrease environmental stimuli.
F. Help identify manifestations of anxiety and relief-connected behaviors.
G. *Health teaching:* teach steps of anxiety reduction (e.g., progressive muscle relaxation breathing exercises, visual imagery).

V. **Evaluation/outcome criteria:** symptoms are diminished.

Panic Disorder

I. **Definition:** Unexpected recurrence of panic attacks with at least four of the following symptoms, which occur abruptly and cause extreme fear.

II. **Assessment**
A. Three acute, terrifying panic attacks within 3-wk period, *unrelated* to marked physical exertion, life-threatening situation, presence of organic illness, or exposure to specific phobic stimulus.
B. Discrete periods of apprehension, fearfulness (lasting from few moments to 1 hr).
C. *Mimics cardiac disease:* dyspnea, chest pain, smothering or choking sensations, palpitations, tachycardia, ↑ BP, dizziness, fainting, ataxia, sweating.
D. Hyperventilation; feelings of unreality (depersonalization), paresthesias.
E. Hot, cold flashes and dilated pupils.
F. Trembling, sense of impending death, fear of becoming insane, fear of losing control.
G. GI and GU frequency.

III. **Analysis/nursing diagnosis**
A. *Ineffective individual coping* related to undeveloped interpersonal processes.
B. *Altered comfort pattern:* distress, anxiety, fear related to threat to security.
C. *Decisional conflict* related to apprehension.
D. *Altered thought processes* related to impaired concentration.

IV. **Nursing care plan/implementation**
A. *Reduce immediate anxiety* to more moderate and manageable levels.
   1. Stay *physically close* to reduce feelings of alienation and terror.
   2. *Communication approach:* calm, serene manner; short, simple sentences; firm voice to convey that nurse will provide external controls.
   3. *Physical environment:* remove to smaller *quiet* room to minimize stimuli.
B. Provide *motor outlet* for diffuse energy generated at high anxiety levels (e.g., moving furniture, scrubbing floors).
C. Administer *anti-anxiety medications* as ordered to ↓ panic reaction.
D. *Health teaching:* recommend more effective methods of coping.

V. **Evaluation/outcome criteria:** can endure anxiety while searching out its causes.

Obsessive-Compulsive Disorder

I. **Definition:** Preoccupation with intrusive recurrent thoughts and behaviors that are extremely distressing to the person or interfere with normal life pattern.

II. **Assessment**
A. *Obsessions:* persistent, involuntary, intrusive *thoughts, images, ideas,* or *desires* that may be trivial or morbid (e.g., fear of germs; doubts as to performance of an act; thoughts of hurting family member, death, suicide). Person knows that these thoughts and urges are irrational.
B. *Compulsions:* uncontrollable, persistent urge to perform repetitive, stereotyped *behaviors* that provide relief from unbearable anxiety (e.g., handwashing, counting, touching, checking and rechecking doors to see if locked, elaborate dressing and undressing rituals. Tension may be relieved by the repetitive act.

III. **Analysis/nursing diagnosis**
A. *Ineffective individual coping* related to:
   1. *Intellectualization* and *avoidance* of awareness of feelings.
   2. Limited ability to express emotions (may be disguised or delayed).
   3. Exaggerated feelings of *dependence* and *helplessness.*
   4. High need to *control* self, others, and environment.
   5. Rigidity in thinking and behavior.
   6. Poor ability to tolerate anxiety and depression.
B. *Social isolation* and *impaired social interaction* related to:
   1. Resentment.
   2. Self-doubt.
   3. Exclusion of pleasure.

IV. **Nursing care plan/implementation**
A. *Accept* rituals permissively (excessive handwashing, for example); stopping or interrupting ritual will increase anxiety. However, limit-setting is necessary.
B. *Avoid* criticism or "punishment," making demands, or showing impatience with client. Give a great deal of positive feedback.
C. *Allow* extra time for slowness and client's need for precision.
D. Provide distraction in attempt to decrease need to perform ritual; *redirect* client's actions into substitute outlets (e.g., activities requiring precision and repetition) to discharge pent-up energy associated with anxiety.
E. *Protect* from rejection by *others.*
F. *Protect* from *self-inflicted* harm.
G. Engage in nursing therapy *after* the ritual is over, when client is most comfortable.
H. *Health teaching:* teach how to prevent health problems related to rituals (e.g., use rubber gloves, hand lotion with excessive handwashing).

V. **Evaluation/outcome criteria:** avoids situations that increase tension and thus reduces need for ritualistic behavior as outlet for tension.

Phobic Disorders

I. **Definition:** A phobic disorder is an intense, *irrational, persistent* fear in response to *external* object, activity, or situation.

    A. **Examples of specific phobias**

        1. *Agoraphobia*—fear of being alone or in public places

        2. *Claustrophobia*—fear of closed places

        3. *Acrophobia*—fear of heights

        4. *Mysophobia* (example of simple phobia)—fear of germs

        5. *Social phobias:* fear of situations that may be humiliating or embarrassing.

        6. *Hydrophobia*—fear of water

        7. *Thanatophobia*—fear of death

        8. *Nyctophobia*—fear of darkness

        9. *Gynophobia*—fear of women

        10. *Kakorrhaphiophobia*—fear of failure

II. **Concepts and principles**—*Dynamics: repression, displacement* of anxiety from original source onto avoidable, *symbolic*, external, and specific object (or activity or situation); i.e., phobias help person control intensity of anxiety by providing specific object to attach it to, which he or she can then avoid.

III. **Assessment:** same as for panic disorder symptoms; fear that someone or something will harm them.

IV. **Analysis/nursing diagnosis:** *social isolation;* avoidance; irrational *fear* out of proportion to actual danger; *defensive coping* with high need to control self, others, environment.

V. **Nursing care plan/implementation**—promote psychological and physical calm:

    A. *Use systematic desensitization*—never force contact with feared object or situation.

    B. Give *positive reinforcement.*

    C. *Health teaching:* progressive relaxation, meditation, biofeedback training, or other behavioral conditioning techniques.

VI. **Evaluation/outcome criteria:** significant decrease in phobic response (i.e., able to come into contact with feared object with lessened degree of physiologic and emotional symptoms of severe anxiety states).

Acute Stress Disorder and Posttraumatic Stress Disorder

I. **Definition:** Development of anxiety symptoms following an excessively distressing serious life event and experienced with terror, fear, and helplessness.

II. **Assessment**

    A. *Acute stress disorder:* symptoms occur *within 1 mo* of extreme stressor; includes dissociative symptoms (i.e., depersonalization, emotional detachment, dazed appearance, amnesia).

    B. *Posttraumatic stress disorder:* symptoms occur *after 1 mo.*

    C. *Precipitant:* severe traumatic event (natural or manmade disaster) that is not an ordinary occurrence; e.g., rape, fire, flood, earthquake, tornado, bombing, plane crash, war, torture, kidnapping.

    D. Self-report of reexperiencing traumatic incident; intrusive memories (e.g., flashbacks).

    E. Numb, unresponsive, detached, estranged reaction to external world (unable to feel tenderness, intimacy); withdrawal from others.

    F. Change in sleep pattern (e.g., insomnia, recurrent dreams, nightmares), memory loss, hyperalertness (startle response).

    G. Guilt rumination about survival.

    H. Avoids activities reminiscent of trauma; phobic responses.

    I. Difficulty with task completion and concentration.

    J. Depression.

    K. Increased irritability may result in unpredictable, explosive outbursts.

    L. Impulsive behavior, sudden life-style changes.

III. **Analysis/nursing diagnosis**

    A. *Posttrauma response* related to overwhelming traumatic event.

    B. *Fear* related to environmental stressor.

    C. *Sleep pattern disturbance* related to fear and rumination.

    D. *Decisional conflict (impaired decision making)* related to perceived threat to personal values and beliefs.

    E. *Guilt* related to lack of social support system.

    F. *Altered feeling states:* emotional lability related to diminished sense of control over self and environment.

IV. **Nursing care plan/implementation**

    A. *Crisis counseling*

        1. *Listen* with concern and sympathy.

        2. Ease way for client to *talk out* the experience and express fear.

        3. Help client to become *aware* and to *accept* what happened. Be nonjudgmental.

    B. *Health teaching:* suggest how to resume concrete activity and how to reconstruct life with available social, physical, and emotional resources. Help make contact with friends, relatives, and other resources.

V. **Evaluation/outcome criteria:** can cry and express anger, loss, frustration, and despair; begins process of social and physical reconstruction.

Anxiety-Related Disorders

Dissociative Disorders

I. **Definition:** Inappropriate use of defense mechanisms (e.g., maladaptive denial) in meeting life's demands and roles related to overwhelming stressors and inadequate or ineffective support systems. Characterized by disturbances or alterations in consciousness, memory, or identity.

II. **Assessment**

    A. *Dissociative amnesia:* partial or total inability to recall the past; occurs during highly stressful events; client may have conscious desire to escape but be unable to accept escape as a solution; uses *repression.*

B. *Dissociative fugue:* client not only forgets previous identity but also *flees* from stress.

C. *Dissociative identity disorder:* client exhibits two or more complete personality systems, each very different from the other; alternates from one personality to the other without awareness of change (*one* personality *may* be aware of others); each personality has well-developed emotions and thought processes that are in conflict; uses *repression*.

D. *Depersonalization disorder:* loss of sense of self; feeling of self estrangement (as if in a dream); fear of going insane.

▶ III. Analysis/nursing diagnosis

A. Sudden *alteration in:*

   1. *Memory: short- and long-term memory loss* (can't recall important personal events) related to repression.

   2. *Personal* and *social identity* (e.g., in amnesia: forgets own identity; becomes another identity) related to intense anxiety.

B. *Confusion* related to use of repression.

C. *Spiritual despair* related to conversion of conflict into physical or mental flights.

D. *Sensory-perceptual alteration* of external environment related to repression and escapism.

E. *Altered meaningfulness* (hopelessness, helplessness, powerlessness) related to lack of control over situation.

▶ IV. Nursing care plan/implementation:

A. *Remove* client from immediate environment to reduce pressure.

☞ B. *Alleviate* symptoms using *behavior-modification* strategies.

C. *Divert* attention to topics other than symptoms (e.g., not remembering names, addresses, and events).

D. Encourage *socialization* rather than isolation.

E. *Avoid* sympathy, pity, and oversolicitous approach.

F. *Health teaching:* teach families to avoid reinforcing dissociative behavior; teach client problem solving, with goal of minimizing stressful aspects of environment.

▶ V. Evaluation/outcome criteria: recall returns to conscious awareness; anxiety kept within manageable limits.

Somatoform Disorders

I. Definition: involuntary, physical complaints or symptoms *without* demonstrable organic findings or identifiable physiologic bases; involve psychological factors or nonspecific conflicts.

▶ II. General assessment

A. *Precipitant:* major emotional, interpersonal stress.

B. Occurrence of secondary gain from illness.

C. Types of somatoform disorders

   1. *Body dysmorphic* disorder—preoccupation by a normal-appearing person who perceives body defect or excessive concern over actual minor defect.

   2. *Pain* disorder—preoccupation with pain that cannot be accounted for through diagnostic evaluation; or if there is related organic pathology, complaints are grossly excessive.

   3. *Somatization* disorder (see p. 115).

   4. *Conversion* disorder (see p. 115).

   5. *Hypochondriasis* (see p. 115).

▶ III. General analysis/nursing diagnosis

A. *Fear* related to loss of dependent relationships.

B. *Powerlessness* related to chronic resentment over frustration of dependency needs.

C. *Altered feeling states:* inhibition of anger, which is discharged physiologically and is related to control of anxiety.

D. *Impaired judgment* related to denial of existence of any conflicts or relationship to physical symptoms.

E. *Altered role performance:* regression related to not having dependency needs met.

▶ IV. General nursing care plans/implementation

A. Long-term goals

   1. Develop interests *outside* of self. Introduce to new activities and people. Provide *diversional* activities.

   2. Facilitate experiences of increased feelings of *independence* and self-reliance.

   3. Increase *reality* perception and *problem-solving ability*.

   4. Emphasize *positive* outlook and promote positive thinking. Reassure that symptoms are anxiety-related, not a result of physical disease.

   5. Develop mature ways for meeting *affection* needs.

B. Short-term goals

   1. *Prevent* anxiety from mounting and becoming uncontrollable by recognizing symptoms, for early intervention. Evaluate behaviors to rule out physical illness. Give prescribed anti-anxiety meds.

   2. *Environment:* warm, caring, supportive interactions, especially during diagnostic work-up, instill hope that anxiety can be mastered.

   3. Encourage client to *express* somatic concerns, anxiety and dependency needs verbally. Encourage awareness of body processes as manifestations of anxiety.

   4. Refocus after acknowledging that physical complaints are real.

   ☞ 5. Develop ability to *relax* rather than ruminate or worry. Help find palliative relief through *anxiety reduction* (e.g., slower breathing, exercise).

   6. *Health teaching*

      a. Relaxation training as self-help measures.

      b. Increase knowledge of appropriate and correct information on physiologic responses that accompany anxiety.

▶ V. General evaluation/outcome criteria

A. Does not isolate self.

B. Discusses fears, concerns, conflicts that are self-originated and not likely to be serious.

C. Decides which aspects of situation can be overcome and ways to meet conflicting obligations.
D. Looks for things of importance and value.
E. Deliberately engages in new activities other than ruminating or worrying.
F. Talks self out of fears.
G. Decrease in physical symptoms; is able to sleep, feels less restless.
H. Makes fewer statements of feeling helpless.
I. Can freely express angry feelings in *overt* way and not through symptoms.

Somatization Disorder

I. **Definition:** Conversion of mental states or experiences into bodily symptoms associated with anxiety. Repeated, multiple, vague, or exaggerated physical complaints of several years' duration *without* identifiable physical cause; clients constantly seek medical attention, undergo numerous tests; at risk for unnecessary surgery or drug abuse.

II. **Assessment**
  A. Onset and occurrence: teen years, more common in women.
  B. Reports illness most of life.
   1. *Neuromuscular* symptoms: fainting, seizures, dysphagia, difficulty walking, back pain, urinary retention.
   2. *Gastrointestinal* symptoms: nausea, vomiting, flatus, food intolerance, constipation or diarrhea.
   3. *Female reproductive* symptoms: dysmenorrhea, hyperemesis gravidarum.
   4. *Psychosexual* symptoms: sexual indifference, dyspareunia.
   5. *Cardiopulmonary* symptoms: palpitations, shortness of breath, chest pain.
   6. *Rule out:* Multiple sclerosis, systemic lupus erythematosus, porphyria, hyperparathyroidism.
  C. Appears anxious and depressed.

III. **Analysis/nursing diagnosis**
  A. *Anxiety* related to threat to security and inability to meet role expectations.
  B. *Self-care deficit* related to development of physical symptoms to escape stressful situations.
  C. *Impaired social interaction* related to inability to accept that physical symptoms lack a physiologic basis.
  D. *Body image disturbance* and *altered role performance* related to passive acceptance of disabling symptoms.

Conversion Disorder

I. **Definition:** Loss or alteration in physical functioning that suggests a physical disorder.
  Sudden symptoms of *symbolic* nature developed under *extreme* psychological stress (e.g., war, loss, natural disaster) that *disappear* through hypnosis. Symptoms allow person to avoid an activity or situation that is perceived as threatening and anxiety provoking and

allows person to gain support that otherwise might not be obtained.

II. **Assessment**
  A. *Neurologic* symptoms: paralysis, aphonia (loss of voice), tunnel vision, seizures, blindness, paresthesias, anesthesias.
  B. *Endocrinologic* symptoms: pseudocyesis (false pregnancy).
  C. Hysterical, dependent *personality profile:* exhibitionistic dress and language; self-indulgent; suggestible; impulsive, forms global impressions and hunches; little capacity to concentrate, integrate, and organize thoughts or plan action or outcomes; little concern for symptoms, despite severe impairment ("*la belle indifférence*").

III. **Analysis/nursing diagnosis**
  A. Prolonged *loss or alteration of physiologic processes* related to severe psychological stress and conflict that results in disuse, atrophy, contractures. *Primary gain*—internal conflict or need is kept out of awareness; there is a close relationship in time between stressor and occurrence of symbolic symptoms.
  B. *Impaired social interaction:* chronic sick role related to attention seeking.
  C. *Noncompliance* with expected routines related to *secondary gain*—avoidance of an upsetting situation, with support obtained from others.
  D. *Impaired adjustment* related to *repression* of feelings through somatic symptoms, *regression, denial* and *isolation,* and *externalization.*
  E. *Ineffective individual coping;* e.g., daydreaming, fantasizing, superficial warmth and seductiveness related to inability to control symptoms voluntarily or to explain them by known physical disorder.

Hypochondriasis

I. **Definition:** *Exaggerated* concern for one's physical health; *unrealistic* interpretation of signs or sensations as abnormal; *preoccupation with fear* of having serious disease *despite* medical reassurance of no diagnosis of physical disorder.

II. **Assessment**
  A. Preoccupation with symptoms; sweating, peristalsis, heartbeat, coughing, muscular soreness, skin eruptions.
  B. Occurs in both men and women in adolescence, 30s, or 40s.
  C. History of long, complicated shopping for doctors and refusal of mental health care.
  D. *Organ neurosis* may occur (e.g., cardiac neurosis).
  E. Personality trait: *compulsive.*
  F. Prevalence of anxiety and depression.
  G. *Controls* relationships through physical complaints.

III. **Analysis/nursing diagnosis**
  A. *Personal identity disturbance* related to perception of self as ill in order to meet needs for dependency, attention, affection.
  B. Displaced *anxiety* related to inability to verbalize feelings.
  C. *Fear* related to not being believed.

D. *Powerlessness* related to feelings of insecurity.
E. *Altered role performance:* disruption in work and interpersonal relations related to regression and need gratification through preoccupation with fantasized illness; related to control over others through physical complaints.

Study and Memory Aids

Characteristics of Anxiety Disorders

Avoidance	**D**isplacement, denial
Nervous (ANS symptoms)	**I**ntellectualization
Xenophobia, etc.	**S**ymbolism
Indigestion	**O**bsessions
Externalization	**R**epression, regression
Tachycardia	**D**ependence
Yearnings: unmet needs for attention, affection	**E**xcessive worry, fears
	Ritualistic
	Social isolation

Glossary

acrophobia   Fear of heights.

agoraphobia   Fear of open spaces or public places from which escape might be difficult or embarrassing; fear of being out of control when in a public place, e.g., shopping mall, classroom, restaurant.

anxiety   A *vague,* widespread, unpleasant subjective feeling of apprehension, uneasiness, helplessness, and uncertainty that is *not* related to a specific object. It is a normal alerting and protective response that occurs as a result of unmet expectations, a threat (*real* or *imagined*) to a person's biologic, psychologic, or social integrity, self-esteem or identity, or a loss of control. *Physiologic* manifestations are: increased pulse and respirations, perspiration, and a feeling of "butterflies." There are also cognitive, perceptual, emotional, and behavioral manifestations. See Chapter 1.

body dysmorphic disorder   A somatoform disorder where there is preoccupation with an imagined or exaggerated defect in physical appearance (e.g., an individual perceives the size of his or her nose as larger than it is).

claustrophobia   Fear of confined spaces (e.g., elevators).

compulsion   An uncontrollable, persistent, repetitive, intru-

Summary of Key Points

Care of a Patient Who Is Anxious

1. Help patient to *identify* anxiety ("I see you are tapping your toes. Are you feeling anxious now?").
2. Help patient *connect* with behaviors that bring *relief* ("What has helped before to make you feel better when you were anxious?").
3. Assist patient to describe what *caused* the anxiety.
4. Provide a calm *environment,* with physical activities (e.g., walking).
5. Use *relaxation* techniques, including breathing awareness and progressive muscle relaxation.

Care of a Patient with Panic Disorder

1. Provide physical presence, in small, quiet room.
2. Reduce environmental stimulation (noise, lights).
3. Administer anti-anxiety medications.

Care of a Patient with an Obsessive-Compulsive Disorder

1. *Negotiate limits* as to *length* of time patient can engage in rituals; however, it is important to differentiate limit setting from *punishment.*
2. *Avoid* interrupting ritualistic behaviors, which patients use to handle anxiety.
3. Give positive feedback—a lot!

Care of a Patient with Phobic Disorder

1. Use behavior modification; relaxation techniques, meditation, and biofeedback training.

2. Do *not* force contact with feared object.
3. Main coping mechanisms involved are: *repression, displacement, symbolism.*

Care of a Patient with Posttraumatic Stress Disorder

1. Approach: nonjudgmental; help patient to express feelings and feel safe.
2. Suggest group or 1:1 therapy for severe anxiety related to flashbacks and poor relationships (home, work) that follow natural disasters (e.g., war, rape, mugging, incest, accidents, fire).

Care of a Patient with Dissociative Disorder

1. *Avoid* focusing on symptoms related to repression of names, places, and events.
2. Use behavior modification approaches.
3. Reduce isolation.

Care of a Patient with Somatoform Disorder

1. *Long-term goals:* foster feelings of self-reliance and *independence;* encourage outside interests.
2. *Short-term goals:* help patient to *verbalize* concerns rather than through body processes. Teach relaxation methods. Give prescribed anti-anxiety meds.

sive, irrational urge to perform an anxiety-reducing ritualistic *action*. The act is often contrary to ordinary wishes or standards (e.g., compulsion to steal).

conversion disorder Loss or alteration of physical function (e.g., vision, mobility) as a result of stress, which is usually *symbolically* linked to a need or psychological conflict at an unconscious level, with *no* demonstrable underlying medical condition (e.g., an individual experiences paralysis when forced to go to combat). The symptom allows the individual to avoid an activity or situation that is perceived as threatening and anxiety provoking, and to gain support from the environment, which the individual feels may not be given otherwise.

delusion An irrational belief not influenced or changed by reason or contrary experience. A thought disorder.

depersonalization disorder An alteration in the perception or experience of self in which one's usual sense of reality is temporarily lost or changed; repeated feelings of being an outside observer of one's own body or thoughts, as if one is detached, in a dreamlike state. May lead to withdrawal.

dissociation An unconscious mechanism that is used to avoid anxiety by pushing out of conscious awareness (by *repression*) anxiety-provoking feelings, thoughts, or events.

dissociative amnesia Inability to remember information that is related to physical or emotional trauma (formerly called *psychogenic amnesia*).

dissociative fugue A sudden, geographic move (physical flight), after which the individual does not remember how he or she got to the new location, and is also usually unable to remember personal identity or history (formerly called *psychogenic fugue*).

dissociative identity disorder The existence of two or more separate personalities in one individual; often caused by physical, emotional, and/or sexual abuse in childhood, and resultant overwhelming or repeated anxiety-producing situations without effective coping mechanisms in place (formerly called *multiple personality disorder*).

generalized anxiety disorder Excessive worry and anxiety concerning many things, lasting for at least 6 months, without presence of phobias, posttraumatic stress, or obsessive-compulsive disorders.

homophobia Irrational fear of homosexuals and homosexuality, usually stemming from myths and stereotypes.

hypochondriasis State of morbid preoccupation with a belief that *serious* illness exists despite negative results on medical tests (somatic concerns); minor symptoms are perceived as serious.

la belle indifférence ("beautiful indifference") Inappropriate, incongruent lack of concern about the seriousness of one's symptoms. Seen in *psychogenic amnesia* and *conversion disorder.*

malingering *Deliberate* (conscious and voluntary) faking or exaggeration of illness or injury in order to avoid an unpleasant situation, to obtain financial benefit, or to control the environment, situation, or circumstances.

obsession Preoccupation with persistent, often irrational ideas, urges, beliefs, or images (related to contamination by dirt, germs; orderliness, religion, sexual behavior, violence, doubts about own behavior) that *cannot* be banished by logic or will and require therapeutic intervention (e.g., an

honors student who persistently fears failure on exams despite a "straight A" academic record).

panic disorder Unexpected but recurrent attacks of intense fear and uneasiness that peak within minutes.

phobia *Irrational, persistent*, abnormal, and *morbid* dread or fear of external object or situation *displaced* from unconscious conflict (e.g., acrophobia, agoraphobia, claustrophobia, homophobia, social phobia, xenophobia).

posttraumatic stress disorder (PTSD) Characteristic acute, chronic, or delayed symptoms of intense fear, terror, and helplessness that occur after an unusually stressful event (e.g., accident, earthquake, fire, abuse, war combat). The individual may relive the traumatic event through flashbacks and nightmares, or may avoid stimuli associated with the traumatic event.

primary gain Obtaining relief from anxiety through physical symptoms stemming from a physical ailment; occurs *unconsciously*, to keep an internal need or conflict out of conscious awareness.

secondary gain *Additional* benefit as a result of calling attention to physical symptoms, to get sympathy and support, and to *avoid* anxiety-provoking events, people, or places. Does not include relief from anxiety, which is a *primary* gain.

social phobia Fear of negative evaluation by others (e.g., fear of doing something embarrassing—like saying something foolish—in front of others).

somatization Expressing emotional stress through physical reaction (e.g., headaches, backache, stomachache).

somatoform disorder Expression of anxiety as physical symptoms, usually involving sensory-motor functions.

splitting Seeing people or events as either positive or negative, good or bad.

xenophobia Fear of strangers.

Questions

1. A patient is seen in the emergency department with symptoms of panic disorder. While assessing the patient, the nurse would be able to support this diagnosis when the patient says:
   1. "I am always sick; I must have a bad heart, like my parents."
   2. "Listen . . . Moses is talking to me through that bush!"
   3. "I don't sleep at night because I have too much work to do, writing six novels that will make me lots of money and bring me fame as well."
   4. "I was in the park when my heart suddenly began to beat very fast. I became unsteady on my feet and started to breathe very fast, with sweat pouring out of me."

2. A patient is unable to stop dressing and undressing many times throughout the day. The nurse determines that this behavior is a(an):
   1. Delusion.
   2. Compulsion.
   3. Obsession.
   4. Phobia.

3. A patient who continuously checks windows and doors

throughout the night says to the nurse, "Do you think I'm foolish to check so much?" Before responding, the nurse needs to understand that the patient is:

1. Expressing his own concern about the compulsive checking.
2. Purposefully putting the nurse "on-the-spot."
3. Asking for help in stopping the ritualistic behavior.
4. Testing the nurse to see if the nurse thinks this repetitive behavior is rational.

4. For which physical problems should the nurse assess an anxious patient with a handwashing ritual?
   1. Integumentary problems.
   2. Cardiac arrhythmias.
   3. Respiratory distress.
   4. Urinary retention.

5. What purpose does ritualism serve for a patient who has an obsessive-compulsive disorder?
   1. To relieve anxiety, as a form of self-help.
   2. To avoid decision making.
   3. To practice perfectionism as a goal.
   4. To provide structure.

6. What type of activity is most therapeutic for a patient with ritualistic behavior?
   1. Playing a card game.
   2. Doing embroidery.
   3. Watching TV.
   4. Going for a walk.

7. The nurse determines that a patient's preoccupation with intrusive thoughts of germs is a(an):
   1. Anxiety attack.
   2. Compulsion.
   3. Delusion.
   4. Obsession.

8. What is the most therapeutic nursing approach for a patient who has an obsessive-compulsive handwashing disorder?
   1. Protect the patient's hands with gloves.
   2. Provide distraction.
   3. Put lotion on the hands.
   4. Ignore the behavior.

9. The nurse needs to know that the probable effect of a permissive nursing approach in letting a patient engage in ritualistic behavior (such as cleaning the room several times a day) will be to:
   1. Increase the patient's awareness of the irrationality of the behavior.
   2. Reduce the patient's anxiety.
   3. Reinforce the delusion.
   4. Increase the patient's responsiveness to the nurse's suggestions by building trust.

10. A patient is referred to the outpatient department for maladaptive behavior related to fear of crowds. Which treatment modality should the nurse anticipate will be the most effective for this patient?
    1. Reality therapy.
    2. Group therapy.
    3. Crisis intervention.
    4. Behavior therapy. — desensitzed tech + positive reinforcement

11. A patient reports that he is always scared, but cannot clearly identify his fears. The nurse should determine that this behavior is most likely due to anxiety, which can be differentiated from phobias in that:

1. Phobias are nonspecific; anxiety is specific.
2. Anxiety is nonspecific; phobias are specific.
3. Phobias are more intense than anxiety.
4. Anxiety is more intense than phobia.

12. What coping mechanism used by a patient who has acrophobia is the nurse likely to encounter during interactions?
    1. Suppression.
    2. Regression.
    3. Displacement.
    4. Compensation.

13. What are the implications for patient care when a person with a history of claustrophobia is scheduled for an MRI?
    1. Provide a staff person for interaction.
    2. Provide earphones to listen to music during the procedure.
    3. Provide reading material as distraction during the procedure.
    4. Provide detailed explanations right before the procedure.

14. What is the best treatment modality for a patient with phobic behavior?
    1. Group therapy to discuss the patient's fears.
    2. Behavior modification to desensitize the patient's reactions.
    3. 1:1 relationship therapy to reduce social isolation.
    4. Forcing the patient to face fears.

15. A person is admitted to the in-patient psychiatric unit for symptoms that include refusal to leave the house, anger, hopelessness, depression, recurrent nightmares, and suicidal ideation. He is a veteran of the Korean War. He relates a history of unemployment, domestic problems, and polysubstance abuse. The nurse should know that these symptoms indicate a medical diagnosis of:
    1. Panic reaction.
    2. Somatoform disorder.
    3. Posttraumatic stress disorder.
    4. Agoraphobia.

16. Following a severely stressful experience, the patient's behavior indicates a nursing diagnosis of altered identity and recall. Which disorder is characterized by this diagnosis?
    1. Somatization disorder.
    2. Dissociative disorder.
    3. Generalized anxiety disorder.
    4. Conversion disorder.

17. What would be the focus of the preliminary nursing care plan for a patient admitted to the unit with a tentative diagnosis of somatization disorder?
    1. Explaining that the perceived physical symptoms are not related to physical causes.
    2. Evaluating behaviors to help the MD rule out the existence of any physical illness.
    3. Promoting participation in group activities.
    4. Encouraging the patient to discuss the history of the physical complaints.

18. Which nursing approach would be therapeutic for a patient who is preoccupied with body symptoms, even though diagnostic tests show no problems?

1. Point out to the patient that the diagnostic workup was normal.
2. Listen and ask the patient to elaborate on the symptoms.
3. Refocus the patient, after acknowledging that the complaints seem real to the patient.
4. Ignore the verbalized complaints, but suggest that the patient write them down.

Answers/Rationale

1. **(4)** Signs and symptoms of panic disorder include tachycardia, ataxia, hyperventilation, and diaphoresis. [*Note:* Other symptoms of panic disorder are elevated BP, dyspnea, paresthesia, GI and GU frequency, with feelings of impending doom. Symptoms appear suddenly and without an identifiable cause.] The statement in **No. 1** is more characteristic of *somatization disorder,* in which there is a long history of anxiety being expressed as a physical condition. The statement in **No. 2** describes auditory and visual hallucinations, which are common in *schizophrenia.* The statement in **No. 3** is descriptive of *bipolar* disorder, manic type, in which there is typically an exaggerated sense of importance that may be delusions of grandeur. **AS, 7, PsI**

2. **(2)** By definition, compulsion refers to insistent, repetitive, intrusive urges to perform an *act* that is contrary to ordinary conscious wishes or standards (such as constant changing of clothes). A delusion (**No. 1**) is an irrational *belief.* Obsession (**No. 3**) refers to a persistent, uncontrollable *urge, idea,* or *thought* that cannot be banished by logic or will. Phobia (**No. 4**) refers to irrational, persistent, morbid, and abnormal *fears* (e.g., claustrophobia, acrophobia, xenophobia). **AN, 7, PsI**

3. **(1)** The person who is compulsive is usually aware of irrational behaviors but cannot stop them. The patient is not focused on the nurse (**Nos. 2 and 4**); rather, the patient is questioning the behavior himself, as a first step, *before* asking for assistance (**No. 3**). **AN, 7, PsI**

💡 *Test-taking tip:* When two options seem good, select the one that usually *precedes* the other in *sequential* order.

4. **(1)** The underlying problem in compulsive disorders—such as ritualistic handwashing—is chronic anxiety, which needs to be discharged. The result of excessive ritualistic handwashing is itchy, excoriated skin and hives or rashes (integumentary system). Skin integrity is threatened. Cardiac irregularities (**No. 2**) and respira-

tory distress (**No. 3**) are not typically seen, although tachycardia and tachypnea can occur when the anxiety is at a *moderate* or *severe* level. Urinary retention (**No. 4**) is not associated with this compulsive behavior. More typically, anxiety disorders result in urinary *frequency.* **AS, 1, PhI**

5. **(1)** Repetitive actions are a form of self-help in an obsessive-compulsive disorder; they relieve built-up tension before anxiety escalates into a panic stage. **Nos. 2 and 4** are both incorporated into **No. 1**, as *examples* of ways repetitive acts (ritualism) are used to provide relief from anxiety. By keeping things the same through ritualism, decision making is reduced (**No. 2**), thereby reducing anxiety. The unknown, another source of anxiety, can by reduced by providing structure (**No. 4**), such as a predictable, ritualistic routine. Ritualistic behaviors *are* a perfectionistic tendency; however, in this case, perfectionism is not a goal (**No. 3**), but an *aspect* of the ritualistic behavior. **PL, 7, PsI**

6. **(2)** The theory behind what makes embroidery the best answer can be summarized by mental imagery. Picture what is involved in embroidery: you see a needle, a thread, and a pattern. A person doing embroidery engages in an exact, precise, repetitive activity. Someone being that exact, that precise, is engaging in a ritualistic behavior, which is what is needed here as a form of *self-help.* This will help discharge pent-up energy associated with anxiety; consequently, the person can then "let go" and be more amenable to ideas, suggestions, and the next step in the treatment process. A card game (**No. 1**) involves decision making: which card to play next? The patient with obsessive-compulsive behavior (i.e., with ritualistic behavior) *cannot* make decisions easily. Television (**No. 3**) doesn't discharge built up anxiety by a ritualistic behavior. A walk (**No. 4**) is not relevant to a person with ritualistic behavior problems; walking is therapeutic for any anxiety-related disorder. **IMP, 3, PsI**

💡 *Test-taking tips*
• Use the process of *elimination.* Eliminate **No. 1** because it involves decision making, and **No. 3** because it doesn't discharge pent-up energy associated with anxiety, and **No. 4** because it is not especially relevant for ritualistic behaviors.
• Use *mental imagery* to picture what the activity entails (**No. 2**).

7. **(4)** By definition, an obsession relates to preoccupation with a persistent, involuntary *urge, idea, thought,* belief, or image that cannot be banished by logic or will (e.g., obsession with one's weight, as in anorexia nervosa). Preoccupation with germs is not a symptom of an anxiety attack (**No. 1**). Compulsion (**No. 2**) refers to a persistent, uncontrollable urge to repeatedly perform an *act* that is contrary to ordinary behavior. A delusion (**No. 3**) is an irrational *belief* (e.g., delusions of grandeur or persecution). **AN, 7, PsI**

8. **(2)** Distraction can serve as *prevention,* and prevention is usually a *priority* intervention. In this case, if distracted, the patient may not *need* to stop and wash hands as frequently. **Nos. 1 and 3** offer *protection*

Key to Codes

Nursing process: AS = Assessment; **AN** = Analysis; **PL** = Planning; **IMP** = Implementation; **EV** = Evaluation. (See Appendix E for explanation of nursing process steps.)

Category of human function: 1 = Protective; **2** = Sensory-Perceptual; **3** = Comfort, Rest, Activity, and Mobility; **4** = Nutrition; **5** = Growth and Development; **6** = Fluid-Gas Transport; **7** = Psychosocial-Cultural; **8** = Elimination.

Client need: SECE = Safe, Effective Care Environment; **PhI** = Physiologic Integrity; **PsI** = Psychosocial Integrity; **HPM** = Health Promotion/Maintenance.

from skin excoriation resulting from the frequent hand-washing that occurs with obsessive-compulsive behavior; but because they are *similar* examples of how to protect the hands in this case, it is not possible to choose one over the other, suggesting that there may be a better answer (prevention, **No. 2**). It is not therapeutic to *ignore* this behavior (**No. 4**), as it may result in harm, such as skin excoriation. **PL, 1, PsI**

💡 *Test-taking tip:* When two options are *too similar*, and one is not included in the other, look for another answer.

9. **(2)** Ritualistic behaviors are used to relieve anxiety, as a form of self-help. Until more adaptive means to reduce anxiety are learned, anxiety may escalate if ritualistic acts are not allowed. **No. 1** is incorrect because patients who are obsessive-compulsive are typically intelligent people who recognize that their behavior is unreasonable but are unable to stop it. Allowing the room-cleaning ritual serves primarily to *release* tension, rather than reinforcing the irrational belief (**No. 3**) that repetitive cleaning will ameliorate conflict, guilt, or insecurity. Relief of anxiety is the immediate, short-term purpose of a permissive approach, not building trust (**No. 4**). **EV, 7, PsI**

10. **(4)** Phobias are most effectively treated with desensitizing techniques and positive reinforcement, which are two important aspects of behavior therapy. Reality therapy (**No. 1**) is most commonly used with patients who are confused, have schizophrenic disorders, or exhibit chronic withdrawal patterns (from long-term institutionalization). Group therapy (**No. 2**) is not appropriate as the initial intervention for a person who is afraid of crowds. *Desensitization* to people is most important (a little stimulus at a time!). Crisis intervention (**No. 3**) is not called for in phobias, which develop over time, rather than being sudden and short-term. **PL, 7, PsI**

11. **(2)** There *are* specific areas of morbid fear or phobia: e.g., agoraphobia, acrophobia, claustrophobia, xenophobia. Anxiety is a free-floating, more general feeling not readily connected with a specific source. **No. 1** is incorrect because it is the opposite of the correct difference between phobias and anxiety. **Nos. 3 and 4** are not correct because *both* phobias and anxiety (especially at a severe and panic level) can be intense, pervasive, and debilitating, with serious impact on activities of daily living. **AN, 7, PsI**

12. **(3)** In phobic behavior, the original source of pain and/or conflict has been pushed out of awareness and displaced onto something or someone that in itself is not realistically dangerous. *Repression* is also an operant psychodynamic mechanism underlying phobic behavior, *not* suppression (**No. 1**) or regression (**No. 2**). Compensation (**No. 4**) is not an underlying mechanism in phobic behavior. **AN, 7, PsI**

13. **(2)** *Distraction* is what is needed to keep anxiety level down for a person who gets very anxious in tight, crowded spaces; music is the best, most direct source of distraction. **No. 1** is incorrect because the staff person is attending to the MRI procedure and is *not* in the room to interact with the patient. Reading (**No. 3**), al-

though a form of distraction, requires free arms to hold the material and therefore cannot be used during an MRI. Detailed, *prior cognitive* input of information (**No. 4**) will not help deal with *feelings* of anxiety *during* the procedure. **PL, 7, PsI**

14. **(2)** This involves an *action*. With behavior modification, the person is exposed to the feared stimulus a little bit at a time, until the person no longer has a fear response attached to that stimulus. **Nos. 1 and 3** involve *talk*, not the desired *action*. In phobic behavior, lack of social interaction is not the central problem. Force (**No. 4**) is not therapeutic. (For example, you wouldn't throw a person who is afraid of water into a swimming pool!) **PL, 7, PsI**

💡 *Test-taking tip:* Look for a pattern and focus on the option that is *not* like the others: two options involve talk (**Nos. 1 and 3**) and one involves action (**No. 2**).

15. **(3)** In all likelihood, the patient experienced unusually traumatic, war-related events that were followed by recurrent nightmares (or flashbacks). Adjustment to civilian life is often impaired (problems at home and at work), which results in maladaptive coping means (polysubstance abuse, feelings of hopelessness, depression, and suicide). Panic reaction (**No. 1**) is characterized by physical symptoms (e.g., dyspnea, palpitations, choking feelings) that develop abruptly and peak within 10 minutes. Patients with somatoform disorders (**No. 2**) have *physical* symptoms of illness, without any physiologic/organic cause. Although fear of leaving the house is a common characteristic of agoraphobia (**No. 4**), the other behaviors described in the scenario are characteristic of the bigger, more comprehensive problem of posttraumatic stress. **AN, 7, PsI**

16. **(2)** A dissociative disorder occurs when an individual blocks off from awareness a particular aspect of life, due to overwhelming anxiety. In one type of dissociative disorder, dissociative amnesia, a cluster of recent events is "forgotten," but can return to awareness. In another type, depersonalization, the individual can also experience feelings of detachment from his or her emotional self. Somatization disorder (**No. 1**) is characterized by a history of many physiologic complaints with no apparent physical cause. Generalized anxiety disorder (**No. 3**) is characterized by chronic, persistent feelings of apprehension and dread without a specific cause. Conversion disorder (**No. 4**) is a type of somatization disorder that is characterized by a loss of function (e.g., paralysis, blindness, coordination) that is caused by an unconscious mental process, symbolically representing an underlying conflict or need. **AN, 7, PsI**

17. **(2)** Until diagnostic tests are completed, the nursing role in care of patients with possible somatization disorder is to observe and record behaviors, and to support the patient through the diagnostic tests. **No. 1** is inappropriate because the nurse doesn't *know* whether the physical symptoms are real until the diagnostic tests are completed; and because the symptoms *may seem real* to the patient, despite the lack of physical findings. Group activities (**No. 3**) may be part of the care plan *later* in the treatment process. Discussing the patient's

history (**No. 4**) is part of the medical exam; the focus of nursing care is generally on the "here-and-now" rather than the "there-and-then." Focusing on past complaints may only serve to reinforce the symptoms, especially if it is determined that the symptoms are not related to physical causes. **PL, 7, PsI**

18. (3) It is important that the nurse realize that the physical complaints are real to the patient. When physical conditions are ruled out by diagnostic tests, these complaints are viewed as manifestations of anxiety, related to dependency needs. The nurse should allow the patient to talk about *other* concerns, to help the patient express anxiety and dependency needs. Pointing out the lack of evidence of physical conditions (**No. 1**) will probably result in even more anxiety for the patient. Focusing on the symptoms (**No. 2**) will only reinforce them. Ignoring the symptoms (**No. 4**) only avoids the problems. **IMP, 7, PsI**

Conditions in Which Psychological Factors Affect Medical Condition

Chapter Outline

Conditions in Which Psychological Factors Affect Medical Condition

Psychophysiologic Illnesses

Psychophysiologic illnesses are stress-related and occur in various organs and systems, whereby emotions are expressed by affecting body organs (mind-body interaction).

I. **Concepts and principles** related to psychological factors affecting medical conditions:
   A. Majority of organs involved are usually under control of *autonomic* nervous system.
   B. **Coping mechanisms** related to *alexithymia* (inability to consciously experience and express emotions).
      1. *Repression* or *suppression* or *denial*— pushing of unpleasant emotional experiences out of awareness.
      2. *Introjection*—illness seen as punishment.
      3. *Projection*—others blamed for illness.
      4. *Conversion*—intrapsychic conflicts where physical symptoms rather than underlying emotional stresses are emphasized.
      5. *Regression*—reverting to earlier developmental mode of need gratification through attention seeking, dependency, and need for security; an attempt to reduce overwhelming anxiety.
   C. Clients often exhibit the following underlying *needs in excess:*
      1. Dependency (these clients tend to have visceral disorders like ulcerative colitis).
      2. Attention.
      3. Love.
      4. Success (these clients tend to have hard-driving personality [Type A] and often develop peptic ulcers).
      5. Recognition.
      6. Security.
   D. Need to distinguish between:
      1. *Factitious disorders*—physical *or* psychological symptoms that the person produces intentionally to feign illness and assume sick role. The behavior is voluntary but presumed to be out of his or her control (like repetitive compulsive disorder).
      2. *Conversion disorder*—affecting *sensory* systems that are usually under *voluntary* control; generally *non–life-threatening;* symptoms are *symbolic* solution to anxiety; *no* demonstrable *organic* pathology.
      3. *Somatization disorder*—multiple, recurrent, vague, or exaggerated physical complaints over several years, *without* identifiable physical causes.
      4. *Psychophysiologic* illnesses—under *autonomic* nervous system control; have structural *organic* changes; may be life-threatening.
      5. *Hypochondriasis*—preoccupation with the fear or belief that one has a serious disease in spite of medical reassurances to the contrary.
   E. **General stress adaptation syndrome (GAS)**— The objectively measurable structural and chemical changes produced in the body when stress affects the whole organism. According to Selye, the individual's response to stress has *three* stages: *alarm reaction, resistance,* and *exhaustion.* Selye's theory states that stress depletes capacity to cope, thereby making the individual under stress more vulnerable to illness.
   F. A *decrease in emotional security* tends to produce an *increase in symptoms.*
   G. When treatment is confined to physical symptoms, emotional problems are *not* usually relieved.

II. Assessment

A. Persistent psychological factors may produce structural *organic* changes resulting in *chronic diseases,* which may be *life-threatening* if untreated (see Selye's **General stress adaptation syndrome**, above).

B. *All* body systems are affected:
1. Skin (e.g., *pruritus* and dermatitis).
2. Musculoskeletal (e.g., *backache,* muscle cramps, and rheumatism).
3. Respiratory (e.g., *asthma,* hiccups, and hay fever).
4. Gastrointestinal (e.g., *ulcers,* ulcerative colitis, irritable colon, heartburn, constipation, and diarrhea).
5. Cardiovascular (e.g., paroxysmal tachycardia, *migraines,* palpitations, and *hypertension*).
6. Genitourinary (e.g., dysuria and *dysmenorrhea*).
7. Endocrine (e.g., hyperthyroidism).
8. Nervous system (e.g., general fatigue, anorexia, and exhaustion).

C. Certain *pre-morbid personality traits* and coping styles have been associated with specific *medical conditions,* e.g., ulcerative colitis with excessive dependency needs; respiratory illnesses with difficulty in crying; hypertension with problems in expressing anger.

III. Analysis/nursing diagnosis: *Ineffective individual coping* related to inappropriate need-gratification through illness (i.e., actual illness used as means of meeting needs for attention and affection). Absence of life experiences that gratify needs for attention and affection. Maladaptive health behaviors affecting medical condition.

IV. Nursing care plan/implementation in disorders in which psychological factors affect medical conditions:

A. **Long-term goal:** release of feelings through verbalization and activity outlets.
1. Help clients *express their feelings,* especially anger, hostility, guilt, resentment, or humiliation, which may be related to such issues as sexual difficulties, family problems, religious conflicts, and job difficulties. Help clients recognize that, when stress and anxiety are not released through some channel such as verbal expression, the body will release the tension through *"organ language."*
2. Provide *outlets* for release of tensions and diversions from preoccupation with physical complaints.
   a. Provide social and recreational activities to decrease time for preoccupation with illness.
   b. Encourage clients to use physical and intellectual capabilities in constructive ways.
3. Help clients feel *in control* of situations and be as independent as possible.

B. **Short-term goals**
1. Take care of *physical* problems during acute phase.

2. Assess precipitating stressors.
3. *Remove* client from anxiety-producing stimuli.

C. Prompt attention in meeting clients' *basic needs* (food, sleep, hygiene, activity), to gratify appropriate needs for *dependency, attention,* and *security.*

D. Maintain an attitude of *acceptance, respect* and *concern;* clients' pains and worries are very real and upsetting to them; do *not* belittle the symptoms. Do not say, "There is nothing wrong with you" because *emotions do* in fact *cause* somatic disabilities.

E. *Treat organic* problems as necessary, but without undue emphasis (that is, do *not* reinforce preoccupation with bodily complaints).

F. *Protect* clients from any disturbing stimuli; help the healing process in the acute phase of illnesses (e.g., myocardial infarct).

G. Be *supportive;* assist clients to bear painful feelings through a helping relationship while assessing precipitating stressors.

H. *Health teaching*
1. Teach how to express feelings.
2. Teach more effective ways of responding to stressful life situations (e.g., stress management techniques).
3. Teach the family supportive relationships.

V. Evaluation/outcome criteria: can verbalize feelings more fully.

💡 Study and Memory Aids

Characteristics of Psychophysiologic Illnesses

1. ↓ security → ↑ symptoms
2. ↑ psychological stress → ↑ physical reactions
3. ↑ needs { dependency / attention / love / recognition / security

Glossary

alexithymia   Inability or difficulty in consciously expressing or describing feelings, or being aware of one's emotions or moods.

psychophysiologic illness   A medical condition with mind-body interaction (i.e., emotional and physical aspects) with observable organic impairment (e.g., hives, pruritus, low back pain, asthma, hypertension, ulcerative colitis, migraines); stress-related physiological response affecting medical condition.

🔑 Summary of Key Points

Psychological Factors Affecting Medical Condition (Psychophysiologic Illness)

1. There is a *relationship* between intrapsychic conflict, anxiety, stress, and psychophysiologic illness (Selye's general stress adaptation syndrome).
2. There are *precipitating stressors* that contribute to the development of psychophysiologic illness.
3. There are predisposing factors: *biologic* factors (endocrine, genetic, target organs, psychoneuro-immunology); *psychological* factors (type A personality; personality characteristics related to specific physiologic disorders).
4. *Nursing goals:* help patient to consciously *experience* and *express* feelings; teach stress management (relaxation techniques); meet *basic* needs (physical aspects of care) and needs for *dependency, attention,* and *security.*

Questions

1. What is the immediate, short-term nursing goal that is appropriate to meet the needs of a patient who has a psychophysiologic illness?
   1. Providing interpersonal support while assessing precipitating stressors.
   2. Exploring alternative approaches to coping with the effect of accumulated stress (e.g., relaxation and meditation exercises).
   3. Helping the patient to consciously experience emotions and communicate feelings.
   4. Providing information about the mind-body relationship in the illness.
2. In planning appropriate nursing interventions, the nurse needs to take into account which coping mechanisms that are commonly used by individuals with psychophysiologic illness?
   1. Repression, denial.
   2. Denial, reaction formation.
   3. Compensation, suppression.
   4. Regression, displacement.
3. The nurse should base the nursing care plan for a patient with a psychophysiologic illness on the knowledge that the basic difference between psychophysiologic illness and hypochondriasis is that in psychophysiologic illness there is:
   1. Real pain.
   2. An emotional cause.
   3. A physical cause.
   4. A possibility of a life-threatening course.
4. In planning appropriate activities for the patient with ulcerative colitis, the nurse will need to be aware that the personality traits most frequently encountered in patients who develop ulcerative colitis are:
   1. Carefree and confident.
   2. Perfectionistic and hard-driving.
   3. Sensitive and dependent.
   4. Hostile and volatile.
5. What would be important to include in the nursing care plan for a person with a physical illness in which psychogenic factors play a significant causative role (such as asthma, ulcer, or arthritis)?
   1. Increase stimulation whenever possible, to provide distraction.
   2. Accept the patient's behavior and encourage expression of feelings.
   3. Ignore the physical symptoms.
   4. Avoid focusing on feelings, as the symptoms will tend to increase.
6. A patient is admitted to the hospital for acute exacerbation of ulcerative colitis, with a recent weight loss of 15 pounds as a result of frequent diarrhea. Given this disorder, what activities would be most appropriate for this patient?
   1. Solitary activities that involve hands-on skills, rather than intellectual abilities.
   2. Activities that are restful and minimize exertion.
   3. Activities that encourage socialization, to decrease isolation.
   4. Group experiences that facilitate increased self-awareness of conflicting feelings.
7. In assessing a patient who has been diagnosed with irritable colon, the nurse should be aware that symptoms related to psychophysiologic illness mostly affect organs controlled by:
   1. The central nervous system.
   2. The autonomic nervous system.
   3. The voluntary nervous system.
   4. The peripheral nervous system.
8. A patient has developed a psychophysiologic illness. The nurse learns that the patient recently lost a position as a high-level executive at a major corporation after an error in judgment which cost the corporation significant loss of profits and angered the stockholders. The patient's family reveals that the patient took this event as a personal failure that deserves punishment. Which coping mechanism should the nurse determine that the patient is probably using?
   1. Projection.
   2. Repression.
   3. Dissociation.
   4. Introjection.

Answers/Rationale

1. **(1)** Since there is a relationship between intrapsychic conflict, anxiety, stress, and psychophysiologic illness, an *immediate short-term nursing goal* is for the nurse to assess stressors that may be related to the illness. **No. 2** would be appropriate as an *intermediate* goal, not immediate. **No. 3** is a *long-term* goal. Cognitive input (**No. 4**) will not help in modifying the stress response and trying new ways to express emotions that have been pushed out of awareness. **PL, 7, PsI**

💡 *Test-taking tip:* The word *assess*, is key to choosing the *immediate, short-term goal.*

2. **(1)** These are primary ego defenses related to the inability to consciously experience feelings and express emotions (alexithymia). The other options are only partially correct: denial (**No. 2**), suppression (**No. 3**), and regression (**No. 4**) *are* commonly associated with psychophysiologic illness; however, reaction formation (**No. 2**), compensation (**No. 3**), and displacement (**No. 4**) are not. **AN, 7, PsI**

3. **(4)** The psychophysiologic response (either hypofunction or hyperfunction) can create actual tissue changes that can lead to a life-threatening condition (e.g., a bleeding ulcer). **Nos. 1, 2, and 3** are incorrect because they can occur in *both* hypochondriasis and psychophysiologic illnesses. **AN, 1, PhI**

4. **(3)** Individuals with a condition in which the colon is involved (a visceral disorder) tend to have a premorbid personality of unresolved conflicts between dependence and independence. Individuals with a carefree, confident personality (**No. 1**) tend to be secure individuals who are *not* predisposed to stress-related visceral disorders. Perfectionistic, hard-driving personalities (**No. 2**) tend to be linked with *peptic* ulcers. Those who externalize aggressive feelings (**No. 4**) are also less likely to experience conditions with visceral changes such as ulcerative colitis. **AS, 7, PsI**

5. **(2)** *Acceptance* is the first step in helping a patient with stress-related conditions. It is important to allow, accept, and encourage expression of feelings that may be linked

to conditions such as asthma, ulcer, or arthritis. The premorbid personality in these patients appears to be that of unexpressed *aggression* and hostility, resulting from unresolved conflicts between needs for *dependence/passivity* and independence. Other unexpressed feelings may be strong desires for *protection* and *security,* yet they fear rejection or engulfment. Rest is usually desirable, *not* stimulation (**No. 1**), due to fatigue from feelings of anxiety and fear. All physical symptoms must be explored, *not* ignored (**No. 3**), and need to be evaluated for medical management. Primary causes must be ruled out. Avoiding focusing on feelings (**No. 4**) is the opposite of the best response, *encouraging* expression of feelings. **PL, 7, PsI**

💡 *Test-taking tip:* When in doubt, consider two contradictory options, and choose the one that focuses on *acceptance* and *feelings.*

6. **(2)** Patients with psychophysiologic illnesses, such as ulcerative colitis, need activities that keep emotional stresses and fatigue to a minimum. The immediate priority is treating the *medical* condition (diarrhea, weight loss). Hands-on activities (**No. 1**) have no bearing on *either* the physical manifestations or the personality traits (dependence/independence conflicts) that are often associated with this psychophysiologic condition. Increased socialization (**No. 3**) is not a specific goal for this condition, and would not address the patient's *medical* condition. Fostering self-awareness (**No. 4**) is *not* an appropriate *immediate* goal, given the physical symptoms of this patient at this time. Developing self-awareness and resolving conflicts that may aggravate this stress-related condition would be *long-term* goals. **PL, 3, PhI**

7. **(2)** The majority of organs involved in psychophysiologic illnesses are under control of the autonomic nervous system, the branch of the nervous system that is not controlled voluntarily or consciously. Examples: skin (dermatitis and pruritus), lungs (asthma), stomach (ulcer), colon (ulcerative colitis). The central nervous system (**No. 1**) refers to the brain and spinal cord in general, not to a specific branch of the system that controls organs. The voluntary nervous system (**No. 3**) controls the striated (skeletal) muscles, not the smooth muscles (as in most organs affected). The peripheral nervous system (**No. 4**) refers generally to nerves and ganglia beyond the brain and spinal cord, not to a specific system that controls organs. **AS, 8, PhI**

8. **(4)** The patient seems to feel that he or she deserves punishment—the psychophysiologic illness—for this error; seeing illness as punishment describes *introjection.* While projection (**No. 1**) and repression (**No. 2**) may be underlying mechanisms of psychophysiologic illness, they do not match the description in this case. Dissociation (**No. 3**) is not a common underlying coping mechanism in psychophysiologic illness. **AS, 7, PsI**

Key to Codes

Nursing process: AS = Assessment; **AN** = Analysis; **PL** = Planning; **IMP** = Implementation; **EV** = Evaluation. (See Appendix E for explanation of nursing process steps.)

Category of human function: 1 = Protective; **2** = Sensory-Perceptual; **3** = Comfort, Rest, Activity, and Mobility; **4** = Nutrition; **5** = Growth and Development; **6** = Fluid-Gas Transport; **7** = Psychosocial-Cultural; **8** = Elimination.

Client need: SECE = Safe, Effective Care Environment; **PhI** = Physiologic Integrity; **PsI** = Psychosocial Integrity; **HPM** = Health Promotion/Maintenance.

Schizophrenia and Related Psychotic Disorders

Chapter Outline

- Schizophrenia
- Delusional Disorder
  - Paranoid Schizophrenia
- Study and Memory Aids

- Glossary
- Summary of Key Points
- Questions
- Answers/Rationale

Schizophrenia

Schizophrenia is a group of interrelated disorders characterized by disturbances in form and *content* of *thought* (loosening of associations, delusions, and hallucinations), *mood* (blunted, flattened, or inappropriate affect), perception (loss of reality), *sense of self and relationship to the external world* (loss of ego boundaries, autistic thinking, and withdrawal), and *behavior* (bizarre, apparently purposeless, and stereotyped activity or inactivity). The term means "splitting of the mind," alluding to the discrepancy between the content of *thought processes* and their emotional expression; used to be confused with "multiple personality" (dissociative disorder).

Half of the clients in mental hospitals are diagnosed as schizophrenic; many more schizophrenics live in the community. The onset of symptoms for this disorder generally occurs between 15 and 27 years of age. Causes, psychodynamics, and psychopathology are still a matter of controversy although a combination of biologic, psychosocial, and environmental factors are implicated.

I. **Common subtypes** of schizophrenia (without clear-cut differentiation):
  A. **Catatonic type:** marked psychomotor disturbance—muscle tension, with rigidity, waxy flexibility, posturing (*stupor*); mutism; violent rage outbursts, negativism, and frenzied activity (*excitement*). Marked decrease in involvement with environment and in spontaneous movement. Require careful supervision to prevent injury, promote nutrition, and *avoid* demands.
  B. **Disorganized type** (previously called **hebephrenic**): disordered thinking ("word salad"), inappropriate *affect* (blunted, silly), *regressive* behavior, *incoherent* speech, preoccupied and withdrawn.
  C. **Paranoid type:** disturbed perceptions leading to disturbance in thought content (delusions) of *persecutory, grandiose,* or hostile nature; projection is

key mechanism, with religion a common preoccupation.
  D. **Residual type:** continued difficulty in thinking, mood, perception, and behavior *after* schizophrenic episode.
  E. **Undifferentiated type:** *unclassifiable* schizophreniclike disturbance with *mixed* symptoms of delusions, hallucinations, incoherence, gross disorganization.
II. **Concepts and principles** related to schizophrenic disorders
  A. **General**
    1. *Symbolic* language expresses schizophrenic's life, pain, and progress toward health; all symbols used have meaning.
    2. *Physical care* provides media for relationship; nurturance may be initial focus.
    3. *Consistency, reliability,* and *empathic* understanding build trust.
    4. *Denial, regression,* and *projection* are key defense mechanisms.
    5. Anxiety gives rise to distorted thinking.
    6. Attempts to engage in verbal communication may result in tension, apprehensiveness, and defensiveness.
    7. Person *rejects real world* of painful experiences and *creates fantasy* world through illness.
  B. **Withdrawal**
    1. Withdrawal from and resistance to forming relationships are attempts to reduce *anxiety* related to:
      a. Loss of ability to experience satisfying human relationships.
      b. Fear of rejection.
      c. Lack of self-confidence.
      d. Need for protection and restraint against potential destructiveness of *hostile* impulses (toward self and others).

127

e. Confusion caused by overwhelming environmental stimuli.

2. *Ambivalence* results from need to approach a relationship and need to avoid it.

    a. *Cannot* tolerate swift emotional or physical *closeness.*

    b. Needs *more time* than usual to establish a relationship; time *to test* sincerity and interest of nurse.

3. Avoidance of client by others, especially staff, will reinforce withdrawal, thereby creating problem of *mutual withdrawal* and fear.

C. Hallucinations

1. It is possible to replace hallucinations with satisfying interactions.

2. Person can relearn to focus attention on real things and people.

3. Hallucinations originate during *extreme* emotional stress when unable to cope.

4. Hallucinations are real to client.

5. Client will react as the situation is perceived, *regardless* of reality or consensus.

6. Concrete experiences, *not* argument or confrontation, will correct sensory distortion.

7. Hallucinations are *substitutes* for human relations.

8. Purposes served by or expressed in falsification of reality:

    a. Reflection of problem in inner life.

    b. Statement of criticism, censure, self-punishment.

    c. Promotion of self-esteem.

    d. Satisfaction of instinctual strivings.

    e. *Projection* of unacceptable unconscious content in disguised form.

9. Perceptions *not* as *totally* disturbed as they seem.

10. Client attempts to restructure reality through hallucinations to *protect remaining ego integrity.*

11. Hallucinations may result from a variety of psychological and biologic conditions (e.g., extreme fatigue, drugs, pyrexia, and organic brain disease).

12. Person needs to feel free to describe his perceptions if he or she is to be understood by the nurse.

III. Assessment of schizophrenic disorders

  A. Eugene Bleuler described four classic and *primary symptoms* as the *"four As"*:

    1. *Associative looseness:* impairment of logical thought progression, resulting in confused, bizarre, and abrupt thinking.

    2. *Affect:* exaggerated, apathetic, blunt, flat, inappropriate, inconsistent feeling tone that is communicated through face and body posture.

    3. *Ambivalence:* simultaneous, conflicting thoughts, ideas, drive, feelings or attitudes toward person or object.

      a. Stormy outbursts.

      b. Poor, weak interpersonal relations.

4. *Autism: withdrawal* from external world; preoccupation with own fantasies, needs, and idiosyncratic thoughts. Loss of interest in others. *Autistic disorder* is different from autism as an element of schizophrenia in that autistic disorder is distinguished *from childhood* by its *early* onset and *lack* of delusions, hallucinations, incoherence or loosening of associations.

    a. *Delusions:* false, fixed beliefs, not corrected by logic; a defense against intolerable feeling. The two most common delusions are:

      (1) *Delusions of grandeur:* conviction in a belief related to being famous, important, or wealthy.

      (2) *Delusions of persecution:* belief that one's thoughts, moods, or actions are controlled or influenced by strange forces or by others.

    b. *Hallucinations:* false sensory impressions without observable external stimuli.

      (1) *Auditory:* affecting hearing (e.g., hears voices).

      (2) *Visual:* affecting vision (e.g., sees snakes).

      (3) *Tactile:* affecting touch (e.g., feels electric charges in body).

      (4) *Olfactory:* affecting smell (e.g., smells rotting flesh).

      (5) *Gustatory:* affecting taste (e.g., food tastes like poison).

    c. *Ideas of reference:* clients interpret cues in the environment as having reference to them. Ideas *symbolize guilt, insecurity,* and *alienation;* may become delusions, if severe.

    d. *Neologisms:* making up new words or condensing words into one.

    e. *Depersonalization:* feelings of strangeness and unreality about self or environment or both; difficulty in differentiating boundaries between self and environment.

  B. *Regression:* extreme *withdrawal* and social isolation.

  C. *Prodromal or residual symptoms*

    1. Social isolation, *withdrawal.*

    2. Marked impairment in *role* functioning (e.g., as student, employee).

    3. Markedly *peculiar* behavior (e.g., collecting garbage).

    4. Marked impairment in personal *hygiene.*

    5. *Affect:* blunt, inappropriate.

    6. *Speech:* vague, overelaborate, circumstantial, metaphorical.

    7. *Thinking:* bizarre ideation or reverting to magical thinking, e.g., *ideas of reference,* "others can feel my feelings."

    8. Unusual *perceptual* experiences, e.g., sensing the presence of a force or person not physically there.

IV. Analysis/nursing diagnosis

  A. *Sensory-perceptual alterations* related to inability to define reality and distinguish the real from the unreal (hallucinations, illusions) and misinterpretation of stimuli.

B. *Altered communication process* with inability to *verbally* express needs and wishes related to difficulty with processing information and unique patterns of speech (e.g., word salad, clang association, echolalia).

C. *Altered thought processes* related to intense anxiety and blocking (delusions).

D. *Altered feeling states* related to anxiety about others (*inappropriate emotions*).

E. *Self-care deficit* with *inappropriate* dress and poor physical hygiene related to perceptual or cognitive impairment.

F. *Altered judgment* related to lack of trust, fear of rejection, and doubts regarding competence of others.

G. *Altered self-concept* related to *feelings of inadequacy* in coping with the real world.

H. *Body image disturbance* related to inappropriate use of defense mechanisms.

I. *Disorganized behaviors:* impaired relatedness to others, related to withdrawal, distortions of reality, and lack of trust.

J. *Diversional activity deficit* related to personal ambivalence.

V. Nursing care plan/implementation in schizophrenic disorders

A. General
1. Set *short-range* goals, realistic to client's levels of functioning.
2. Use *nonverbal* level of communication to demonstrate concern, caring, and warmth, as client often distrusts words. Building *trust* is primary.
3. Help client tolerate nurses' presence and learn to *trust* nurses enough to move out of isolation and share painful and often unacceptable (to client) feelings and thoughts.
4. Set climate for free expression of *feelings* in whatever mode, without fear of retaliation, ridicule, or rejection.
5. Seek client out in his or her own fantasy world. Try reflecting observations of client's behavior in order to facilitate disclosure of his perceptions. Recognize and acknowledge *feelings* underlying the hallucination or other sensory experience rather than focusing on the *content*.
6. Try to understand meaning of symbolic language; help client communicate less symbolically.
7. Provide *distance*, as client needs to feel safe and to observe nurses for sources of threat or promises of security.
8. Anticipate and accept negativism; do *not* personalize.
9. *Avoid* joking, abstract terms, and figures of speech when client's thinking is literal.
10. Give antipsychotic medications.

B. Withdrawn behavior (with *catatonia* as an extreme example)

1. **Long-term goal:** develop satisfying interpersonal relationships.
2. **Short-term goal:** help client feel safe in *one-to-one* relationship and prevent hazards of immobility.
3. Attend to *nutrition* (*diet:* high fiber, fluids), *elimination, exercise,* hygiene, and signs of physical illness.
4. Seek client out at every chance, and establish some bond. *Build trust.*
   a. Stay with client, in silence.
   b. Initiate talk when client is ready.
   c. Draw out, but do *not* demand, response.
   d. Do *not* avoid the client.
5. Use *simple language,* specific words.
6. Use an *object* or *activity* as medium for relationship and socialization; initiate activity.
7. Focus on *everyday* experiences.
8. *Delay* decision making.
9. Accept one-sided conversation, with silence from the client; *avoid* pressuring to respond.
10. *Accept* the client's outward attempts to respond and inappropriate social behavior, without remarks or disdain; teach social skills.
11. *Avoid* making demands on client or exposing client to failure.
12. *Protect* from aggressive persons and from impulsive attacks on self and others.
13. Add structure to the day; tell the client, "This is your 9 A.M. medication."
14. *Health teaching:* assist family to understand client's needs, to see small sign of progress; teach client to perform simple tasks of self-care in order to meet own biologic needs.

C. Hallucinatory behavior
1. **Long-term goal:** establish satisfying relationships with *real* persons.
2. **Short-term goal:** interrupt *pattern* of hallucinations.
3. Provide a *structured* environment with routine activities. Use *real* objects to keep client's interest or to stimulate new interest (e.g., in painting or crafts).
4. *Protect* against injury to self and others resulting from listening to "voices."
5. *Short, frequent* contacts initially, increasing social interaction gradually (one person → small groups).
6. Ask client to describe experiences as hallucinations occur.
7. Respond to anything real the client says, e.g., with acknowledgment or reflection. Focus more on *feelings, not* on delusional, hallucinatory *content*.
8. *Distract* client's attention to something real when client hallucinates. If client is experiencing an illusion, provide corrective interpretation of actual stimuli.
9. *Avoid* direct confrontation about the falseness of the hallucination; do not argue, but listen.
10. *Clarify* who "they" are:

a. Use personal pronouns, *avoid* universal and global pronouns.
b. Nurse's own language needs to be clear and unambiguous.

11. Use one sentence, ask only one question, at a time.
12. Encourage *consensual validation* (check out perceptions with others). Point out that experience is not shared by you; voice doubt.
13. *Health teaching*
    a. Recommend more effective ways of coping (e.g., consensual validation).
    b. Advise that highly emotional situations be avoided.
    c. Explain the causes of misperceptions.
    d. Recommend methods for reducing sensory stimulation.
    D. **Delusions:** See **Nursing care plan/implementation** in following section.

⋈ VI. **Evaluation/outcome criteria**
    A. Small behavioral changes occur (e.g., eye contact, better grooming).
    B. Evidence of beginning trust in nurse (e.g., keeps appointments).
    C. Initiates conversation with others; participates in activities.
    D. Decreases amount of time spent alone.
    E. Demonstrates appropriate behavior in public places.
    F. Articulates relationship between feelings of discomfort and autistic behavior.
    G. Makes positive statements.

Delusional Disorder

Paranoid Schizophrenia

Paranoid disorders have a concrete and pervasive delusional system, usually *persecutory. Projection* is a chief coping mechanism of this disorder.

I. **Concepts and principles** related to paranoid disorders
    A. Delusions are attempts to cope with stresses and problems.
    B. May be a means of allegorical or symbolic communication and of testing others for their trustworthiness.
    C. *Interactions* with others and activities *interrupt* delusional thinking.
    D. To establish a rational therapeutic relationship, gross distortions, misorientation, misinterpretation, and misidentification need to be overcome.
    E. Delusional people have *extreme need* to maintain self-esteem.
    F. False beliefs cannot be changed without first changing experiences.
    G. A delusion is held because it *performs a function.*
    H. When people who are experiencing delusions become at ease and comfortable with people, delusions will not be needed.

I. Delusions are misjudgments of reality based on a series of mental mechanisms: (1) *denial,* followed by (2) *projection,* and (3) *rationalization.*
J. There is a *kernel of truth* in delusions.
K. Behind the anger and suspicion in a paranoid, there is a *lonely, terrified* person who *feels vulnerable* and *inadequate.*

⋈ II. **Assessment** of paranoid disorder
    A. Chronically *suspicious,* distrustful (thinks "people are out to get me"). Tends to see others as bad, wrong, or dangerous.
    B. Distant, but *not* withdrawn.
    C. Poor insight; blames others (*projects*).
    D. Misinterprets and *distorts reality.*
    E. Difficulty in admitting own errors; takes pride in intelligence and in being correct (*superiority*).
    F. Maintains false persecutory belief despite evidence or proof (may refuse food and medicine, insisting they are poisoned).
    G. Literal thinking (*rigid*).
    H. Dominating and *provocative.*
    I. Hypercritical and intolerant of others; *hostile,* quarrelsome, and aggressive.
    J. *Very sensitive* in perceiving minor injustices, errors, and contradictions.
    K. Evasive.

⋈ III. **Analysis/nursing diagnosis**
    A. *Severe anxiety* related to projection of threatening, aggressive impulses and misinterpretation of stimuli.
    B. *Ineffective individual coping* related to lack of trust, fear of close human contact.
    C. *Impaired cognitive functioning* related to rigidity of thought.
    D. *Chronic low self-esteem* related to feelings of inadequacy.
    E. *Impaired social interaction* related to lack of tender, kind feelings, feelings of grandiosity and/or persecution.
    F. *Altered thought processes* related to lack of insight.

⋈ IV. **Nursing care plan/implementation** in paranoid disorder:
    A. **Long-term goals:** gain clear, correct perceptions and interpretations through corrective experiences.
    B. **Short-term goals**
        1. Help client recognize distortions, misinterpretations.
        2. Help client feel safe in exploring reality in brief, non-demanding contacts.
    C. Help client learn to *trust self;* help to develop self-confidence and ego assets through positive reinforcement.
    D. Help to *trust others.*
        1. Be *consistent* and *honest* at all times.
        2. *Do not whisper, act secretive, or laugh* with others in client's presence when he or she cannot hear what is said.
        3. Do *not* mix medicines with food.
        4. Keep promises.
        5. Let client know ahead of time what he or she can *expect* from others.

6. Give *reasons* and careful, complete, and repetitive explanations.
7. Ask permission to contact others.
8. Consult client first about all decisions concerning him or her.

E. Help to *test reality*.
1. Present and repeat reality of the situation.
2. Do *not* confirm or approve distortions.
3. Help accept responsibility for own behavior rather than project.
4. *Divert* from delusions to reality-centered focus.
5. Let client know when behavior does not seem appropriate.
6. Assume nothing and leave no room for assumptions.
7. *Structure* time and activities to limit delusional thought, behavior.
8. Set limit for *not* discussing delusional content.
9. Look for *underlying needs* expressed in delusional content.

F. Provide *outlets* for anger and aggressive drives.
1. *Listen* matter-of-factly to angry outbursts.
2. *Accept* rebuffs and abusive talk as symptoms.
3. *Do not* argue, disagree, or debate.
4. *Allow* expression of negative feelings without fear of punishment.

G. Provide *successful group experience*.
1. *Avoid* competitive sports involving close *physical* contact.
2. Give *recognition* to skills and work well done.
3. Utilize managerial talents.
4. Respect client's intellect and engage in activities with others requiring *intellect* (e.g., chess, puzzles, and Scrabble).

H. *Limit* physical contact.
I. *Health teaching*: teach a more rational basis for deciding whom to trust by identifying behaviors characteristic of trusting and trustworthy people.

▶◀ V. **Evaluation/outcome criteria**
A. Able to differentiate trustworthy from untrustworthy people.
B. Growing self-awareness; able to share this awareness with others.
C. Accepts others without need to criticize or change them.
D. Open to new experiences.
E. Able to delay gratification.

💡 Study and Memory Aids

Schizophrenia: assessment—"Four As"

Associative looseness: *thinking* disorder (delusions)
Affect: *feeling, mood* disorder
Ambivalence: *interpersonal* relationship disorder
Autism: *perception* and *communication* disorder

Schizophrenia: mental status assessment —"COAST MAP"

Consciousness: distractible
Orientation: disoriented to time and place
Activity: hyperactivity or retarded; bizarre, stereotyped movements
Speech: neologisms
Thought: disturbed in progression and content—flight of ideas, *loose associations, delusions of persecution, thought broadcasting* (ideas and thoughts are being transmitted to others), *thought insertion* (others can put thoughts into person's mind), *thought withdrawal* (thoughts can be taken from the person's mind)

Memory: intact
Affect and mood: wide swings in mood, or flat
Perception: auditory hallucinations

Source: Caroline N. *Emergency Care in the Streets* (5th ed). Boston: Little, Brown, 1995. pp 908–909.

Give antipsychotic medications to ↑ reality orientation and ↓ perceptual disturbances

Glossary

ambivalence   Coexisting *contradictory* (positive and negative) emotions, desires, or attitudes toward an object, person, or action (e.g., love-hate relationship) resulting in the inability to make, or difficulty in making, choices when faced with decisions, emotions, and relationships (e.g., approach-avoidance conflict).

associative looseness   A thought disorder and communication pattern characterized by unrelated words or phrases, with little connection between one thought and the next.

autism   Self-preoccupation and absorption; withdrawal into one's own internal world (needs, fantasies, language) and inner experiences, with a complete *exclusion of reality* and loss of interest in and appreciation of others.

autistic thought   Assigning private meanings, originating within the individual, to words, events, and relationships that are *not* shared by others.

catatonia   Type of schizophrenia characterized by psychomotor behavior disturbance; an unresponsive state (mute or negativistic behavior) related to fear of loss of impulse control, involving either extreme agitation (**catatonic excitement**) or rigid immobile posture (**catatonic stupor**) in which person seems unaware of the environment and may resist efforts to be moved.

clang association   A speech pattern in which sound governs the choice of words; e.g., words that rhyme are put together; punning. Seen most often in schizophrenia, mania, or autism.

concreteness   Literal interpretation of words due to difficulty with abstract thinking.

⚷ Summary of Key Points

Schizophrenic Disorders

General

1. In order to intervene appropriately (provide *corrective* information in all cases of illusions; express *doubt* with others), know the difference between *hallucinations* (sensory perceptions *without* external stimuli), *illusions* (*real* stimuli are misinterpreted), and *delusions* (false, fixed beliefs).
2. Most common *characteristic behaviors:* withdrawn, aloof; bizarre; disorganized; autistic (retreat to a fantasy world); hypersensitivity to sound, sight, and smell.
3. Characterized by disturbed *affect* (feelings): negativistic, flat, blunt, and/or inappropriate.
4. *Thought disorders* are common: confused, chaotic, delusional.
5. *Social relations* are impaired: difficulty relating to others; lack of social awareness; inability to trust; ambivalence (love/hate feelings).

Withdrawn Behavior (Autism, Catatonic Schizophrenia)

1. Initiate brief, nondemanding, structured 1:1 activities to build trust.
2. Provide stimulation from recreational and other milieu activities to increase opportunities for socialization.
3. Assist client to meet basic needs (sleep, nutrition, personal hygiene).

Hallucinatory/Delusional Behavior (Paranoid Schizophrenia)

1. Focus on *reality* orientation.
2. *Avoid* arguing; merely state that your viewpoint is *different*.
3. Express *doubt* regarding patient's altered perceptions.
4. Give *feedback* about observable behavior. Encourage contact with others (rather than solitary activities), for providing opportunities for feedback.
5. Respond clearly and honestly.
6. Respond to underlying *feeling or* message (e.g., fear).
7. Encourage patient to *validate*.
8. Build trust by being *consistent*.
9. Do *not* avoid or ignore patient.

delusion   A false, fixed *belief* that is contrary to what others think of as real and that cannot be influenced or changed by logic; arises out of individual's needs and is maintained in spite of evidence or facts to the contrary (e.g., delusions of grandeur, persecution).

echolalia   Exact, automatic repetition of another's words.

echopraxia   Imitating other's actions, e.g., body position.

hallucination   *False sensory perception* that does not have an actual external stimulus. May be due to chemicals or inner needs, and may occur in any of the five senses. Seen in psychosis and cognitive disorders.

ideas of reference   Interpret cues in the environment that external events have reference to self; false beliefs that other people or messages from the media (TV, radio, or newspaper) are directly referring to the client.

magical thinking   According to Piaget, it is a primitive, prelogical thinking disorder based on the belief that one's words, actions, thoughts are powerful enough to exert influence on situations, to produce an outcome that defies normal laws of cause and effect. It is often seen in normal children with a strong sense of imagination.

negativism   Doing the opposite of or resisting what is asked, needed, or required (e.g., not eating; catatonic schizophrenic may resist efforts to move arms).

neologisms   Newly coined words with private meaning that may be related to the individual's conflict; condensed combination of several words not readily understood by others (e.g., "The ridjams frast wolmix"). Found in schizophrenia.

nihilistic delusion   False belief that oneself, part of oneself, or another object *no longer exists.*

paranoid   An adjective indicating feelings of suspicion and persecution; one type of schizophrenia.

primary thought process   Infantile ideas and thoughts that are usually repressed and unconscious.

psychosis   Severe emotional illness characterized by a disorder of *thinking, feeling,* and *action* which includes the following symptoms: loss of contact with reality, bizarre thinking and behavior, perceptual distortion and regression.

schizophrenia   Severe functional mental disorder characterized in general by disturbances in thought, moods, perceptions, interpersonal relationships, and behavior.

secondary thought process   Logical thoughts and ideas that are usually conscious and are under ego control.

somatic delusion   A false belief that all or part of one's body is *impaired.*

tangential communication   A communication pattern in which a main point is obscured by off-the-point verbalizations.

thought broadcasting   The feeling that one's thoughts are being broadcast to others.

thought insertion   The delusion that thoughts that are not one's own are being put into one's mind.

thought withdrawal   The delusion that someone or something is removing thoughts from one's mind.

waxy flexibility   Psychomotor underactivity, in which the individual maintains the posture in which he or she is placed; symptom of catatonic schizophrenia.

word salad   A pattern of communication in which unrelated words are strung together; meaningless mixture of phrases and words, often seen in schizophrenic disorders.

Questions

1. When admitting a patient whose diagnosis is schizophrenia, catatonic type, what is the nursing priority?
   1. Avoid demands and situations requiring decision making. ✓
   2. Administer prn medications.
   3. Introduce the patient to a group activity, to reduce alienation.
   4. Spend 1 hour each day with the patient, to build trust.

2. Which problem will have the highest priority in planning care for a person whose diagnosis is catatonic schizophrenia?
   1. Decreased nutritional intake.
   2. Impaired circulation to pressure areas of the skin. ✓
   3. Brief violent behavior.
   4. Minimal participation in group therapy.

3. When planning care for a patient who is exhibiting withdrawn behavior as part of the schizophrenic process, the nurse needs to be aware that withdrawn behavior provides a means for the patient to:
   1. Keep the family from forcing the patient to do what they insist.
   2. Avoid forming interpersonal relationships.
   3. Cope with confusion caused by environmental stimuli that may be too overwhelming to understand. ✓
   4. Remain preoccupied with delusional thoughts.

4. Which behavioral notation made by the nurse in the chart of a patient with a schizophrenic disorder would alert the next shift of high risk for violence?
   1. "Withdrawn; stays in room; appears preoccupied."
   2. "Asking to leave the hospital; makes frequent phone calls."
   3. "Hallucinations; increased anger and negativism." ✓
   4. "Increased physical activity and talking to all other patients."

5. A young, single woman's behavior has become more and more bizarre and reclusive; she has begun eating with her hands, refuses to bathe or dress, and responds to others with inappropriate grimacing and incomprehensible mumbling. Which nursing diagnosis would be most significant for this patient?
   1. Altered thought processes.
   2. Disturbance in self-esteem.
   3. Social isolation. ✓
   4. High risk for self-directed violence.

6. What would be the most appropriate initial nursing goal when working with a patient with a schizophrenic diagnosis?
   1. Helping the patient to verbalize feelings.
   2. Discouraging strange behavior.
   3. Encouraging self-care.
   4. Building trust. ✓

7. What autistic behavior would the nurse be most likely to see in a patient with a diagnosis of schizophrenia?
   1. Associative looseness.
   2. Affect that is flat and/or inappropriate.
   3. Ambivalence.
   4. Neologism. ✓

8. A patient describes buzzing sensations in his body from transmitters implanted by the CIA. He believes that the secret evidence he has for world salvation is threatening to all world powers. The most appropriate treatment modality for this patient would be:
   1. ECT.
   2. Chemotherapy and 1:1 therapy. ✓
   3. Chemotherapy and group therapy.
   4. Chemotherapy.

9. A patient in a mental health center tells the nurse that a little green man has been placed in her head by the CIA to record all her movements. What would be the most therapeutic action by the nurse?
   1. Acknowledge the fear that the patient must be experiencing, but reaffirm that she is safe at the center. ✓
   2. Encourage the patient to bring these thoughts up during the next one-to-one session.
   3. Put the patient in a room by herself, away from the radio or TV and other external stimuli.
   4. Tell the patient that this is not a real situation.

10. A patient is scaring others when she tells them that she has special powers over people. The nurse recognizes this behavior as:
    1. A delusion. ✓
    2. A threat.
    3. Magical thinking.
    4. A manipulative act.

11. The nurse notices that a young adult male patient on the unit appears remote and suspicious. He is well groomed, and is a loner. From time to time, the patient stares upward and tilts his head to the left while pulling his earlobe downward. The nurse determines that the patient:
    1. May be having auditory hallucinations. ✓
    2. May want attention.
    3. Has bizarre mannerisms.
    4. May want to avoid interaction with others.

12. The nurse suspects the patient is experiencing hallucinations when the patient:
    1. Asks, "Where did these bugs come from? They are crawling on my arms."
    2. Calls a lamppost "Homer."
    3. States, "They are coming to get me."
    4. Says, "I am responsible for the world's salvation."

13. When a patient with a schizophrenic disorder begins to talk about people stealing her children, the nurse should initially:
    1. Tell her that her thoughts are confused.
    2. Question her about the details concerning her missing children.
    3. Focus on her feelings of anxiety and real events. ✓
    4. Tell her that the nurse does not believe her stories.

14. A homeless man was involuntarily admitted to the adult psychiatric unit. He has not eaten in three days, sleeps only a few hours a night, and says that people are trying to steal his belongings. On admission, he told the nurse that the television was sending him special messages to leave the hospital. The nurse would determine that this man is exhibiting:
    1. Ideas of reference.

2. Delusions of grandeur.
3. Circumstantiality.
4. Illusions.

15. Which is likely to be the most therapeutic nursing intervention when working with patients with delusional behavior?
    1. Demonstrate to the patient that the delusion is not real.
    ✓ 2. Emphasize reality-oriented behavior.
    3. Ignore the delusions.
    4. Provide the patient with information about the symptoms.

16. When planning care for a patient newly diagnosed with paranoid schizophrenia, what characteristic of the illness should the nurse keep in mind?
    ✓ 1. The patient will misinterpret stimuli in the environment.
    2. The patient will have insight into own dysfunctional behavior.
    3. Behavior is usually socially appropriate.
    4. Perception of changes in self and environment will be lacking.

17. Which initial nursing action would be best for a patient whose diagnosis is paranoid schizophrenia?
    1. Encourage group activity.
    2. Allow time alone, to help the patient initiate contact.
    ✓ 3. Initiate a short, nondemanding relationship.
    4. Hold in-depth one-to-one counseling sessions.

18. What potential problem should be the first nursing concern when a new patient with paranoid schizophrenia is suspicious, restless, and withdrawn?
    1. Inadequate nutrition.
    2. Disorientation and confusion.
    ✓ 3. Aggressiveness.
    4. Sleep deficit.

19. What intervention by the nurse would be appropriate when a patient on the psychiatric unit complains that his shirt has been stolen?
    1. Ask the patient if he wants help to look for the shirt.
    2. Suggest that the patient keep his clothes locked in a place where others cannot take them.
    3. Tell the patient that stealing is not uncommon in the center.
    4. Write an incident report stating that one item is missing.

20. While working with a patient who is paranoid, the nurse should:
    1. Be sure to shake the patient's hand.
    ✓ 2. Avoid touching the patient.
    3. Only touch the patient on the shoulder.
    4. Provide relaxing daily back rubs.

21. Which initial action should the nurse take when the patient refuses to take her oral medications because "they are dangerous"?
    1. Ask the patient if she would prefer an injection.
    2. Find out why the medicines are dangerous.
    3. Withhold the medications until the patient is more amenable to taking them.
    ✓ 4. Proceed to give the pills to the patient, saying firmly that she needs to take them.

Answers/Rationale

1. **(1)** Early in the hospitalization, stressors need to be avoided, since these patients have difficulty in communicating, interacting, and thinking. **No. 2** is not correct because these patients are usually *on* medications, like *Thorazine* or *Haldol*. These are *not* prn meds. The patient needs to develop trust and a relationship with *one* person before being introduced to a group (**No. 3**). Spending consistent time each day with the patient can be therapeutic, but spending 1 hour (**No. 4**) is too long. **IMP, 7, PsI**

2. **(2)** Impaired circulation due to immobility is the greatest concern. Picture catatonic behavior: immobility—staying in one position indefinitely—is the hallmark. A person with catatonic behavior *may not* eat (**No. 1**), but the most important concern is impaired circulation due to immobility. Behavior (**No. 3**) and group participation (**No. 4**) can be eliminated because they involve socialization, which is higher on Maslow's hierarchy of human needs than physiologic integrity. **AN, 3, PhI**

💡 *Test-taking tip:* When the question asks for the *priority*, think *physiologic* integrity, the first level on *Maslow's* hierarchy of needs.

3. **(3)** Withdrawal is a defense mechanism to move away from stimuli that are confusing because they cannot be processed normally. There are no data presented here about the family (**No. 1**). Nos. 2 and 4 are "spin-off" effects, or *secondary* "benefits" of withdrawal. **PL, 7, PsI**

4. **(3)** These behaviors may be indicative of escalating agitation. Frightening hallucinations may lead to anger and hostility, as well as a violent outburst. The behaviors in **No. 1** do not usually indicate a risk of escalating agitation. The behaviors in **Nos. 2 and 4** are signs of improvement. Increased physical activity does not necessarily mean increased agitated activity. **AS, 7, SECE**

5. **(3)** These behaviors indicate social withdrawal related to deterioration in behavior and inappropriate affect that is common in schizophrenia. There are no descriptive data here to indicate thought disturbance (**No. 1**). Although patients with these behaviors generally have low self-esteem (**No. 2**), this is not the most significant nursing diagnosis requiring immediate intervention. There is no indication here that the patient hears voices

---

Key to Codes

Nursing process: AS = Assessment; **AN** = Analysis; **PL** = Planning; **IMP** = Implementation; **EV** = Evaluation. (See Appendix E for explanation of nursing process steps.)

Category of human function: 1 = Protective; **2** = Sensory-Perceptual; **3** = Comfort, Rest, Activity, and Mobility; **4** = Nutrition; **5** = Growth and Development; **6** = Fluid-Gas Transport; **7** = Psychosocial-Cultural; **8** = Elimination.

Client need: SECE = Safe, Effective Care Environment; **PhI** = Physiologic Integrity; **PsI** = Psychosocial Integrity; **HPM** = Health Promotion/Maintenance.

that may lead to self-destructive behavior (**No. 4**). **AN, 7, PsI**

6. **(4)** Before any therapeutic results can be attained, a trusting nurse-patient relationship must be built. The issues of lack of trust, fear, and ambivalence about relationships are problems that need primary nursing focus. **Nos. 1, 2, and 3** would be appropriate goals *after* trust is built and antipsychotic medication has taken effect; the patient will be more able to express feelings (**No. 1**), control behavior (**No. 2**), and care for self (**No. 3**) *later* in the treatment process. **PL, 7, PsI**

7. **(4)** One of Bleuler's four primary symptoms of schizophrenia is *autistic thinking,* of which *neologism* (invented words) is an example. Autism is defined as preoccupation with thoughts and needs that have private, rather than shared meanings. The other options describe the three *other* primary symptoms of schizophrenia (not autistic behaviors): *associative looseness* (**No. 1**) is characterized by putting together unrelated thoughts; flat/inappropriate *affect* (**No. 2**) is characterized by a monotone voice, a bland expression, or inappropriate laughing when talking about sad or painful topics; *ambivalence* (**No. 3**) is manifested by difficulty with decision making or the existence of two opposing emotions (e.g., fear of getting close to another person while at the same time wanting the closeness). **AS, 7, PsI**

💡 *Test-taking tip:* A way to remember Bleuler's primary symptoms of schizophrenia is the mnemonic tool of the *"four As":* Associative looseness, Affect, Ambivalence, and Autism.

8. **(2)** A combination of chemotherapy and one-to-one therapy will be the *most* therapeutic because in addition to use of drugs in treatment, there is also a need for reality orientation, which comes with the one-to-one relationship. ECT (**No. 1**), or electroconvulsive treatment (also known as EST, electroshock treatment), is a mode that is mostly used to treat depression, *not* delusions. Chemotherapy plus group therapy (**No. 3**) is not good because the patient is not ready for working with a group; the need is for one-to-one *first.* Chemotherapy alone (**No. 4**) is not enough, because drugs alone do not provide the needed reality testing. **IMP, 2, SECE**

💡 *Test-taking tip:* You may have been derailed by the word *chemotherapy,* thinking, *"Chemotherapy . . . that means* conditions related to cancer." Don't be fooled into avoiding options that include the word "chemotherapy" if the condition is not cancer. Pull apart the word: *Chemo* = chemical; *therapy* = treatment. "Chemical treatment" simply means drug therapy.

9. **(1)** The nurse provides support by acknowledging the perceptions that seem real to the patient, and provides reality orientation by pointing out that the nurse's perception is different (safety rather than danger). "Putting off" the patient (**No. 2**) is inappropriate, because an *immediate* intervention is needed. Distraction is needed, rather than isolation (**No. 3**). Confrontational reality orientation (**No. 4**) is too direct and does not build trust. **IMP, 7, PsI**

10. **(1)** A delusion is a fixed false belief; in this case, it is a delusion of grandeur. There is no indication that this "power over other people" is meant to harm others; therefore it cannot be seen as a threat (**No. 2**) or a manipulative act (**No. 4**). A manipulative act is usually a deliberate behavior intended to control others. According to Piaget, magical thinking (**No. 3**) is a primitive, prelogical thinking that is often seen in *normal children* who have a strong sense of imagination. Since no age is mentioned in the question, this option can be eliminated as a correct response. **AN, 7, PsI**

11. **(1)** A typical precursor to auditory hallucination is a position that the patient takes to "sit up and listen" to the voice(s). There are insufficient data presented here to substantiate the determination of a desire for attention (**No. 2**) or interaction (**No. 4**). By definition, a mannerism (**No. 3**) is a repetitive, *involuntary* movement (like lip-smacking), and does not apply to this behavior. **EV, 7, PsI**

12. **(1)** This comment is an example of a visual and tactile hallucination. **No. 2** is an example of an *illusion;* the definition of an illusion is a misinterpretation of an actual external sensory stimuli (the lamppost). **No. 3** is an example of a *delusion* of persecution. **No. 4** is an example of a *delusion* of grandeur. **AN, 7, PsI**

13. **(3)** As an initial intervention, this encourages her to discuss her *feelings,* and *decreases verbalization* of the false belief (delusion). The response in **No. 1** is *not* supportive; **No. 2** reinforces focus on the *delusion;* **No. 4** *decreases* trust. **PL, 7, PsI**

14. **(1)** The patient has false ideas and interpretations of external events (messages on TV), as though they had direct reference to him. The other descriptions (not eating or sleeping and thoughts about people stealing belongings) may be a reality in the life of a homeless person. **Nos. 2, 3, and 4** are incorrect because, by definition, they are *other* types of faulty thought processes that do *not* describe this man's behavior. **AN, 7, PsI**

15. **(2)** By focusing on reality-based topics, the nurse limits the time the patient has to focus on delusional activity. Showing that the delusions are false (**No. 1**) will only serve to increase anxiety, which in turn will increase the use of delusions to defend against the anxiety. The patient *needs* the delusions and will hold on to delusional thoughts even more when attempts are made to disprove them. It is only when anxiety is decreased through treatment (therapeutic relationship) that the patient can let go of the delusions. Delusions should not be ignored (**No. 3**); however, they will be deemphasized by focusing on reality-based topics. Providing information (**No. 4**) is inappropriate because the level of anxiety that accompanies delusional activity will interfere with learning or processing of information. **IMP, 7, PsI**

16. **(1)** Patients with this disorder tend to see others and/or the environment as dangerous, bad, or wrong. These patients *lack* insight (**No. 2**), as do most patients with psychotic disorders. Socially *inappropriate* behavior is common (**No. 3**). The patient *does* perceive (**No. 4**), but misinterprets what is perceived. **PL, 7, PsI**

17. **(3)** Distance and brief contacts that are neither over-

whelming nor threatening are best. A group activity (**No. 1**) is inappropriate, because it would be overwhelming. The nurse *first* needs to build trust slowly, in a one-to-one relationship. The result of leaving the patient alone (**No. 2**) will be avoidance of the patient, which is not therapeutic. Intense contact (**No. 4**) is inappropriate because it would be threatening to a patient with paranoid behavior. **IMP, 7, PsI**

18. (**3**) Due to probable delusional behavior, the patient may misinterpret cues in the environment, perceiving them as threatening; the nurse must therefore watch for aggressive behavior (as a defensive reaction by the patient). Nutrition (**No. 1**) and sleep (**No. 4**) are not typically deficient; hence, assessment of dietary and sleep deficits can be done *following* assessment for potential aggressiveness. *Safety* is a prime concern. Confusion may occur, but not usually disorientation (**No. 2**); moreover, they would not be the primary nursing concern with a paranoid schizophrenic diagnosis. **AN, 7, PsI**

19. (**1**) This response is aimed at keeping the patient from jumping to conclusions. **Nos. 2 and 3** would make the patient feel more insecure and unsafe, by implying that the shirt has indeed been stolen or will be in the future if the patient is not careful. Before concluding and reporting that the shirt is missing (**No. 4**), a careful search needs to be done first. **IMP, 7, PsI**

20. (**2**) This is the *only* option in which there is no physical contact. A patient whose mode of interaction is suspiciousness typically feels threatened by the close physical contact involved in **Nos. 1, 3, and 4.** Touch may often be misinterpreted as feared, unwanted sexual contact or as an aggressive act. The nurse should allow extra personal distance. **PL, 7, PsI**

Test-taking tip: Look at the pattern: Which one is not like the others? Three options involve touching the patient, but one option involves "no touch."

21. (**4**) This response is best because it does not reinforce the paranoid delusion, and the nurse comes across as sounding certain (in a matter-of-fact tone) that the medication is a necessary part of treatment. **No. 1** reinforces the delusion that the pill may be dangerous; moreover, an injection may be more threatening. **No. 2** maintains focus on the delusional belief. **No. 3** is incorrect because the medication *must* be given to relieve paranoid thoughts. **IMP, 7, PsI**

Mood Disorders

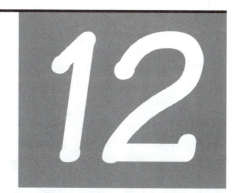

Chapter Outline

- Depressive Disorders
  - Major Depression
  - Dysthymic Disorder
- Bipolar Disorders
  - Manic
  - Depressed

- Study and Memory Aids
- Glossary
- Summary of Key Points
- Questions
- Answers/Rationale

Mood disorders are a group of diagnostic categories that describe a range of emotional disturbances whose essential feature is a substantial decrease in or entire loss of control over mood. Functional mood disorders are subclassified as: (1) *Depressive disorders* (including *major depression* and *dysthymia*) and (2) *Bipolar disorders* (including *mania* and *cyclothymia*). The mood disturbance may occur in a number of patterns of severity and duration, alone or in combination, where client feels extreme sadness and guilt, withdraws socially, expresses self-deprecatory thoughts (*major depression*), *or* experiences an elevated, expansive mood with hyperactivity, pressured speech, inflated self-esteem, decreased need for sleep (*manic episode or disorder*).

These affective disorders should be *distinguished* from *grief*. Grief is *realistic* and proportionate to what has been *specifically* lost and involves *no loss of self-esteem*. There is a *constant* feeling of sadness over a period of 3–12 mo or longer, with good reality contact (no delusions).

Depressive Disorders

A mood disorder with one or more episodes of major depression *without* a history of a manic or hypomanic episode.

Major Depression

Depressed mood and loss of interest or pleasure in life. Other symptoms are listed below.

I. Concepts and principles
A. *Self-limiting* factors—most depressions are self-limiting disturbances, making it important to look for a change in functioning and behavior.
B. *Theories of cause of depression*
    1. Aggression turned inward—*self-anger*.
    2. Response to separation or object *loss*.
    3. *Genetic* and/or *biochemical* basis (Table 12.1).
    4. *Cognitive:* negative mind-set of hopelessness.

    5. *Personality:* negative self-concept, low self-esteem affect belief system and appraisal of stressors.
    6. *Learned helplessness:* environment can't be controlled.
    7. *Behavioral:* loss of positive reinforcement.
    8. *Integrated:* interaction of chemical, experiential, and behavioral variables acting on diencephalon.

▶ II. General assessment
A. *Physical*
    1. Sleep disturbances: Early-morning awakening, *insomnia* at night, increased need for sleep during the day, fatigue.
    2. Constipation.
    3. *Anorexia* with weight loss.
    4. Amenorrhea.
    5. Loss of sexual interest.
    6. *Psychomotor retardation.*
B. *Psychological*
    1. Inability to remember.
    2. Decreased *concentration.*
    3. Slowing or blocking of thought, all-or-nothing thinking.
    4. *Less interest* and involvement with external world and own appearance, difficulty in enjoying activities.
    5. Feeling worse at certain times of day or after any sleep.
    6. Difficulty in enjoying activities.
    7. Monotonous voice.
    8. *Repetitive* discussions.
    9. *Inability to make decisions* due to ambivalence, impaired coping with "practical problems."
    10. Suicidal thoughts.
C. *Emotional*
    1. Loss of self-esteem; feelings of *hopelessness*

TABLE 12.1   THEORIES OF CAUSATIVE FACTORS RELATED TO THE DEVELOPMENT OF DEPRESSION

Biologic	*Psychological*	*Cognitive*	*Sociocultural*
Genetic Possible genetic influence	Dependency	Narrow, negative perspective called "cognitive triad": view of self, world, and the future	Social situations that contribute to feelings of powerlessness and low self-esteem:
Hormonal influence (drop in estrogen and progesterone)	Low self-esteem		Status of minority groups
	Powerlessness		
Biochemical	Ambivalence	Draws conclusions on inadequate or contradictory evidence	Status of women in male-oriented professional and business culture
Impaired neurotransmission of monoamine oxidase (MAO)	Guilt		
High levels of catecholamines (dopamine and norepinephrine)	Lack of support system	Overgeneralizes from one instance	Role loss, such as loss of mother role in empty nest phase
	Severe stress		
Toxic reactions	Lack of clear goals	Focuses on a single detail rather than on the whole	Being the object of cultural stereotypes (e.g., African Americans, aged, Jews)
	Feelings of failure		
	Inability to fulfill expectations	Distortion of long-range consequences, hence bad judgment	

Source: Wilson HS, Kneisl CR. *Psychiatric Nursing* (3rd ed). Redwood City, CA: Addison-Wesley, 1983. p. 371.

and *worthlessness;* shame and self-derogation due to *guilt.*

2. *Irritability,* despair, and *futility* (leading to *suicidal* thoughts).

3. Alienation, *helplessness,* passivity, avoidance, *inertia,* powerlessness.

4. Denied anger; uncooperative, tense, crying, demanding.

5. *Dependent* behavior.

III. Analysis/nursing diagnosis

A. *Altered nutrition* (anorexia) related to lack of interest in food.

B. *Risk for violence* toward self (suicide) related to inability to verbalize emotions.

C. *Sleep pattern disturbance* (insomnia or excessive sleep) related to emotional dysfunctioning.

D. *Self-care deficit* related to disinterest in activities of daily living.

E. *Chronic low self-esteem* with self-reproaches and blame related to feelings of inadequacy.

F. *Altered feeling states* and *meaning patterns* (sadness, loneliness, apathy) related to overwhelming feeling of unworthiness and dysfunctional grieving.

G. *Altered social interaction* related to social isolation and *withdrawal.*

IV. Nursing care plan/implementation

A. Promote sleep and food intake—take nursing measures to ensure the *physical* well-being of the client.

B. Provide steady company to assess *suicidal* tendencies and to diminish feelings of loneliness and alienation.

1. Build trust in a 1:1 relationship.

2. Interact with client on a nonverbal level if that is client's immediate mode of communication; this will promote feelings of being recognized, *accepted,* and understood.

3. Focus on *today,* not the past or far into the future.

4. Reassure that present state is temporary and that client will be protected and helped.

C. Make the *environment* nonchallenging and nonthreatening.

1. Use a kind, firm attitude, with warmth.

2. See that client has *favorite foods;* respond to other wishes and likes.

3. Protect from overstimulation and coercion.

D. Postpone client's *decision making* and resumption of duties.

1. Allow *more time* than usual to complete activity (dressing, eating) or thought process and speech.

2. Structure the environment for client to help reestablish a set schedule and predictable *routine* during ambivalence and problems with decisions.

E. *Provide nonintellectual activities* (e.g., sanding wood). *Avoid* intellectual activities (e.g., chess and crossword puzzles) as thinking capacity at this time tends to be circular.

F. *Encourage expression* of emotions, denial, hopelessness, helplessness, guilt, regret.

1. Provide *outlets for anger* that may be underlying the depression; as client becomes more verbal with anger and recognizes the origin

and results of anger, help client resolve feelings.

2. Allow client to complain and be *demanding* in initial phases of depression.

G. *Discourage redundancy* in speech and thought by redirecting focus from a monologue of painful recounts to an appraisal of more neutral or positive attributes and aspects of situations.

H. Encourage client to *assess own* goals, unrealistic expectations, and perfectionist tendencies.

1. May need to change goals or give up some goals that are incompatible with abilities and external situations.

2. Assist client to recapture what was lost through substitution of goals, sublimation, or relinquishment of unrealistic goals.

  a. Reanchor client's self-respect to other aspects of his or her existence.

  b. Help client free self from *dependency* on one person or single event or idea.

I. Indicate that success is possible and not hopeless.

1. Explore what steps client has taken to achieve goals and suggest new or alternate ones.

2. Set *small, immediate goals* to help attain mastery.

3. Recognize client's efforts to mobilize self.

4. Provide positive reinforcement for client through exposure to activities in which client can experience a sense of *success, achievement,* and *completion* to build *self-esteem* and self-confidence.

5. Help client experience *pleasure;* help client start good relationships in social setting.

J. Long-term goal: to encourage interest in external surroundings, outside of self, to increase and strengthen social relationships.

1. Encourage purposeful activities.

2. Let client advance to activities at own pace (graded task assignments).

3. Gradually encourage activities with others.

K. Health teaching

1. Explain need to recognize highly stressful situations and fatigue as stress factors.

2. Advise that negative responses from others be regarded with minimum significance; explain need to maintain positive self-attitude.

3. Advise occasional respite from responsibilities.

4. Emphasize need for realistic expectation of others.

▶ **V. Evaluation/outcome criteria**

A. Performs self-care.

B. Expresses increased self-confidence; identifies positive attributes and skills in self.

C. Engages in activities with others; accepts positive statements from others.

Dysthymic Disorder

Dysthymia (depressive neurosis) is a chronic (rather than episodic) mood disorder characterized by depressed feeling and loss of interest or pleasure in one's usual activities, but symptoms are not of sufficient severity or duration to be classified as *major depression.* Psychotic features are absent. Diagnosis is made after two years of chronic symptoms. Table 12.2 summarizes the main points of difference between *dysthymia* and *major depression.*

Bipolar Disorders

Bipolar disorders are mood disorders characterized by mood swings, alternating from depression to elation, with periods of relative normality between episodes. Bipolar disorders are subdivided into (a) *manic,* (b) *depressed,* (c) *mixed*—if manic and depressive episodes alternate every few days, (d) *cyclothymia*—alternating periods of hypomania and depression, with mood swings out of proportion to apparent stimuli; less severe than manic and depressive phases of bipolar disorder. Most persons experience a *single* episode of *manic* or *depressed* type; some have *recurrent* depression or recurrent mania or *mixed.* There is increasing evidence that a biochemical disturbance may exist and that most individuals with manic episodes eventually develop depressive episodes.

I. Concepts and principles related to bipolar disorders

A. The psychodynamics of manic and depressive episodes are related to hostility and guilt and the need to relieve internal discomfort of these reactions.

1. *Manic* phase: hostile feelings are *projected* onto others or onto objects in the environment.

2. *Depressive* phase: hostility and guilt are *introjected* toward self.

B. The struggle between unconscious impulses and moral conscience produces feelings of *hostility, guilt,* and *anxiety.*

C. Demands, irritability, sarcasm, profanity, destructiveness, and threats are signs of the *projection of hostility;* guilt is handled through *persecutory delusions* and *accusations.*

D. Feelings of inferiority and fear of rejection are handled by being light and amusing.

E. Both phases, though appearing distinctly different, have the *same objective: to gain attention, approval, and emotional support.* These objectives and behaviors are unconsciously determined by the client; this behavior may be either biochemically determined or *both* biochemically and unconsciously determined.

▶ **II. Assessment** of bipolar disorders

A. Manic and depressed types are *opposite* sides of the *same* disorder.

1. Both are disturbances of mood and self-esteem.

2. Both have underlying aggression and hostility.

3. Both are intense.

4. Both are self-limited in duration.

B. Comparison of mania and depression: Table 12.3.

▶ **III. Analysis/nursing diagnosis**

A. *Risk for injury* related to poor judgment.

B. *Altered nutrition, less than body requirements,* related to inability to sit down long enough to eat.

C. *Sleep pattern disturbance:* lack of sleep and rest related to restlessness, hyperactivity, emotional dysfunctioning.

TABLE 12.2   COMPARISON OF THE TWO DIFFERENT TYPES OF DEPRESSIVE DISORDERS

Dimension	Major Depressive Disorder	Dysthymic Disorder
Cause	Primary disturbance in structure and function of brain and nervous system	Severe, prolonged stress, unresolved conflicts; chronic anxiety, fears, anger
Onset	Rapid and without apparent cause	Gradual
Form of depression	Restlessness and agitation, *or* psychomotor retardation; severe; tends to be worse in morning and better in evening	Mixed; mild to severe; unpredictable mood; usually optimistic in morning and depressed in evening
Sleep	Insomnia after being awakened	Easily awakened, but goes back to deep sleep in morning
Appetite	Anorexia leading to weight loss	Varied (anorexia leading to compulsive eating)
Activity	Chronically tired; needs structure at all times	Occasional energy bursts (feels embarrassed at lack of energy)
Self-esteem	Very low	Fluctuates from high to low
Fears	Intense fear of being alone	Multiple fears about present and future
Decision making	Totally indecisive	O.K. on minor decisions; indecisive on important decisions
Memory	Poor	Unreliable
Contact with reality	Poor; paranoid, self-deprecatory delusions, distorted judgment	Varies

D. *Self-care deficits* related to altered motor behavior due to anxiety (e.g., not able to perform or complete feeding, dressing, grooming activities).

E. *Altered feeling state* (anger), *judgment, thought content* (magical thinking), *thought processes* (altered concentration and problem solving) related to disturbance in self-concept.

F. *Altered feeling states:* mood swings.

G. *Altered attention:* hyperalertness.

H. *Impaired social interaction* related to internal and external stimuli (overload, underload).

◄ IV. **Nursing care plan/implementation**

  A. **Manic**

    1. Prevent *physical* dangers stemming from suicide and exhaustion: promote rest, sleep, and intake of nourishment.

      ☞ a. Use *suicide* precautions.

      b. Reduce outside stimuli or remove to quieter area.

      c. *Diet:* provide *high-calorie beverages, high-protein,* high-carbohydrate soft *finger foods* that can be consumed on the run, without spilling, and do *not* require use of a knife (need to be concerned with safety due to poor judgment).

    2. Attend to client's personal care.

    3. Absorb with understanding and without reproach behaviors such as talkativeness, provocativeness, criticism, sarcasm, dominance, profanity, and dramatic actions.

      a. Allow, postpone, or partially fulfill demands and freedom of expression *within limits* of ordinary social rules, comfort, and safety of client and others.

      b. *Do not* cut off manic stream of talk, as this

increases anxiety and need for release of hostility.

    4. Constructively utilize excessive energies with *activities* that do *not* call for concentration or follow-through.

      a. Outdoor walks, gardening, putting, and ball-tossing are therapeutic.

      b. Exciting, disturbing, and highly *competitive* activities should be *avoided*.

      c. Creative occupational therapy activities promote release of hostile impulses, as does creative writing.

    💊 5. Give tranquilizers as ordered until lithium affects symptoms (*3 wk*); then give lithium carbonate as ordered.

    6. Help client to recognize and express *feelings* (denial, hopelessness, anger, guilt, blame, helplessness).

    7. Encourage realistic self-concept.

    8. *Health teaching:* how to monitor effects of lithium; *when* blood levels are usually drawn; and diet.

      a. In the *acute* phase, blood is drawn 10–14 hr after the last dose is taken tid; then every 2–3 d until 1.6 mEq/L is reached; then once a wk while in the hospital; and then every 2–3 mo to maintain therapeutic blood levels.

      b. The *side effects* to watch for when blood levels are 1.6–2.0 mEq/L are: tremors, nausea, vomiting and diarrhea, polyuria and polydipsia. Side effects with levels *above* 2.0 mEq/L are: motor weakness, ataxia, headaches, edema, and lethargy. *Severe* signs of toxicity are neurologic: twitching,

TABLE 12.3   COMPARISON OF MANIA AND DEPRESSION

	Mania (periods of predominantly and persistently elevated, expansive, or irritable mood)	*Depression* (loss of interest or pleasure in usual activities)
Affect	Lack of shame or guilt Inflated self-esteem; euphoria Intolerance of criticism	Delusions of guilt, anger; anxiety, apathy, denial, helplessness, feelings of doom, hopelessness, loneliness Low self-esteem (self-degradation)
Physiology	Insomnia Inadequate nutrition, weight loss	Insomnia Anorexia, constipation, indigestion, nausea, vomiting → weight loss
Cognition	Denial of realistic danger *Thoughts:* flight of ideas, loose associations, illusions, delusions of grandeur Lack of judgment Distractibility	Self-destructive (preoccupied with suicide); self-blame *Thoughts:* Ambivalent, confused, inability to concentrate Loss of interest and motivation
Behavior	Hyperactivity (social, sexual, work) → irrationality, aggressiveness, sarcasm, exhibitionism, and acting-out in behavior and dress Hostile, arrogant, argumentative, demanding, and controlling *Speech:* rapid, rhyming, punning, witty, pressured	Altered activity level, social isolation Overdependency, underachievement, inability to care for self *Psychomotor retardation* Substance abuse

marked drowsiness, slurred speech, dysarthria, convulsions, delirium, stupor, and coma.

  c. *Health teaching* concerning dietary implications: lithium needs to be taken *with* meals to reduce GI symptoms; urge client to drink *2–3 liters of liquids/day;* patient should *avoid* caffeine, crash diets, self-prescribed low-salt diet, and acids (which increase lithium excretion and reduce drug's effect).

B. Depressed
  1. Take routine *suicide* precautions.
  2. Give attention to *physical* needs for food and sleep and to hygiene needs. Prepare warm baths and hot beverages to aid sleep.
  3. Initiate *frequent* contacts:
     a. *Do not allow long periods of silence* to develop or client to remain withdrawn.
     b. Use a kind, understanding, but emotionally neutral approach.
  4. *Allow dependency* in severe depressive phase. Since dependency is one of the underlying concerns with depressive persons, if nurse allows dependency to occur as an initial response, he or she must plan for resolution of the dependency toward himself or herself as an example for the client's other dependent relationships.
  5. Slowly repeat simple, direct information.

  6. *Assist in daily decision making* until client regains self-confidence.
  7. Select *mild* exercise and diversionary *activities* instead of stimulating exercise and competitive games, as they may overtax physical and emotional endurance and lead to feelings of inadequacy and frustration.
  8. Give antidepressive drugs such as tricyclics.
  9. *Health teaching:* how to make simple decisions related to health care.

V. Evaluation/outcome criteria
  A. *Manic:* speech and activity are slowed down; affect is less hostile; able to sleep; able to eat with others at the table.
  B. *Depressed:* takes prescribed medications regularly; does not engage in self-destructive activities; able to express feelings of anger, helplessness, hopelessness.

💡 Study and Memory Aids

Manic—Interventions

Diet: ↑ calories, ↑ protein, ↑ carbohydrate finger foods
Drugs: give tranquilizers; then lithium carbonate (lag effect)

Depression: general assessment— "FLAT"

Feelings: despair and hopelessness
Low energy
Affect (flat); **A**norexia
Trouble sleeping (insomnia)

Depression assessment: physical

↓ Activity (can also be ↑)
Appetite (anorexia)
Bowels (constipation)
Libido (lack of sexual interest)
Energy (fatigue)
Sleep (insomnia)

Depression assessment: thoughts— "NPO"

Negative (about self, future, others)
Poverty of ideas
Obsessed with suicidal ideation

Depression assessment: mood

"Three Ds" { **D**espair
Dysphoric
"**D**own" }

Nursing goals: "Four Ss"

1. **S**afety (physical well-being)
2. **S**uicide prevention
3. **S**upportive approach
4. **S**ocialization

Manic: mental status exam—"COAST MAP"

Concentration: impaired
Orientation × 3 (time, place, person)
Activity: hyper; inappropriate
Speech: rapid, forced, vulgar, loud
Thought disorder: flight of ideas, delusions of grandeur

Memory: intact
Affect: elated
Perception: may be disturbed

Source: Caroline N. *Emergency Care in the Streets* (5th ed). Boston: Little, Brown, 1995. p 912.

Depression: interventions—"PEER"

Provide for physical needs: nutrition, sleep, hygiene
Express feelings
Exercise and simple activities to ↑ self-esteem
Risk **R**eduction, for suicide

Common antidepressive medications: Tricyclics—"VENT"*

Vivactil
Elavil
Norpramin
Tofranil

*Remember: "Patients need to *vent* (externalize) feelings."

Glossary

affect *External observable* manifestation of emotion (e.g., flat, labile, expansive).

bipolar disorder A subgroup of mood disorders, with at least one episode of manic state (exaggerated, expansive, or elevated mood).

circumstantial speech Person digresses into extraneous and unnecessary details and inappropriate thoughts before communicating a central idea; may serve the purpose of avoiding an emotionally charged area.

clang association A speech pattern in which sounds determine which words are chosen, as in rhyming or punning. Seen in mania, schizophrenia, autism.

cyclothymic A chronic mood disorder of at least two years' duration, characterized by alternating periods of hypomania (elation) and depression (sadness) with normal mood states in between; mood swings are out of proportion to apparent stimuli; however, symptoms are less severe than in manic and depressive phases of bipolar disorder.

depression A persistent emotional condition, ranging from mild sadness to extreme despair; can be an abnormal (morbid) extension of dejection, sadness, and grief, accompanied by feelings of hopelessness, inadequacy, unworthiness, and lowering of functional activity (e.g., can't work or carry on daily activities). Term used as a sign, mood, symptom, syndrome, reaction, state, or illness (e.g., major depression). *Distinguished from grief,* which is realistic and usually in proportion to the loss.

dysthymia A chronic (rather than episodic) mood disorder with an absence of psychotic features; characterized by persistent depression and loss of interest of pleasure in usual activities for at least two years. Tend to feel worse as day progresses. Not as severe as major depression. May have anorexia or overeat; may have insomnia or hypersomnia.

🔑 Summary of Key Points

Assessment of Depressive Phase

Mood	Flat, apathetic, despairing, tearful
Speech	Monosyllabic, monotonous, redundant
Behavior	Slow, tired, may be agitated; ↓ libido; suicidal
Thoughts	Confused, blocking, all-or-nothing thinking
Viewpoint	Negative view (of self, world, future)
Sleep	Trouble sleeping (insomnia)
Appetite	Decreased (anorexia)

Care of a Patient Who Is Depressed

1. Provide for *physical* needs: nutrition, exercise, prevention of constipation, hygiene, adequate rest.
2. Prevent *suicide*.
3. Promote expression of thoughts and feelings (angry, despairing).
4. Initiate frequent contacts: supportive, permissive, concerned approach.
5. Provide a *structured* environment, with limited decision making.
6. Restore socialization: encourage simple activities.
7. *Long-term goal:* enhance *self-esteem*, sense of dignity, and self-worth through purposeful activities and social relationships.

Assessment of Manic Phase

Mood	Elevated, expansive, irritable
Speech	Loud, rapid, forced, rhyming, punning (clang association); vulgar
Behavior	Hyperactive; inappropriate (sexually); distractible
Thoughts	Flight of ideas
Viewpoint	Grandiose (delusions)
Sleep	↓ need
Appetite	Forgets to eat

Care of a Patient Who Is Manic

1. Prevent physical dangers related to hyperactivity and resulting in suicide.
2. Reduce external stimuli; encourage sleep to prevent exhaustion.
3. Offer 3000–4000 calories in finger foods or fluids.
4. Suggest activities that are solo and noncompetitive.
5. Administer prescribed *lithium*. Draw blood level 12 hr after last dose; therapeutic level for acute care = 0.8–1.6 mEq/L; toxic level = > 2.0 mEq/L. *Avoid* dehydration and salt depletion. Give with meals to decrease GI side effects.
6. Set limits; be firm.

May be introverted, brooding, demanding, and self-degrading. See Table 12.2 for differences from depression.

euphoria Exaggerated feeling of physical and emotional well-being *not* related to external events or stimuli. Most often seen in manic phase of bipolar disorder.

mania A pathologic condition characterized by exaggerated euphoric mood, hyperactivity, irritability, and impaired concentration, flight of ideas, grandiosity, and impaired judgment (e.g., buying sprees, sexual indiscretion, inappropriate joking).

mood An *internal, subjectively* experienced emotion or feeling state that is pervasive and influences personality and functioning (e.g., sad, depressed, joyful, angry).

psychomotor retardation A generalized slowing of motor activity that is characteristic of severe depression.

tangential communication Responses that digress or are irrelevant to topic at hand, with a focus on an incidental aspect.

Questions

1. Before planning interventions with patients who direct anger at themselves, the nurse needs to know that this behavior may be a cause of:
   1. Aggression.
   2. Repression.
   3. Sublimation.
   4. Depression.
2. The nurse's initial approach in caring for a patient with major depression would be to:
   1. Encourage the patient to select her own meals.
   2. Involve the patient in group therapy.
   3. Sit silently at the patient's side when she does not feel like talking.
   4. Provide cheerful activities.
3. A teenager is admitted to the psychiatric unit for observation and evaluation of severe depression. During which time period will the patient most likely experience intense melancholia?
   1. Upon awakening in the morning.
   2. At the end of the day.
   3. In the middle of the afternoon.
   4. On weekends.
4. What would be significant for the nurse to assess as contributing factors while interviewing a patient who is depressed?
   1. Family structure.
   2. Reaction to any existing chronic illness or disability.
   3. History of significant losses.
   4. Manifestations of depression.
5. A patient who is depressed has been put on *Elavil* at HS (hour of sleep), and wants to know when the drug will most likely take effect. Which response by the nurse best demonstrates knowledge of this drug's action?
   1. 24–48 hours.

2. 8–10 days.
3. 2–3 weeks.
4. One month.

6. Which physical aspect will be most important for the nurse to assess in a patient with depression?
   1. Sleep patterns.
   2. Bladder function.
   3. Bowel function.
   4. Socialization behaviors.

7. A patient is hospitalized in acute manic phase. During the first few days of caring for this patient, the nurse's primary plan of care needs to include a focus on the patient's degree of:
   1. Exhaustion and decreased nutrition.
   2. Decreased self-esteem and inappropriate grooming.
   3. Flirtatious and provocative behavior.
   4. Demanding and impulsive behavior.

8. Which action should be included in the initial nursing plan of care for a recently admitted patient with bipolar disorder?
   1. Place the patient in a quiet environment.
   2. Put the patient in seclusion.
   3. Ensure that the therapeutic lithium level is reached.
   4. Provide 1:1 supervision.

9. In providing adequate nutrition for a person in manic phase, which would be the best diet consideration?
   1. Finger foods high in protein, such as bananas and peanut butter sandwiches.
   2. Foods high in fiber and low in fats, such as bran muffins and fish.
   3. Liquids, such as cream soup, and pudding.
   4. Foods high in carbohydrates, such as baked potatoes.

10. A middle-aged woman is admitted with a diagnosis of bipolar disorder, manic phase. In the past few days, she has charged $500 worth of makeup, and told her daughter that she is a royal princess and cannot find her diamond crown. During the first day in the mental health unit, this patient enters the recreation area and tells the other patients they must kneel when she is present. The nurse's initial intervention would be to:
    1. Confront the patient about her superior attitude.
    2. Take the patient to a less stimulating area.
    3. Engage the patient in an intense individual session.
    4. Prepare to take the patient to the seclusion room.

11. When a patient in acute manic phase says that she is the President of the United States, the nurse determines that the patient is experiencing:
    1. Delusions of grandeur.
    2. Loose associations.
    3. Tangential communication.
    4. Circumstantial speech.

12. What activity is best for a patient in manic phase?
    1. Volleyball.
    2. Walking with a nurse.
    3. Bingo.
    4. A puzzle.

13. What is the therapeutic serum lithium level for a patient in acute manic phase of a bipolar disorder?
    1. > 2.0 mEq/L.
    2. 0.8–1.6 mEq/L.
    3. 1.0–1.2 mEq/L.
    4. < 1.0 mEq/L.

14. When a patient is on lithium for bipolar disorder, what is especially important for the nurse to teach about the diet?
    1. The diet should be high in fiber.
    2. Fluids should be increased.
    3. The diet should be low in protein.
    4. The diet should include adequate salt.

15. What is the best food to give a patient in manic phase of bipolar disorder?
    1. Barbecued steak.
    2. Turkey burger.
    3. Scrambled eggs.
    4. Broiled fish.

Answers/Rationale

1. **(4)** Anger turned inward is a common cause of depression. Aggression (**No. 1**) is anger turned *outward*. Repression (**No. 2**) is a means of denying anger by pushing it out of conscious awareness; it might be manifested by forced "sweetness." Sublimation of anger (**No. 3**) may involve channeling the anger into a constructive outlet (e.g., shoveling snow) or a socially accepted role outlet (e.g., becoming a police officer). **EV, 7, PsI**

2. **(3)** This option conveys acceptance, with no demands. The key word here is "initial"; showing acceptance is an important *initial* intervention. **No. 1** is incorrect because it involves decision making, which is a problem in major depression. The nurse should provide direction until depression lifts and the patient can participate in more decision making. The greater the depression, the more active and directive the nurse needs to be. **No. 2** is incorrect because a depressed patient needs to start with 1:1 interaction, *not* group therapy. **No. 4** is definitely not good because an attitude of "merry sunshine" ("Good morning! How are you this lovely day?") when a person is depressed usually evokes an angry response. Be matter-of-fact. Avoid an overly cheerful approach. **PL, 7, PsI**

3. **(4)** Weekends tend to be the most difficult time period for teenagers, since that is typically a time when they get together with peers. Loneliness is likely to be accentuated at this time. In the absence of further data regarding the type of depression (major depressive disorder or dysthymic disorder), it is not possible to determine whether melancholy would characteristically be more severe in the morning (**No. 1**) or at the end of the day (**No. 2**). Afternoons (**No. 3**) are not associated

---

Key to Codes

Nursing process: AS = Assessment; **AN** = Analysis; **PL** = Planning; **IMP** = Implementation; **EV** = Evaluation. (See Appendix E for explanation of nursing process steps.)

Category of human function: 1 = Protective; **2** = Sensory-Perceptual; **3** = Comfort, Rest, Activity, and Mobility; **4** = Nutrition; **5** = Growth and Development; **6** = Fluid-Gas Transport; **7** = Psychosocial-Cultural; **8** = Elimination.

Client need: SECE = Safe, Effective Care Environment; **PhI** = Physiologic Integrity; **PsI** = Psychosocial Integrity; **HPM** = Health Promotion/Maintenance.

with increasing loneliness and potentiating depression. **AS, 7, PsI**

4. **(3)** Theories of the causes of depression include unresolved loss (which may be actual, symbolic, interpersonal, economic, or physiologic), as well as "anger turned inward." Family *history* (genetic/biochemical factors), *not* family *structure* **(No. 1)**, is a contributing factor to depression. Chronic illness and disability **(No. 2)** are incorporated in the theory of loss **(No. 3)**, e.g., loss of body function such as loss of mobility due to amputation. Manifestations **(No. 4)** are the signs and symptoms of depression, *not* contributing factors. **AS, 7, PsI**

💡 *Test-taking tips:*

• Eliminate options that do not meet the condition of the question stem (in this case, *contributing factor*); be aware of nuances in terminology.

• Choose the one option **(No. 3)** that incorporates (includes) another option **(No. 2)**; this is a *telescope* answer.

5. **(3)** There is a time lag before a patient will notice any appreciable effects of the medication. **Nos. 1 and 2** are too short a time for the drug to reach a therapeutic level. **No. 4** is longer than usual. **EV, 7, PsI**

6. **(1)** Sleep disturbances (insomnia or hypersomnia) can be both an antecedent factor and a result of a depressive state. Depression can be *potentiated* by sleep deprivation. Bladder function **(No. 2)** is *not* a relevant factor in depressive states. Bowel dysfunction **(No. 3)**, in the form of constipation, may occur when a person is depressed; everything "slows down," including the bowels; however, constipation is not a problem that makes depression *worse*. Socialization behavior **(No. 4)** is *not* a physical aspect, which is called for in the question. **AS, 8, PsI**

💡 *Test-taking tip:* Eliminate as the correct option one that doesn't meet the condition in the question stem (in this case, **No. 4**, "*physical* aspect").

7. **(1)** Although all of the behaviors listed may be displayed by the manic patient, the basic human needs of rest and food (affected by hyperactivity) must be met *first*. **Nos. 2, 3, and 4** are not good choices at *this* time, but can be addressed *later*. **PL, 3, PsI**

💡 *Test-taking tip:* Priority care is usually given to *physical* needs **(No. 1)**. The higher level of basic human needs (according to Maslow, e.g., self-esteem and behaviors related to socialization) are not the priority concern here **(Nos. 2, 3, 4)**.

8. **(1)** External sources of visual and auditory stimulation need to be reduced, to avoid overstimulation or to encourage sleep. Although **Nos. 2 and 4** also refer to a therapeutic environment, seclusion **(No. 2)** and 1:1 supervision **(No. 4)** are not necessary as the *first* goal. Maintenance of serum lithium levels **(No. 3)** is a *later* intervention. **PL, 1, PsI**

9. **(1)** Because of the patient's hyperactivity, the best diet is one that is high in protein and includes foods that are easy to eat during short attention spans. **Nos. 2, 3, and 4** all require longer eating times (the patient must sit down and concentrate on using utensils); also, these op-

tions do not address the nutritional need for increased protein. **IMP, 4, HPM**

10. **(2)** The increased activity in the recreation room may increase the patient's delusions, so the initial intervention would be to remove her to a quiet area. **No. 1** is incorrect because the patient does *not* have a superior attitude, but she is delusional; confrontation is not helpful at this time. **No. 3** is not a good choice because the patient is *not* capable of insight and has a short attention span. **No. 4** is incorrect because seclusion would be used only as a *last resort*, if at all. **IMP, 3, PsI**

11. **(1)** The patient has a false *belief* of great power and prestige, which is a delusion of grandeur. Loose associations **(No. 2)** refer to a lack of clarity and connection between thoughts. Tangential communication **(No. 3)** is the loss of the main topic while speaking, while circumstantial speech **(No. 4)** is the inclusion of many nonessential details; the problem in this case is *not in speaking* but in a false *belief*. **AN, 7, PsI**

💡 *Test-taking tip:* Look at patterns. For an educated guess, select the one that is different (three options deals with *speech;* one with *belief*).

12. **(2)** This is a nonstimulating, 1:1 activity that is noncompetitive and doesn't require concentration; yet it provides an outlet to discharge the high energy level. Volleyball **(No. 1)** is not good because it requires a group, cooperative effort, with a win-lose competitive element; this is all too stimulating for someone who is hyperactive. Bingo **(No. 3)** is not good because it also is too stimulating; it involves concentration and sitting down, which is not usually possible while the patient is manic (especially since there are no data here to indicate that the patient is on lithium medication)! A puzzle **(No. 4)** is not good because it also requires concentration, a problem for a patient who is hyperactive and on-the-go. **IMP, 3, PsI**

13. **(2)** This is the accurate therapeutic range and therefore the only correct option. **No. 1** is the level at which *toxic* reactions occur, not therapeutic. **No. 3**, while *within* the therapeutic range, is *narrower* than the therapeutic range (which is narrow to begin with). **No. 4** is too open-ended, and can move toward too low a level for therapeutic effect. **EV, 1, PhI**

14. **(4)** Because lithium is a salt depleter, it is important to teach the patient to maintain a diet that is adequate in salt (3–6 grams). **Nos. 1, 2, and 3** are not part of an adequate diet when a patient is on lithium. **IMP, 4, HPM**

💡 *Test-taking tip:* The key word is *adequate*. **Nos. 1 and 2** call for an *increase* in the diet. **No. 3** calls for a *decrease* in an item in the diet.

15. **(2)** The person in manic phase needs "finger foods" that can be eaten while "on-the-run," like a sandwich. Steak **(No. 1)** is difficult to eat on-the-run; patients may choke if they don't stop long enough to masticate well. Scrambled eggs **(No. 3)** are also hard to eat "on-the-go," requiring the patient to sit down and use a utensil. Broiled fish **(No. 4)** is also usually eaten sitting down with a fork and even a knife, rather than as "finger food" (additionally, there is no indication that bones have been removed). **IMP, 4, SECE**

Cognitive Disorders

Chapter Outline

- Sensory Disturbance
- Delirium, Dementia, Amnestic and Other Cognitive Disorders
  - Definition and Causes
  - General Concepts and Principles
  - Etiology
  Delirium
  Dementia
  * Alzheimer's Disease
  Amnestic Disorders
  - Assessment
  General
  Delirium
  Dementia
  Alzheimer's Disease
  Amnestic Disorders
  - General Analysis/Nursing Diagnosis

  - General Nursing Care Plan/Implementation
  Specific Emphasis in Care of Patient with Delirium
  Special Emphasis in Care of Patient with Dementia
  Special Emphasis in Care of Patient with Alzheimer's Disease
  - General Evaluation/Outcome Criteria
- Study and Memory Aids
- Glossary
- Summary of Key Points
  - Comparison of Cognitive Impairment in Delirium and Dementia
  - Care of Patient with Alzheimer's Disease
- Questions
- Answers/Rationale

Sensory Disturbance

I. **Types** of sensory disturbance
   A. *Sensory deprivation:* amount of stimuli *less* than required; e.g., isolation in bed or room, deafness, stroke victim.
   B. *Sensory overload:* receives *more* stimuli than can be tolerated; e.g., bright lights, noise, strange machinery, barrage of visitors.
   C. *Sensory deficit:* impairment in functioning of sensory or perceptual processes; e.g., blindness, changes in tactile perceptions.

II. **Assessment**—based on awareness of behavioral changes:
   A. *Sensory deprivation:* boredom, daydreaming, increasing sleep, thought slowness, inactivity, thought disorganization, hallucinations.
   B. *Sensory overload:* same as for sensory deprivation, plus restlessness and agitation, confusion.
   C. *Sensory deficit:* may not be able to distinguish sounds, odors, and tastes or differentiate tactile sensations.

III. **Analysis/nursing diagnosis**—problems related to sensory disturbance:
   A. *Altered thought processes.*
   B. *Confusion.*
   C. *Anger, aggression.*
   D. *Body image disturbance.*
   E. *Sleep pattern disturbance.*

IV. **Nursing care plan/implementation**
   A. *Management of existing* sensory disturbances in:
      1. *Sensory deprivation*
         a. Increase interaction with staff.
         b. Use TV.
         c. Provide touch.
         d. Help clients choose menus that have aromas, varied tastes, temperatures, colors, textures.
         e. Use light cologne or aftershave lotion, bath powder.
      2. *Sensory overload*
         a. Restrict number of visitors and length of stay.
         b. Reduce noise and lights.
         c. Reduce newness by establishing and following routine.

    d. Organize care to provide for extended rest periods with minimal input.

  3. *Sensory deficits*

    a. Report observations about hearing, vision.

    b. May imply need for new glasses, medical diagnosis, or therapy.

B. *Health teaching: Prevention* of sensory disturbance involves *education* of parents during child's growth and development regarding tactile, auditory, and visual stimulation.

  1. Hold, talk, and play with infant when awake.

  2. Provide bright toys with variety of designs for children to hold.

  3. Change environment.

  4. Provide music and auditory stimuli.

  5. Give foods with variety of textures, tastes, colors.

V. Evaluation/outcome criteria

A. Oriented to time, place, person.

B. Little or no evidence of mood or sleep disturbance.

Delirium, Dementia, Amnestic and Other Cognitive Disorders

I. Definition and Causes. These conditions were previously categorized under DSM-III-R as *organic mental disorders* (OMD).

delirium   A *clouded* state of consciousness; decreased sensorium; reduced awareness of environment accompanied by reduced capacity to sustain, shift or focus *attention* to external stimuli. May be a reversible *or* irreversible state, depending on the *underlying* disease process.

dementia   A mental syndrome characterized by sufficient impairment of cognitive abilities to interfere with social or occupational functions. There is a *progression* of impairments: from loss of recent memory, personality changes, and inability to abstract or make judgments, leading to loss of remote memory. There is *no* clouding of consciousness, but delirium may occur in the final stages.

Alzheimer's disease   A form of dementia ("senile dementia" or "presenile dementia") that usually occurs in *late* middle age. A progressive condition of atrophy of the brain and degeneration of the neurons; usually fatal within a few years. As the condition progresses, there is impairment of memory and judgment, loss of interest, and carelessness. Symptoms worsen until disorientation, epileptiform attacks, and contractures develop (from immobility). Diagnosis is made on autopsy based on histopathologic brain changes (plaques, neurofibrillary tangles). Cause is unknown. Treatment trials are ongoing (tacrine [*Cognex*]).

amnestic disorders   A category of mental syndromes in which relatively selective areas of cognition (e.g., short-and long-term memory) are impaired as a result of a specific organic factor.

Delirium, dementia, amnestic and other cognitive disorders are directly attributable to *either:* (a) the *aging process* (such as hypoxia from diminished blood flow; dementias arising in the senium or presenium, including primary degenerative dementia of the *Alzheimer* type; and multi-infarct dementia); (b) *substance-related disorders* (e.g., in the form of over-medication or drug reaction, a toxin or a drug of abuse such as: *alcohol, barbiturates, opioids, amphetamines, phencyclidine* [PCP], *hallucinogens, cannabis, nicotine,* and *caffeine*); (c) *general medical conditions* that may or may not be identifiable (e.g., *metabolic* disturbances such as: hypoglycemia and hypothyroidism; *systemic infections* such as: HIV, encephalitis, pneumonia, brain infection; *postoperative* states; *nutritional* deficiencies; *neurologic* diseases such as Huntington's chorea; *brain trauma* and *brain tumors.*

II. General concepts and principles

A. Cognitive dysfunctions involve impairments of *memory* and ability to *think* and *reason* logically and effectively.

  1. Cognitive impairment may result in disturbances of *consciousness, perception, judgment,* and *language. Intellectual* capacities are diminished (e.g., short concentration, difficulty with abstract thought).

  2. Impairment may be permanent or temporary, progressive or reversible, mild or severe.

  3. Alternative pathways and compensatory mechanisms may develop to show a clinical picture of remissions and exacerbations.

B. *Personality changes*

  1. Loss of ego flexibility; adoption of more rigid attitudes.

  2. Ritualism (*obsessive-compulsiveness*) in activities of daily living.

  3. Hoarding behaviors.

  4. Somatic preoccupations (*hypochondriasis*).

  5. Fearful, restless.

III. Etiology

A. Delirium

  1. Brain trauma.

  2. Brain infections (encephalitis, meningitis).

  3. Systemic infections with fever (e.g., pneumonia).

  4. Seizures related to epilepsy.

  5. Drugs (prescribed medications such as lithium, levodopa; psychoactive substances such as cocaine, alcohol).

  6. Withdrawal reactions from drugs.

  7. Toxins (e.g., heavy metals, carbon monoxide).

  8. Endocrine dysfunction (e.g., hypoglycemia, hypothyroidism).

  9. Organ systems diseases/dysfunctions (e.g., liver or kidney failure, cardiovascular conditions with hypoxia caused by diminished blood flow due to arteriosclerosis.)

10. Postoperative states (e.g., electrolyte imbalance).
11. Brain tumors.
B. Dementia
  1. Age-related (most often seen in elderly).
  2. *Primary dementias.*
    a. *Not* related to *another* disorder (e.g., Huntington's chorea, Parkinson's disease, Pick's disease, Creutzfeldt-Jakob disease).
    b. Dementia, **Alzheimer's** type is a form of primary dementia. Hypothesis:
      (1) Genetics—gene for apolipoprotein-E (apo-E); runs in families; chromosome 19 degenerates with age.
      (2) Slow-acting virus.
      (3) Aluminum—presence of *higher* levels in brains of Alzheimer's on autopsy.
      (4) Acetylcholine loss—reduced levels of the neurotransmitter that is important for memory and cognition.
      (5) Autoimmune response.
      (6) Decreased blood flow to the brain.
      (7) Protein accumulation in the brain.
  3. *Secondary dementias* that *are* related to (i.e., caused by) *another* medical condition or to a drug (e.g., neurosyphilis; multiple sclerosis; brain tumors; amyotrophic lateral sclerosis [ALS]; normal pressure hydrocephalus; Korsakoff's disease; HIV infection; deficiency of vitamin B_{12}, folic acid, or niacin; vascular dementia).
C. Amnestic Disorders
  1. Direct physiologic effects of a general medical condition (e.g., *physical trauma;* or *chronic alcoholism* and associated *thiamine deficiency,* namely **Wernicke-Korsakoff Syndrome;** or due to persisting effects of a *substance* (such as drug of abuse, a medication, or toxin exposure).
  2. Any event or process that results in bilateral damage to certain brain structures.
IV. Assessment
A. General assessment of cognitive impairment
  1. Health history: dietary habits; hearing or vision impairment; history of head trauma; use of medication or psychoactive substance, and alcohol.
  2. Family history.
  3. Assess:
    a. Appearance and hygiene.
    b. Attitude: cooperative or defensive.
    c. Level of consciousness: degree of alertness, attention span.
    d. Memory: immediate, short-term, long-term.
    e. Mood and affect: labile, euphoria, apathy, depression, anger, irritability, anxiety, fearfulness.
    f. Motor activity: agitated or slowed, restless.
    g. Orientation to time, place, situation, and person.

    h. Perception: vision, hearing, ability to recognize objects; illusions; hallucinations.
    i. Ability to abstract.
    j. Ability to do calculations.
    k. Risk of danger to self and others.
    l. Speech: coherence, clarity.
B. Delirium
  1. Distinguishing characteristics:
    a. *Rapid* onset; usually *brief* (hours or days). Usually *reversible.*
    b. Causal relationship to an *underlying medical condition,* to intoxication with or withdrawal from medications or other drugs, or to a combination of these conditions.
    c. Reduced and *fluctuating levels* of awareness (clouded *consciousness*) and intensity, along with *reduced* ability to *focus, sustain or shift attention* ("dysattention"). Some lucid periods during the day.
    d. *Thought processes:* slowed, with inability to think or talk coherently, to reason, or to problem-solve; disorganized thinking.
    e. *Sensory misperceptions* of actual external stimuli (e.g., *illusions*).
    f. *Memory* disturbances, especially for *recent* events.
    g. Mood lability.
    h. Worse at night ("sundowner's syndrome") and sometimes early morning hours ("sunriser's syndrome"); *diurnal variation* is one of the prominent diagnostic signs.
    i. EEG changes.
    j. *Disturbances* in psychomotor activity.
  2. Typical behaviors:
    a. Limited attention span (*diagnostic feature:* cannot repeat sequential string of information such as digit span).
    b. Disturbed *sleep-wake* cycle.
    c. *Disorientation* to time and place (*not* person).
    d. Confusion.
    e. *Visual hallucinations* are most common.
    f. *Emotional* disturbances: fearfulness and anxiety; apathy may follow; agitation, restlessness, anger; euphoria.
    g. *Speech:* slurred or incoherent.
C. Dementia
  1. Distinguishing characteristics:
    a. Non-fluctuating symptoms.
    b. Impaired *short-* and *long-term memory.*
    c. *Multiple and global cognitive deficits:* impairment of intellectual function, reasoning, judgment, abstract thinking. *No* clouding of consciousness.
    d. Personality and emotional changes that cause problems at work and with social relationships.
    e. May be permanent or reversible, depending on underlying pathology; usually *gradual* onset; most often affects the elderly.
    f. Sleep disturbances.

g. Dementia is differentiated from *pseudo-dementia* (depression) in the elderly; however, depression may be present in dementia.

Dementia	*Pseudodementia*
Gradual onset of symptoms	Time of onset can be identified
Denies, conceals, or minimizes cognitive deficits	No attempt to cover up memory loss; complains of poor memory and intellectual performance; ruminates over problems
Global cognitive and intellectual deficits	Primary cognitive impairment: memory disturbance
Affect: labile, superficial	Affect: consistently *depressed*; appears sad, worried
Cognitive deficits *precede* depression	Cognitive deficits *follow* depressive symptoms

2. Typical behaviors:
  a. *Early* stages or *mild* cases: *memory impairment* is evidenced by forgetfulness, e.g., names, phone numbers, directions, appointments (*short-term* memory affected at first).
  b. *Advanced* stages or *severe* cases: may forget own name or be unable to identify closest significant others (*long-term* memory is impaired).
  c. Reasoning, judgment, and impulse control impairment affects: *hygiene* and appearance; *compliance with the law* (e.g., steals or drives the wrong way); decisions (e.g., withdraws money for unwise investments); *social behavior* (e.g., out-of-character *lewd* gestures or comments) due to loss of inhibitions; *orientation* (i.e., is disoriented and confused).
  d. Abstract thinking is compromised; inability to plan, organize, or sequence; avoids new tasks; cannot perform complex tasks even if familiar. *Diagnostic feature: cannot learn new* information (e.g., a list of words) *nor retain, recall, or recognize* information.
  e. *Aphasia, agnosia,* and *apraxia* can occur.
  f. Personality changes: premorbid traits are *accentuated* or *altered* (e.g., may become excessively jealous or suspicious); irritable, resistant to change, compulsive in an effort to control the deficits.
  g. Emotional changes: labile affect; fearful, anxious, and depressed due to awareness (in early stages) of failing faculties.
  h. Uses *confabulation* to cover memory loss.
  i. Restlessness (wanders), especially at night; disoriented.
D. Alzheimer's disease (Table 13.1)
  1. Distinguishing characteristics:
    a. Dementia symptoms *progressively worsen* over 1–10 yr.
    b. May lead to *death* within 2 yr; average du-

ration from onset of symptoms to death: 5–7 yr.
    c. *Irreversible* loss of cerebral function due to cortical atrophy, neuritic plaques, neurofibrillary tangles, and neuronal degeneration (confirmed by neuropathologic and histologic findings on autopsy).
    d. Onset is *insidious;* early onset (ages 40–65); late onset (after age 65); most frequently occurs between ages 65 and 70 yr.
    e. Cognitive deficits *not* due to CNS or systemic conditions or induced by substances.
  2. Typical behaviors:
    a. Progressive decline in *intellectual capacity* (i.e., recent *and* remote memory, *judgment*), *affect,* motor coordination (*apraxia*), loss of *social* sense (inhibitions); *apathy or restlessness, wandering* (especially at night; may become lost).
    b. *Early stage:* subtle changes in personality reported by family and close friends; *forgetting* names and appointments; misplacing things; difficulty in concentrating and handling everyday or personal activities (e.g., writing a check); attempts to conceal forgetfulness; becomes apathetic, withdrawn, depressed.
    c. *Moderate to severe stage:* problems with speech (*aphasia*), recognition of familiar objects (*agnosia*); *disorientation* to self (even to parts of *own* body); extreme personality changes (*agitation, violence, paranoia*).
    d. *Late stage:* severe disorientation; severe agitation; psychotic symptoms (hallucinations, delusions); loss of ability for: self-care, talking, or walking; stupor; coma; death, usually caused by *infection* (e.g., pneumonia), *malnutrition,* or *dehydration.*
E. Amnestic disorders
  1. Distinguishing characteristics:
    a. Impaired *short-* and *long-term* memory; may be more successful in retrieving remote information than with recent recall.
    b. *Retrograde* amnesia (loss of memory *before* onset of illness) and *anterograde* amnesia (inability to establish new memory *after* onset of illness) is usually accompanied by lack of insight, *denial* or *rationalization* about the deficit.
    c. *Severe* memory impairment *without* other significant impairments of cognitive functioning (i.e., *without* aphasia, apraxia, or agnosia).
    d. *Diagnostic feature:* memory impairment is *always* manifested by impairment in the ability to learn *new* information, and sometimes problems remembering previously learned information or past events.
  2. Typical behaviors:
    a. *Confabulation,* whereby inaccurate, untrue information is aimed at filling in memory lapses.

Table 13.1 ◧ **ASSESSMENT OF ALZHEIMER'S DISEASE: 10 SIGNS**	

Sign	*Example*
1. **Recent memory loss**	Repeatedly asking the same question
2. **Disorientation** (time and place)	Getting lost
3. **Difficulty performing familiar tasks**	Forgetting to serve dinner after making it
4. **Poor judgment**	Forgetting to watch a child and leaving the house
5. **Language difficulty**	Forgetting words; using inappropriate words
6. **Misplacing objects**	Putting objects in inappropriate places, like eyeglasses in the freezer
7. **Problems with abstract thinking**	Inability to write a check or sign name because forgot how to write numbers and/or alphabet
8. **Labile mood and rapid behavior changes**	Changing quickly from calm to rage, to smiles, to tears
9. **Personality changes**	Irritability, suspiciousness, fearfulness
10. **Loss of initiative**	Passivity

b. Disorientation to place and time, but *rarely* to self. Appears bewildered or befuddled.

c. *Memory disturbance:* sufficiently severe to cause marked impairment in social or occupational functioning, and represents a significant decline from previous level of functioning. May require *supervised living* situation to ensure nutrition and care.

d. Lack of insight into own memory deficit; may *explicitly deny* the presence of severe memory impairment despite evidence to the contrary.

e. *Altered personality* function: apathy, lack of initiative, emotional blandness, shallow range of expression.

◧ **V. General analysis/nursing diagnosis**

A. *Altered thought and knowledge processes* related to misperceptions, forgetfulness, confusion, and disorientation; and to destruction of cerebral tissue resulting in inability to process, synthesize, and utilize information to make judgments and transmit messages.

B. *Risk for injury* related to decreased cognitive functioning, evidenced by wandering from premises, and to altered motor behavior (hyperactivity).

C. *Impaired verbal communication* related to poverty of speech and withdrawal behavior, progressive neurologic losses, and cerebral impairment.

D. *Self-care deficit* (feeding, bathing/hygiene, dressing, toileting) related to physical impairments (poor vision, lack of coordination) and forgetfulness.

E. *Sleep pattern disturbance* related to confusion, resulting in disorientation at night ("sundowner's syndrome").

F. *Altered attention and memory* related to progressive neurologic losses (recent memory loss progresses to remote memory loss and eventually extends to global memory loss).

G. *Sensory-perceptual alterations:* illusions and hallucinations (visual, auditory, kinesthetic, gustatory, tactile, olfactory).

H. *Altered conduct/impulse processes* (irritability and aggressiveness) related to neurologic impairment.

I. *Altered nutrition,* more or less than body requirements, related to confusion.

J. *Altered role performance* related to decreased intellectual competence, difficulty in focusing attention (distractibility), delusions (e.g., ideas of reference, alien control, nihilistic, self-deprecation, grandeur), somatic preoccupations.

K. *Impaired social interactions* related to altered thought processes, confused or disoriented state; impaired intellect and memory, sensory/perceptual alterations; loss of body functions, self-care deficit; emotional lability, fear, anxiety, depression; panic/rage reaction; self-concept disturbance; social isolation, apathy; impaired verbal communication.

◧ **VI. General nursing care plan/implementation**

See also interventions for **Confusion/disorientation** in Chap. 7, pp. 91–92.

A. Long-term goals

　1. *Optimize* general level of functioning.

　2. *Minimize regression* related to cognitive and memory impairment; *avoid* unnecessary dependence.

　3. When symptoms are *reversible:* rehabilitate through retraining and re-education program as a *priority;* offer hope for recovery in the future.

　4. When symptoms are *irreversible:*

　　a. *Avoid* insightful explorations to prevent excessive anxiety, irritability, rage, or depression.

　　b. Encourage *family* to seek continued *support* as needed to maintain own emotional and physical well-being.

B. Short-term goals and interventions

☞ **1.** Maintain *physiologic* well-being:

　a. *Nutrition/hydration:* monitor food intake and fluid and electrolyte balance.

　b. Bowel/bladder functions: set up routine for toileting.

c. Normal *day/night* sleep patterns: promote relaxation with back rubs; allow walking until tired; eliminate naps.

d. *Hygiene* (bathing, grooming): set up schedule to accommodate alertness phases.

e. *Infection* prevention (e.g., pneumonia).

f. *Mobility*/exercise during the day for socialization and physical therapy.

2. Ensure a *safe* environment: provide continuous observation when agitated; institute security measures to prevent wandering and inadvertent self-harm.

3. Promote *reality orientation*

a. Provide *structure* and *consistency* (e.g., *routine,* schedules) to increase security and diminish stress.

b. *Continuously orient* to time, place, situation, and person (especially at night); reinforce reality-oriented comments.

c. Keep room well lighted, to reduce misperceptions (e.g., illusions).

d. Optimize perception by ensuring that glasses, hearing aids, and other *assistive devices* are used and functioning.

e. Provide easy-to-read big clocks and calendars (with date, day, season, weather) in open view. Provide reality-orientation board with name of facility, city, and state to enhance optimal memory function and orientation.

f. Encourage family to visit and bring *familiar personal belongings.*

g. Keep environment the *same* as much as possible (i.e., assign *same staff* as often as possible, *same* room, *same* placement of furniture).

h. If patient begins to mumble incoherently, redirect by providing a familiar task (e.g., folding towels, stirring batter) to provide direction for disorganized thoughts and to rechannel anxiety-producing energy.

4. Promote *cognitive, memory, and perceptual* functioning

a. Provide cognitive and sensory stimulation by using *associative patterns* to improve recall (through repetition, summarizing, and focusing); *allow time* to talk and to complete projects; break down tasks into *individual steps* and ask patient to do them one at a time (e.g., "Here are your glasses.... Take them out of the case.... Put the glasses on.")

b. Maintain adequate environmental stimulation (e.g., *music* therapy; television; use of *colors* to promote identification and direction and to enhance recent memory; *pet/plant* therapy sessions to enhance the senses and support memory function; *celebration* of special events or holidays to enhance memory and demonstrate caring.)

c. Use *concrete* language to minimize confusion.

d. Allow *reminiscence* and life review through photo albums (even when redundant) to maintain remote memory and help with situational low self-esteem.

e. Arrange pictures of familiar objects, utensils, foods, pets, or flowers with appropriate identifying label, to stimulate memory and cognition.

f. Place *familiar* and *cherished* objects in the patient's room (e.g., family photos, quilt, vase) to enhance memory and promote comfort.

5. Enhance *socialization* as tolerated

a. Brief, frequent contacts, due to short attention span.

b. Provide familiar, pleasurable, simple activities (e.g., old-time movie) to provide enjoyment.

c. Recreational therapy, without overtaxing; learn of interests and assess skills.

d. Give recognition for each accomplishment.

6. Promote *effective communication*

a. Give clear instructions; *repeat* with *same* wording. Repetition reinforces communication.

b. Face patient and speak slowly; eliminate sensory overload due to distracting, background stimuli (e.g., group noise).

c. Use gestures and pictures to supplement verbal comments (e.g., "Do you want your coat?" while holding coat in front of patient).

d. Incorporate orientation cues into contacts (e.g., "I am Jack, your nurse. It's time for lunch.").

e. Limit choices.

f. Change topics when patient becomes agitated.

g. Use gentle touch with care (e.g., hold hand), and only if preceded by telling the patient what will be done. Touch is a physical expression of caring and empathy.

h. Correct misperceptions carefully. Do *not* argue or *agree* with the patient regarding misperceptions, *or* ask patient to explain illusions and hallucinations.

i. Follow conversational cues from topics initiated by patient.

j. *Avoid* demands; make requests; *avoid* power struggles.

k. Ask questions that can be answered with a "yes" or "no" (e.g., "Are you cold?"). Ask only *one* simple question or make only one simple, short statement at a time (no more than 5–6 words at a time) to decrease confusion, promote concentration, and increase attention span (e.g., "That door leads to the bathroom.")

7. Reinforce *compensatory coping mechanisms*

a. Recognize importance of *confabulation.*

b. *Avoid:* contradicting, arguing, challenging,

and openly confronting the patient's use of denial, hoarding of food, redundancy in speech.

8. Health education

a. When feasible, provide explanations to patient about the condition.

b. Provide information to family members about care; reinforce doctor's explanations of cause and prognoses.

c. Give *specific* instructions for diet, medication, and treatment; how to use many sensory approaches to learn new information (when feasible); how to use existing knowledge and habitual approaches to deal with new situations.

C. Specific emphasis in care of patient with **delirium** (in addition to **General nursing care plan/implementation**)

1. Determine all possible contributing factors to decreased sensorium (e.g., hypoxia, electrolyte imbalance such as sodium and potassium deficits; renal, hepatic, cardiac, respiratory conditions; pain; malnutrition, vitamin deficiency; effects of drug therapy).

2. Carry out treatments to correct the dysfunctions

a. Maintain adequate hydration, electrolytes, nutrition, vitamins.

b. Give O_2 as ordered.

3. Assess medication effects and restructure medication schedule as necessary, to increase alertness and subsequent cognition and social interactions.

4. Promote 4–6 h of sleep at night.

5. Use simple terms and a clear, *modulated* voice tone to explain procedures; soft, too-low voice tones may be inaudible to patient with a hearing deficit.

6. Ensure that patient uses dentures, hearing aids, or eyeglasses when needed, to enhance the senses and reduce frustration and confusion.

D. Specific emphasis in care of patient with **dementia** (in addition to **General nursing care plan/implementation,** p. 151–152)

1. Maintain appropriate level of physical activity to prevent hazard of immobility and sensory overload.

2. Limit wandering to within prescribed safe areas only.

a. Identify potential causes of wandering (e.g., medication schedules, attention-seeking behaviors, avoidance of stressful procedures).

b. Secure ID information to ensure safe return to residence if patient wanders away.

3. Reduce resistance to self-care activities through patience and a pleasant, gentle demeanor and tactful humor.

4. Serve simple, easy-to-eat meals to decrease amount of time required to sit, thereby minimizing restlessness and agitation.

5. If patient wakes up at night, reorient in calm, soothing manner, to avoid precipitating extreme agitation.

6. *Health teaching:* review post-discharge needs such as medication and safety precautions; refer family to community resources for respite care.

E. Specific emphasis in care of patient with **Alzheimer's disease**

1. Care is primarily *symptomatic, consistent, supportive* (counseling and working with family to reduce family's stress).

a. Open, gentle, friendly, relaxed approach, as these patients often "mirror" the affect of those around them.

b. Maintain *routine* and *structure,* rather than variety, and schedule changes as these patients have difficulty in coping with changes in routine due to short-term memory deficits and labile emotions. Routine that is *consistent* supports memory function and orientation and reduces confusion and frustration.

c. Recommend day care and respite care when the patient is severely confused.

2. Speak in clear, *lower-pitched* voice, rather than high-pitched ones which create anxiety in these patients.

3. Use *simple* topics and *concrete* language rather than abstractions or slang (e.g., say "It's time to sleep," rather than, "It's time to hit the sack"), as patients with Alzheimer's lose the ability to understand abstract or slang remarks, and become confused and frustrated. *Avoid* sensory overload; support positive interactions.

4. Offer *distraction* rather than reasoning when behavior is socially inappropriate or stereotypic (e.g., rubs hands or taps tabletop with fingers).

5. Use strategies (e.g., distraction) and responses (e.g., empathy) that reduce or avoid agitation and aggression, to protect patient and others from injury.

6. Give prescribed low-dose antipsychotic (e.g., *Haldol*) if agitation is not manageable by other means. Assess effectiveness of tranquilizers (dosage and time may need to be adjusted) if patient is sleepy during the day or has paradoxical agitation.

7. Demonstrate patience when patient hesitates before initiating or responding to comments or requests. Anticipate needs to avoid frustration.

8. *Health teaching*

a. Educate the family about what to do when patient is *confused and wanders:* keep bed in low position at night to prevent falls; keep in supervised setting; lock exits and dangerous areas; place an identification band on wrist.

b. Educate about the effects of the disease on short-term memory and cognition (capabilities and limitations), to promote realistic expectations and reduce family's frustrations.

c. Teach strategies to enhance memory, decrease confusion, facilitate communication (e.g., via structure and routine, reminiscence sessions, patience).

d. Teach the family to *decrease stimulation* and to focus patient on *task* at hand when patient exhibits *rage* reaction. Inform the family that patients with Alzheimer's disease experience emotional lability not only from the effects of the disease in areas of the brain that control mood and affect, but also from overwhelming frustration and powerlessness.

e. Educate the family that the patient can *no longer* engage in *conversation* in *social situations,* to help family avoid demands that may agitate the patient unnecessarily.

f. Inform the family that the patient may use *confabulation* in social situations to hide memory deficits, *not* as an attempt to lie. Teach the family *not* to argue or disagree as that would antagonize the patient.

g. Suggest that the family engage in reminiscence sessions about the past rather than "here-and-now" conversations, as this provides a positive experience to help patient get in touch with familiar feelings and engage in more meaningful interactions.

VII. **General evaluation/outcome criteria**

A. To the extent possible, symptoms occur *less* frequently and are less severe in areas of: emotional lability and appropriateness; false perceptions; self-care ability; disorientation, memory, and judgment; and decision making.

B. Able to preserve optimum level of functioning and independence (for stage of condition) while allowing basic needs to be met.

C. Physical well-being is maintained.

D. Stays relatively calm and noncombative when upset or fearful. Responds favorably to *reminiscence* activities with staff, peers, and family.

E. Accepts own irritability and frustrations as part of illness; interacts with increased comfort during social interactions in accordance with capabilities.

F. Asks for assistance with self-care activities; participates in some basic decisions about ADL (food and clothing); sits through meals and activities for longer periods of time without agitation or restlessness.

G. Knows and adheres to daily routine; knows own nurse, location of room, bathroom, clocks, calendars; follows repeated, concrete directions.

H. Uses *supportive community services* (e.g., respite care for family).

I. Family understands condition and participates in care.

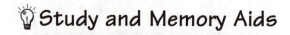

Study and Memory Aids

Dementia: key points

- Problems with multiple cognitive defects: short- and long-term memory, judgment, abstract thinking
- Result: confusion
- Changes may be progressive and irreversible

Most common areas of difficulty in dementia—"JOCAM"

Judgment (poor; socially inappropriate behavior)
Orientation (*disorientation*; illusions; confused)
Confabulation ("stories" to fill in memory gaps)
Affect (labile; quarrelsome, angry, withdrawn, depressed)
Memory (poor for: names, recent events)

Glossary

agnosia   Impaired ability to *recognize* or understand familiar words, objects, symbols, or people despite intact *sensory* function. Can be acoustic or auditory, tactile, or visual, or may be *somatagnosia* (disturbance in recognition of own body parts).

agraphia   Total or partial inability to express thoughts in *writing*, due to organic cerebral pathology.

aphasia   *Language* loss, disturbance, or impairment; deterioration of language function; e.g., difficulty in producing names of people or objects; incorrect use of words, with excessive use of terms of *indefinite reference* ("thing," "it").

apraxia   Impaired ability to carry out purposeful *motor* activities despite intact motor abilities, sensory function, and comprehension of the required task; e.g., inability to draw a form or figure in two or three dimensions, inability to use utensils.

cognition   The mental process that includes all aspects of knowing, thinking, learning, remembering, judging, and problem solving.

confabulation   A compensatory coping mechanism used in cases of memory loss to fill in gaps in memory; characterized by responses that sound plausible but are not factual. Most often seen in "organic" mental disorders, as opposed to functional mental disorders.

delirium   A clouded state of consciousness; decreased sensorium and reduction in clarity of awareness, accompanied by a reduced capacity to shift, focus, and sustain attention to environmental stimuli. Acute brain syndrome, with rapid onset; usually reversible with early treatment of underlying medical condition. Specific precipitating stressors (e.g., drug, toxin) are usually identifiable.

dementia   Chronic, progressive brain syndrome, with gradual onset; may be irreversible with global cognitive and intellectual deficits that *precede* depression. Precipitating stressors may or may not be identifiable. Person tends to

🔑 Summary of Key Points

Comparison of Cognitive Impairment in Delirium and Dementia

	Delirium	Dementia
Cause	Underlying *medical* condition (e.g., brain trauma; brain infections like encephalitis; epilepsy; endocrine dysfunction; postoperative reaction; electrolyte imbalance; fever; liver, cardiovascular, kidney disease or dysfunction); *substance intoxication* or *withdrawal*; or *toxin exposure* (e.g., carbon monoxide, heavy metal)	May or may not be related to underlying medical condition; autoimmune response; chromosome 19 degeneration with age; slow-acting virus; acetylcholine loss.
Onset	Rapid (hours, days)	Gradual
Prevalence	More common in very young and elderly; patients in ICU and CCU; severely burned patients	Age related: most often affects elderly
Duration	Brief (hours, days); usually reversible	Progressive (over months, years); may be irreversible
Level of consciousness	Clouded consciousness. Fluctuating levels of awareness, with some daytime lucidity; worse at night and early morning	Normal. Stable course through 24 hr
Thoughts	*Disordered* thinking	Impaired *abstract* thinking and impaired judgment
Speech	Commonly affected; slurred and incoherent	Rarely affected in *early* stages; aphasia in *late* stages
Memory	Poor, especially for recent events	Progressive loss, starting with short-term, then long-term
Perception	Sensory misperceptions (e.g., visual hallucinations, often vivid and frightening)	Sensory misperceptions are rare
Mood	Mood swings	Personality changes or exaggeration of typical personality
EEG	Changes noted	No changes
Levels of activity	Either abnormally reduced or increased	Usually normal
Orientation	Disoriented as to *time* (*sundowner's syndrome*) and sometimes to *place*, but *not* to person	May be disoriented

Care of Patient with Alzheimer's Disease: Key Points

1. Care is primarily symptomatic, consistent, supportive (counseling and working with family to reduce family's stress).

2. Recommend day care and respite care when patient is confused.

3. When patient is *confused and wanders:* keep bed in low position at night to prevent falls; keep in supervised setting; lock exits and dangerous areas.

deny, *conceal,* or minimize cognitive deficits; may become *angry* when unable to respond correctly to questions.

dysgraphia Impaired ability to *write.*

dysnomia Impaired ability to *name* objects.

echolalia Automatic repetition (*echoing*) of phrases or words that are heard.

executive functions Cognitive abilities that involve planning, organizing, sequencing, and abstracting.

labile affect   Rapid changes in mood or emotion, unrelated to external stimuli.

organic mental disorders   Now classified by DSM-IV as *delirium, dementia, and amnestic and other cognitive disorders;* a class of disorders characterized by disturbances in cognition, memory, emotions, and motivation.

palilalia   Repeating *sounds* or words over and over with increasing rapidity.

pica   Ingestion of a nonnutritive substance.

pseudodementia   A psychiatric condition that *mimics* dementia; the mood disorder *depression* is most often the cause. Person appears sad, worried, consistently depressed. Cognitive deficits (i.e., memory disturbance) *follow* depressive symptoms; ruminates over problems; *complains* of poor memory and intellectual performance.

sundowner's syndrome   A prominent diagnostic sign of delirium that refers to diurnal variation, when delirium is more pronounced at night.

Questions

1. In planning interventions for a patient with Alzheimer's disease, the nurse is aware that the most frequent emotional expression by the patient will be:
    1. Lability.
    2. Euphoria.
    3. Irritability.
    4. Depression.
2. A family has recently placed a patient on an Alzheimer's unit for long-term care. On the first visit to the patient, a family member asks the nurse why the patient will not talk and wonders if perhaps the patient is upset about being there and should be cared for at home after all. What is the nurse's best response?
    1. "This is part of the illness. There is nothing you can do."
    2. "I'm sure the family has made the right decision for all concerned."
    3. "This must be difficult for you both."
    4. "Are you feeling guilty about bringing a member of your family here?"
3. In the early afternoon, a person with Alzheimer's disease complains to the nurse that there has been nothing to eat all day. The nurse knows that this patient did eat breakfast and lunch. The nurse recognizes that this behavior indicates:
    1. Loss of recent memory.
    2. Feelings of deprivation, with food symbolizing love.
    3. Confabulation as a coping mechanism.
    4. Loss of remote memory.
4. In planning care for a patient with advanced Alzheimer's disease, it is reasonable to expect that the patient will:
    1. Be oriented as to time, place, and person.
    2. Remember his wedding day.
    3. Be able to dress himself.
    4. Want to go home.
5. Which progression of symptoms best describes Alzheimer's disease?
    1. Urinary incontinence, wandering off, forgetfulness.
    2. Difficulty in ambulation, inability to manage tasks, speech impairment.
    3. Forgetfulness, inability to select proper clothing, inability to walk.
    4. Speech impairment, forgetfulness, death.
6. For which signs and symptoms would the nurse observe a patient who is diagnosed with Korsakoff's psychosis?
    1. Loss of memory and confabulation.
    2. Self-destructiveness.
    3. Delusions of persecution and phobias.
    4. Delusions of grandeur.
7. Which nursing diagnosis is of primary concern for a patient who has developed delirium?
    1. Risk for injury.
    2. Risk for violence.
    3. Altered nutrition, less than body requirements.
    4. Sleep pattern disturbance.
8. The nurse should recognize that the patient is exhibiting signs of delirium, rather than the early stages of dementia, when the assessment reveals:
    1. Cognitive impairment.
    2. Impaired speech.
    3. Anxiety.
    4. Loss of short-term memory.
9. The nurse should recognize that the patient is exhibiting signs of dementia, rather than depression, when the assessment reveals:
    1. Confabulation.
    2. Apathy.
    3. Changes in personality.
    4. Withdrawal from socialization.
10. Which activity would be best to provide for a person with dementia?
    1. Playing chess.
    2. Watching an old movie.
    3. Attending a bingo game.
    4. Playing Scrabble.
11. What is the main goal of therapy for patients who have dementia?
    1. To minimize the steady decline.
    2. To avoid confusion.
    3. To promote interpersonal relationships.
    4. To optimize functioning.
12. Which is the most important intervention when working with a patient who has dementia?
    1. Encouraging physical exercise.
    2. Reinforcing the patient's thoughts.
    3. Giving anti-anxiety medications.
    4. Using short sentences and simple words.
13. The plan of nursing care for a person with dementia would include:
    1. Focus on the "here-and-now," rather than on the past.
    2. A variety of new experiences to keep the patient stimulated.
    3. Assignment of different caregivers for the patient in order to avoid personnel burnout.
    4. Adherence to a consistent daily routine.
14. In planning care for elderly patients with delirium, when should the nurse anticipate that the patients will

need the most supervision because of increasing confusion?
1. Morning.
2. Midday.
3. Night.
4. Late afternoon.

15. Redundancy in recounting the past is a characteristic of dementia. When a patient hospitalized with dementia tells the same story over and over again about the whole family baking holiday cookies for the carolers every year, which would be the most appropriate response by the nurse?
1. "What does your family do nowadays for winter holidays?"
2. "What else did you traditionally do to prepare for the holidays?"
3. "That seems to bring back good memories for you. How about joining me in making fudge for the staff-patient party?"
4. "That sounds like it was very enjoyable, but let's talk about what you want to do now."

16. A patient with dementia is incontinent, and avoids eye contact with the nurse when discovered. Which response by the nurse is most therapeutic?
1. "How can I help you avoid these accidents?"
2. "You can call one of the staff to help you."
3. "Don't wait so long next time when you need to go to the bathroom."
4. "This must be upsetting to you. I'll help you change clothes."

17. An elderly person with dementia is admitted to a board-and-care home. The patient's recent history includes confusion, wandering away, and increasing carelessness about personal grooming. The nurse understands that personality changes will most likely manifest as:
1. Negativistic behavior.
2. Dependent behavior.
3. Suspicious behavior.
4. Regressive behavior.

Answers/Rationale

1. **(1)** Lability, meaning variability of mood or emotion, is a frequent manifestation in Alzheimer's disease. The mood can at one time be euphoria **(No. 2)**, at another time depression **(No. 4)**; irritability **(No. 3)** is also a common response to the patient's own inability to cope with activities of daily living. **AS, 7, PsI**

💡 *Test-taking tip:* Look for the "umbrella" option. Here, *all* four are applicable, but the *general* term (lability) covers them all.

2. **(3)** This *open-ended* response allows for elaboration and catharsis; it is a form of support. **No. 1** closes off the opportunity for the family to voice any additional feelings or concerns. **No. 2** is *closed-ended* (a conversation "stopper") and offers a value judgment; it gives the nurse's opinion, which is not even solicited. **No. 4** puts words ("guilty") into the family member's mind. It is an

attempt to *analyze* what the person might have implied, and is therefore not therapeutic. A question that can be answered by "yes" or "no" is also an example of non-therapeutic communication. **IMP, 7, PsI**

3. **(1)** Loss of recent memory is one of the characteristic signs and symptoms of Alzheimer's disease. **No. 2** is too analytic, with insufficient data to support this conclusion. Confabulation **(No. 3)** *is* a common coping mechanism to *fill in* memory gaps; in this case, however, the problem described is the *loss* of recent memory, *not how* the person *copes* with the loss. Remote memory loss **(No. 4)** is the *opposite* of the correct answer. **AN, 7, PsI**

4. **(4)** It is realistic to expect that the patient will want to go home, or will think he is home. **Nos. 1 and 2** can be eliminated because *disorientation* and *loss* of memory are two cardinal symptoms that *get worse* as the condition becomes *advanced*. **No. 3** is reasonable to expect in the *early* stages of Alzheimer's disease, but not in the advanced stage. **EV, 7, PsI**

💡 *Test-taking tip:* Note key words that define the condition, to enable you to eliminate three of these options. The *key words* are "advanced" and "reasonable to expect."

5. **(3)** Forgetfulness is usually the *first* symptom observed in Alzheimer's disease. **Nos. 1 and 4** are incorrect because, although forgetfulness appears, it is *not listed first* in the progression of symptoms. **No. 2** does *not* include forgetfulness and therefore can be eliminated. **AN, 7, PsI**

💡 *Test-taking tip:* The *key word* in this question is "progression" of symptoms; this asks for the *sequence* of symptoms, not just what the symptoms might be.

6. **(1)** Loss of memory and confabulation are characteristic of an amnestic disorder like Korsakoff's psychosis. See Chap. 14 on substance-related disorders for Korsakoff's. Self-destructiveness **(No. 2)** is not a characteristic of Korsakoff's. Delusions **(Nos. 3 and 4)** are more characteristic of paranoid disorder. **AS, 7, PsI**

7. **(1)** *Safety* is the main concern, as a *result* of impaired judgment and sensory misperceptions (illusions and hallucinations) that often are part of delirium. The patient may fall, wander off, or sustain an accidental injury. Aggressive, destructive behavior **(No. 2)** is *not* as common as *accidental* injury to self. Nutritional deficiencies **(No. 3)**—malnutrition, thiamine deficiencies—are *one cause* of cognitive impairment, not a result of it. Although a disturbed sleep-wake cycle **(No. 4)** is com-

Key to Codes

Nursing process: AS = Assessment; **AN** = Analysis; **PL** = Planning; **IMP** = Implementation; **EV** = Evaluation. (See Appendix E for explanation of nursing process steps.)

Category of human function: 1 = Protective; 2 = Sensory-Perceptual; 3 = Comfort, Rest, Activity, and Mobility; 4 = Nutrition; 5 = Growth and Development; 6 = Fluid-Gas Transport; 7 = Psychosocial-Cultural; 8 = Elimination.

Client need: SECE = Safe, Effective Care Environment; **PhI** = Physiologic Integrity; **PsI** = Psychosocial Integrity; **HPM** = Health Promotion/Maintenance.

mon with delirium, it is *not* the *main* concern; *safety* is the top priority. **AN, 1, SECE**

8. **(2)** Speech is commonly affected in delirium (slurred, incoherent), but rarely affected in early dementia. Cognitive impairment (**No. 1**) (e.g., impaired judgment) and loss of short-term memory (**No. 4**) occur in *both* conditions. Anxiety (**No. 3**), an early sign of delirium, may *also* occur in dementia, when the patient becomes aware of memory loss and cognitive impairment (confusion, disorientation). **AN, 7, PsI**

9. **(1)** Due to memory loss, the individual with dementia attempts to cover up by using the coping mechanism of confabulation. Those who are depressed make little attempt to hide the loss of memory. See **pseudodementia** glossary definition on p. 156; also see Chap. 16, p. 202 for differences between depression and dementia. Apathy (**No. 2**) is more typical of *depression* than dementia; *anxiety* is more characteristic of dementia. Changes in personality (**No. 3**) are exhibited in *both* dementia and depression. In dementia, the individual may become suspicious and irritable, whereas in depression, the behavior is one of sadness and apathy. Withdrawal (**No. 4**) is more commonly seen in *depression.* **AN, 7, PsI**

10. **(2)** An old movie allows the person to reminisce. A person with dementia needs to go back and focus on the past because the memory functions for past events better than for recent ones; the person feels better about him- or herself when memory is intact. Playing chess (**No. 1**) and Scrabble (**No. 4**) involves intellectual ability (which is often diminished) and the ability to concentrate (which those with dementia usually cannot do). Bingo (**No. 3**) requires seeing (visual acuity), hearing (auditory acuity), and hand-eye coordination—the very things that may be affected in dementia. Second, the game is time-pressured; the person has to hear the letters and numbers called, see them on the card, and pick up and place the marker. When this sequence takes too long, it is not a good feeling for someone with dementia! Last, Bingo is not a good choice because it is a "win or lose" game, with only one or two winners; if the person doesn't win, he or she loses; this psychosocial stressor results in decreased self-esteem. **PL, 3, PsI**

Test-taking tip: Look at patterns. When in doubt, focus on the option *not* like the others. Here, three involve games (**Nos. 1, 3, and 4**) and one (**No. 2**) is *not* a game; three (**Nos. 1, 3, and 4**) involve *active* interaction and a response, while one is passive (**No. 2**). Both patterns point to **No. 2** as the one that is different.

11. **(4)** The therapy goal needs to be individualized so that each patient, with varying degrees of impaired functioning, achieves the *best level that individual patient can attain.* In maximizing individual function, the steady decline can then be minimized (**No. 1**) and/or slowed down; minimizing decline is desirable, but it occurs as a result of optimizing functioning (**No. 4**). Confusion needs to *minimized,* but cannot be altogether *avoided* (**No. 2**). Promoting relationships (**No. 3**), while seemingly desirable, is not a realistic goal and is certainly not the *main* goal given the common characteristics of dementia (including confusion). **PL, 7, PsI**

Test-taking tip: When two goals seem appropriate, choose the one which *leads to* the other, as optimizing functioning (**No. 4**) leads to minimized decline (**No. 1**).

12. **(4)** It is important to minimize confusion and promote even minimal interaction through simple, rather than complex, communication. Encouraging physical exercise (**No. 1**) is *not the most important* intervention for a patient whose clinical manifestations are *primarily* problems of memory, judgment, and orientation. *Reality orientation* is needed, *not* reinforcement (**No. 2**) of the altered thought patterns that are characteristic of dementia. Anti-anxiety medications (**No. 3**) are not always appropriate for dementia. **IMP, 7, PsI**

13. **(4)** Consistency provides stability and minimizes the confusion seen in dementia. Focusing on the *past,* rather than the present (**No. 1**), is commonly a source of satisfaction, since the person has difficulty relating to the present. Variety (**No. 2**) is the opposite of the correct response—routine. Assigning different caregivers (**No. 3**) provides variety, which is not therapeutic when a patient needs consistency and routine. **PL, 7, PsI**

14. **(3)** Decreased visibility and altered perception at night adds to the already existing confusion that is characteristic of an elderly patient with delirium. This evening confusion is called "sundowner's syndrome." Morning (**No. 1**), midday (**No. 2**), and late afternoon (**No. 4**) are not critical time periods requiring increased supervision for elderly patients with delirium. **IMP, 2, PsI**

15. **(3)** This response acknowledges positive past experiences, yet brings the focus back to the present, with a similarly pleasurable activity. **No. 1** focuses on the family, rather than the *patient.* **No. 2** is not therapeutic because it focuses only on the past, not what the patient is experiencing now (most probably sadness). **No. 4** is similar to the correct response (**No. 3**), but it is open-ended and calls for a decision, which may be difficult for a person with dementia. **IMP, 7, PsI**

16. **(4)** The most therapeutic approach is to focus on solving the problem at hand (wet clothes), "here-and-now," while acknowledging feelings. It may not be realistic to tell this patient to "avoid these accidents" (**No. 1**) or "don't wait so long" (**No. 3**). **No. 2** avoids taking care of the situation "here-and-now." **IMP, 7, PsI**

Test-taking tip: Better psychosocial answers focus on the "here-and-now" and on feelings.

17. **(4)** Regressive behavior (a return to previous traits) is a compensatory mechanism that patients in this situation may employ when memory, speech, and cognitive abilities are deteriorating. Negativistic (**No. 1**) and dependent (**No. 2**) behaviors may be *examples* of regressive behavior, as exaggerations of earlier behaviors, but they are *both* covered by the correct response, regression. Suspicious behavior (**No. 3**) is part of paranoid behavior, and it is not common. There are *no data* here to indicate that suspicious behavior is part of this patient's previous behaviors (and if it were, then it would also be covered by regression). **AN, 7, PsI**

Test-taking tip: Choose the "umbrella" option that covers the other options; in this case, **No. 4** covers the other examples of previous behaviors.

Substance-Related Disorders

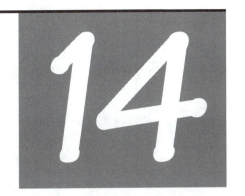

Chapter Outline

Introduction

Definition: ingesting in any manner a chemical that has an effect on the body.

Major Substances Used for Mind Alteration

See Table 14.1.

▶ **I. General assessment**
  A. *Behavioral* changes exist while under the influence of substance.
  B. Engages in regular *use* of substance.
    1. *Substance abuse*
      a. Pattern of *pathologic* use (i.e., day-long intoxication; inability to stop use, even when contraindicated by serious physical disorder; overpowering need or desire to take the drug despite legal, social, or medical problems); daily need of substance for functioning; repeated medical complications from use.
      b. *Interference* with social, occupational functioning.
      c. Willingness to obtain substance by any means, including illegal.
      d. Pathologic use for more than 1 month.
    2. *Substance dependence*
      a. More severe than substance abuse; body *requires* substance to continue functioning.
      b. *Physiologic dependence* (i.e., either develops a *tolerance*—must increase dose to obtain desired effect—or has *physical withdrawal symptoms* when substance intake is reduced or stopped).
      c. Person feels it's impossible to get along without drug.
  C. Effects of substance on *central nervous system* (CNS).
II. General analysis: Only in recent years has substance abuse been viewed as an illness rather than moral delinquency or criminal behavior. The disorders are very complex and little understood. There are physiologic, psychologic, and social aspects to their *causality, dynamics, symptoms,* and *treatment,* where personality disorder has a major part.
  A. *Physiologic aspects:* current unproven theories include "allergic" reaction to alcohol, disturbance in metabolism, genetic susceptibility to dependency, and hypofunction of adrenal cortex. There are *organic effects* of chronic excessive use.
  B. *Psychological aspects:* disrupted parent-child relationship and family dynamics; deleterious effect on ego function.
  C. *Social and cultural aspects:* local customs and attitudes vary about what is excessive.
  D. *Maladaptive behavior* related to:
    1. *Low self-esteem.*
    2. Anger.
    3. *Denial.*

Table 14.1 ● **MAJOR SUBSTANCES USED FOR MIND ALTERATION**

Official Name	Usual Single Adult Dose/Duration	Legitimate Medical Uses (Present and Projected)	Short-Term Effects	Long-Term Effects
Alcohol—whiskey, gin, beer, wine	1½ oz. gin or whiskey; 12 oz. beer/2–4 hr	Rare: sometimes used as a sedative (for tension)	CNS depressant; relaxation (sedation); euphoria; drowsiness; *impaired* judgment, reaction time, coordination, and emotional control; frequent aggressive behavior and driving accidents	Diversion of energy and money from more creative and productive pursuits; habituation; possible obesity with chronic excessive use; irreversible damage to brain and liver; addiction with severe withdrawal illness (DTs) with heavy use; many deaths
Caffeine—coffee, tea, cola, No-Doz	1–2 cups, 1 bottle, 5 mg/2–4 hr	Mild stimulant Treatment of some forms of coma	CNS stimulant; increased alertness; reduction of fatigue.	Sometimes insomnia, restlessness, or gastric irritation; habituation.
Nicotine (and coal tar) —cigarettes, cigars	1–2 cigarettes/1–2 hr	None (used as an insecticide)	CNS stimulant; relaxation or distraction.	Lung (and other) cancer, heart and blood vessel disease, cough, etc; higher infant mortality; many deaths; habituation; diversion of energy and money; air pollution; fire.

Sedatives
Alcohol—see above

Barbiturates—*Amytal, Nembutal, Seconal, Phenobarbital*	50–100 mg	Treatment of insomnia and tension Induction of anesthesia	CNS depressants; sleep induction; relaxation (sedation); sometimes euphoria; drowsiness; *impaired* judgment, reaction time, coordination, and emotional control; relief of anxiety/tension; muscle relaxation.	Irritability, weight loss, addiction with severe withdrawal illness (like DTs); diversion of energy and money; habituation, addiction.
Glutethimides (*Doriden*)	500 mg			
Chloral hydrate	500 mg			
Meprobamate (*Miltown, Equanil*)	400 mg/4 hr[a]			

Stimulants
Caffeine—see above

Nicotine—see above

Amphetamines *Benzedrine Methedrine Dexedrine*	2.5–15.0 mg	Treatment of *obesity,* narcolepsy, fatigue, depression	CNS stimulants; increased energy and alertness; reduction of fatigue; loss of appetite; insomnia; often euphoria; talkativeness; grandiosity; ↑ T, BP, P; weight loss; dry mouth.	Restlessness, weight loss, toxic psychosis (mainly paranoid); diversion of energy and money; habituation; extreme irritability, toxic psychosis.

Table 14.1 ● **MAJOR SUBSTANCES USED FOR MIND ALTERATION (CONTINUED)**

Official Name	Usual Single Adult Dose/Duration	Legitimate Medical Uses (Present and Projected)	Short-Term Effects	Long-Term Effects
Cocaine	Variable/4 hr[a]	Anesthesia of the eye and throat	Sudden death related to MI or respiratory arrest.	Seizures, CVA, TIA; nasal septum deterioration, brain's pleasure center no longer capable of responding to natural pleasures. May take up to several months to restore brain's balance.
Tranquilizers				
Chlordiazepoxide (*Librium*)	5–25 mg	Treatment of anxiety, tension, alcoholism, neurosis, psychosis, psychosomatic disorders, and vomiting	Selective CNS depressants; relaxation, relief of anxiety/tension; suppression of hallucinations or delusions, improved functioning	Sometimes drowsiness, dryness of mouth, blurring of vision, skin rash, tremor; occasionally jaundice, agranulocytosis, or death
Phenothiazines				
Thorazine	10–50 mg			
Compazine	5–10 mg			
Stelazine	2–5 mg			
Reserpine (*Rauwolfia*)	0.1–0.25 mg/4–6 hr[a]			
Marijuana or Cannabis[b]	Variable: 1 cigarette or pipe, or 1 drink or cake (India)/4 hr[a]	Treatment of depression, tension, loss of appetite and high BP	Relaxation, euphoria, increased appetite, some alteration of time perception, possible impairment of judgment and coordination; mixed CNS depressant-stimulant	Usually none; possible diversion of energy and money; habituation; occasional acute panic reactions
Antidepressants				
Ritalin	5–10 mg	Treatment of moderate to severe depression	Relief of depression (elevation of mood), stimulation	Basically the same as tranquilizers above
Imipramine HCl (*Tofranil*) amitriptyline HCl (*Elavil*)	25 mg, 10 mg			
MAO inhibitors (*Nardil, Parnate*)	10 mg, 15 mg/4–6 hr[a]			
Narcotics (Opiates, Analgesics)				
Opium	10–12 "pipes" (Asia)/4 hr[a]	Treatment of severe pain, diarrhea, and cough	CNS depressants; sedation, euphoria, relief of pain, impaired intellectual functioning and coordination	Constipation, loss of appetite and weight, temporary impotency or sterility; habituation, addiction with unpleasant and painful withdrawal illness
Heroin	Variable: bag or paper with 5–10% heroin			
	10–15 mg			
Morphine	15–30 mg			
Codeine	1 tablet			
Percodan	50–100 mg			
Demerol	2.5–40 mg			
Methadone	2–4 oz. (for euphoria)/4–6 hr[a]			
Cough syrups (*Cheracol, Hycodan, Romilar,* etc.)				

continues

Table 14.1 ☞ Major Substances Used for Mind Alteration (Continued)

Official Name	Usual Single Adult Dose/Duration	Legitimate Medical Uses (Present and Projected)	Short-Term Effects	Long-Term Effects
Hallucinogens				
LSD	150 µg/10–12 hr	Experimental study of mind and brain function; enhancement of creativity and problem solving; treatment of alcoholism, mental illness, and the dying person; chemical warfare	Production of visual imagery, increased sensory awareness, anxiety, nausea, impaired coordination; sometimes consciousness expansion	Usually none; sometimes precipitates or intensifies an already existing psychosis; more commonly can produce a panic reaction
Psilocybin	25 mg			
STP	6 mg			
DMT				
Mescaline (peyote)	350 mg/12–14 hr			
PCP				
Miscellaneous				
Glue, gasoline, and solvents	Variable	None except for antihistamines— used for allergy— and amyl nitrite for fainting	When used for mind alteration generally produces a "high" (euphoria) with impaired coordination and judgment	Variable: some of the substances can seriously damage the liver or kidney, and some produce hallucinations
Amyl nitrite	1–2 ampules			
Antihistamines	25–50 mg			
Nutmeg	Variable/2 hr			
Nonprescription "sedatives" (*Compoz*)				
Catnip				
Nitrous oxide				

*a*Time given pertains to all drugs listed.

*b*Hashish or charas is a more concentrated form of the active ingredient THC (tetrahydrocannabinol) and is consumed in smaller doses, analogous to vodka–beer ratios.

Key: LSD = lysergic acid diethylamide; MAO = monoamine oxidase; PCP = phencyclidine.

Copyright © Joel Fort, M.D., author of *Alcohol: Our Biggest Drug Problem* (McGraw-Hill) and *The Pleasure Seekers* (Grove Press); founder, The National Center for Solving Special Social & Health Problems—FORT HELP and the Violence Prevention Program, San Francisco; and formerly Lecturer, School of Criminology, University of California, Berkeley, and Consultant, World Health Organization. Used by permission.

4. Rationalization.
5. Social isolation.
6. A rigid pattern of coping.
7. Poorly defined philosophy of life, values, mores.

☒ **E. Analysis/nursing diagnosis in acute phase** of abuse, intoxication:

1. *Risk for injury* related to impaired coordination, disorientation, and altered judgment (worse at night).
2. *Risk for violence:* self-directed or directed at others, related to misinterpretation of stimuli and feelings of suspicion or distrust of others.
3. *Sensory-perceptual alterations:* visual, kinesthetic, tactile, related to intake of mind-altering substances.
4. *Altered thought processes* (delusions, incoherence) related to misinterpretation of stimuli.
5. *Sleep pattern disturbance* related to mind-altering substance.
6. *Ineffective individual coping* related to inability to tolerate frustration and to meet basic needs or role expectations, resulting in unpredictable behaviors.
7. *Noncompliance* with abstinence and supportive therapy, related to inability to stop using substance because of dependence and refusal to alter life-style.
8. *Impaired communication* related to mental confusion or CNS depression related to substance use.
9. *Impaired health maintenance management* related to failure to recognize that a problem exists and inability to take responsibility for health needs.

Alcohol Use Disorders: Abuse and Dependence

Alcohol dependence is a chronic disorder in which the individual is unable, for physical or psychological reasons or both, to refrain from frequent consumption of alcohol in quantities that produce intoxication and disrupt health and ability to perform daily functions.

I. Concepts and principles

    A. Alcohol affects cerebral cortical functions:

        1. Memory.

        2. Judgment.

        3. Reasoning.

    B. Alcohol is a *depressant:*

        1. Relaxes the individual.

        2. Lessens use of repression of unconscious conflict.

        3. Releases inhibitions, hostility, and primitive drives.

    C. Drinking represents a tension-reducing device and a relief from feelings of insecurity. Strength of drinking habit equals degree of *anxiety* and *frustration intolerance.*

    D. Alcohol abuse and dependence is a *symptom* rather than a disease.

    E. Underlying fear and anxiety, associated with inner conflict, motivate the alcoholic to drink.

    F. Alcoholics can *never* be cured to drink normally; cure is to be a "sober alcoholic," with total abstinence.

    G. The spouse of the alcoholic often unconsciously contributes to the drinking behavior because of own emotional needs (*co-alcoholic* or *co-dependent*).

    H. Intoxication occurs with a blood alcohol level of 0.08% or above. *Signs of intoxication* are:

        1. Incoordination.

        2. Slurred speech.

        3. Dulled perception.

    I. *Tolerance* occurs with alcohol dependence. Increasing amounts of alcohol must be consumed in order to obtain the desired effect.

II. Assessment

    A. *Vicious cycle:* low tolerance for coping with frustration, tension, guilt, resentment → uses alcohol for relief → new problems created by drinking → new anxieties → more drinking.

    B. Coping mechanisms used: primarily *denial,* with *rationalization* and *projection.*

    C. *Complications* of abuse and dependence:

        1. Alcohol withdrawal delirium (*delirium tremens* [*DTs*]) (Figure 14.1): result of nutritional deficiencies and toxins; requires *sedation* and constant watchfulness against unintentional *suicide* and *convulsions.*

            a. *Impending* signs (within 8–12 h):

                (1) *CNS:* marked nervousness and restlessness, increased irritability; gross tremors of hands, face, lips; weakness.

                (2) *Cardiovascular:* increased BP, tachycardia, diaphoresis.

                (3) *Depression.*

                (4) *Gastrointestinal:* nausea, vomiting, anorexia.

            b. *Actual* (within 24–48h): *serious* symptoms of mental confusion, convulsions, hallucinations (visual, auditory, tactile). Without cure, *15–20% may die.*

        2. Wernicke-Korsakoff syndrome: a neurologic disturbance manifested by confusion, ataxia, eye movement abnormalities, and memory impairment. Other problems include:

            a. Disturbed vision.

            b. Mind-wandering.

            c. Stupor and coma.

        3. Alcohol amnestic syndrome (Korsakoff's psychosis): degenerative neuritis due to *thiamine* deficiency.

            a. Impaired thoughts.

            b. Confusion, loss of sense of time and place.

            c. Use of confabulation to fill in severe memory loss.

            d. Follows episode of *Wernicke's encephalopathy.*

        4. *Polyneuropathy:* sensory and motor nerve endings are involved, causing pain, itching, and loss of limb control.

        5. Others (Table 14.2): *gastritis, esophageal varices, cirrhosis, pancreatitis, diabetes,* pneumonia, REM sleep deprivation, *malnutrition.*

III. Analysis/nursing diagnosis

    A. *Risk for self-directed violence:* tendency for *self-destructive* acts related to intake of mind-altering substances.

    B. *Altered nutrition, less than body requirements,* related to a lack of interest in food.

    C. *Defensive coping* related to tendency to be *domineering* and critical, with difficulties in *interpersonal* relationships.

    D. *Conflict with social order* related to *extreme dependence* coupled with resentment *of authority.*

    E. *Spiritual distress* or general dissatisfaction with life related to *low frustration* tolerance and demand for immediate need satisfaction.

    F. *Dysfunctional behaviors* related to tendency for *excess* in work, sex, recreation, marked *narcissistic* behavior.

    G. *Social isolation* related to use of coping mechanisms that are primarily *escapist* (e.g., *denial*).

IV. Nursing care plan/implementation

    A. Detoxification phase

        1. Administer *adequate sedation* to control anxiety, *insomnia,* agitation, *tremors.*

        2. Administer *anticonvulsants* to prevent *withdrawal seizures.*

        3. *Control nausea* and *vomiting* to avoid massive GI bleeding or rupture of esophageal varices.

        4. *Assess fluid* and *electrolyte balance* for dehydration (may need IV fluids) or overhydration (may need a diuretic).

        5. Reestablish *proper nutrition: high protein* (as long as no severe liver damage), carbohydrate (CHO), *vitamins C and B* complex.

        6. Provide *calm, safe environment:* bedrest *with rails,* well-lit room to reduce illusions; constant supervision and reassurance about fears and *hallucinations,* assess depression for *suicide potential.*

    B. Recovery-rehabilitation phase

        1. Encourage participation in *group* activities.

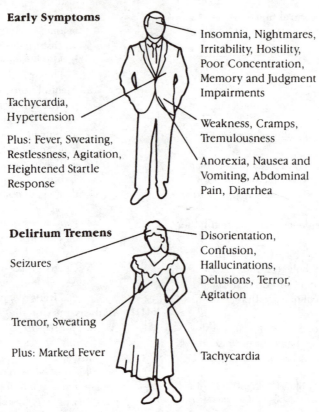

Early Symptoms

Insomnia, Nightmares, Irritability, Hostility, Poor Concentration, Memory and Judgment Impairments

Tachycardia, Hypertension

Plus: Fever, Sweating, Restlessness, Agitation, Heightened Startle Response

Weakness, Cramps, Tremulousness

Anorexia, Nausea and Vomiting, Abdominal Pain, Diarrhea

Delirium Tremens

Seizures

Disorientation, Confusion, Hallucinations, Delusions, Terror, Agitation

Tremor, Sweating

Plus: Marked Fever

Tachycardia

FIGURE 14.1   SYMPTOMS ASSOCIATED WITH ALCOHOL WITHDRAWAL (From Wilson HS, Kneisl CR: *Psychiatric Nursing* (2nd ed.) Menlo Park, CA: Addison-Wesley, 1983, p. 388.)

2. *Avoid sympathy* when client tends to rationalize behavior and seeks special privileges—use acceptance and a *nonjudgmental*, consistent, firm, but kind approach.
3. *Avoid* scorn, contempt, and moralizing or punitive and rejecting behaviors.
4. Do *not* reinforce feelings of worthlessness, self-contempt, hopelessness, or low self-esteem.

C. Problem behaviors
  1. *Manipulative*—be firm and consistent; *avoid* "bid for sympathy."
  2. *Demanding*—set limits.
  3. *Acting out*—set limits, enforce rules and regulations, strengthen impulse control and ability to delay gratification.
  4. *Dependency*—place *responsibility* on client; *avoid* advice-giving.
  5. *Superficiality*—help client make realistic self-appraisals and expectations in lieu of grandiose promises and trite verbalizations; encourage formation of lasting interpersonal relationships.

D. Common reactions among staff
  1. *Disappointment*—instead, set realistic goals, take one step at a time.
  2. *Moral judgment*—instead, support each other.
  3. *Hostility*—instead, offer support to each other when feeling frustrated from lack of results.

E. Refer client from hospital to **community resources** for follow-up treatment with social, economic, and psychological problems, as well as to self-help groups, in order to reduce "revolving door" situation in which client comes in, is treated, goes out, and comes in again the next night.
  1. *Alcoholics Anonymous (AA)*: a self-help group of addicted drinkers who confront, instruct, and support fellow drinkers in their efforts to stay sober one day at a time through fellowship and acceptance.
  2. *Alanon*: support group for *families* of alcoholics. *Alateen*: support group for *teenagers* when parent is alcoholic.
  3. *Aversion therapy*: client is subjected to revulsion-producing or pain-inducing stimuli at the same time client takes a drink, to establish alcohol rejection behavior. Most common is *Antabuse* (disulfiram), a drug that produces intense headache, severe flushing, extreme nausea, vomiting, palpitations, hypotension, dyspnea, and blurred vision when alcohol is consumed while person is taking this drug.
  4. *Group psychotherapy*: the goals of group psychotherapy are for the client to give up alcohol as a tension reliever, identify cause of stress, build *different means for coping* with stress, and accept drinking as a serious symptom.

Table 14.2	MEDICAL PROBLEMS TO WHICH ALCOHOLICS ARE PARTICULARLY SUSCEPTIBLE
Condition	*Contributing Factors*
Subdural hematoma	Frequent falls Impaired clotting mechanisms
Gastrointestinal bleeding	Irritant effect of alcohol on the stomach lining (leading to *gastritis*) Impaired clotting mechanisms *Cirrhosis* of the liver, leading to engorgement of esophageal veins (*esophageal varices*)
Pancreatitis	Indirect effect of alcohol on the pancreas
Hypoglycemia (diabetes)	Damage to the liver, which normally mobilizes sugar into the blood
Pneumonia	Aspiration of vomitus occurring during intoxication and coma Suppression of immune system by alcohol
Burns	Relative insensitivity to pain occurring during intoxication Falling asleep with a lit cigarette while intoxicated
Hypothermia	Insensitivity to extremes of temperature while intoxicated Falling asleep outside in the cold
Seizures	Effect of withdrawal from alcohol
Dysrhythmias	Toxic effects of alcohol on the heart
Cancer	Mechanism not known (perhaps related to suppression of the immune system), but alcoholics are 10 times more likely than the general population to develop cancer
Sleep disturbance	REM sleep deprivation
Malnutrition	Poor eating habits

Source: Caroline N. *Emergency Care in the Streets* (5th ed). Boston: Little, Brown, 1995. P. 695.

F. *Health teaching*
1. Improved coping patterns to tolerate increased stress.
2. Substitute tension-reducing strategies.
3. Prepare in advance for difficult, painful events.
4. How to reduce irritating or frustrating environmental stress.
5. Provide dietary counseling.

◄► V. **Evaluation/outcome criteria:** everyday living patterns are restructured for a satisfactory life without alcohol; demonstrates feelings of increased self-worth, confidence, and reliance.

Other Substance-Related Disorders

I. **Concepts and principles**
A. *Three* interacting key factors give rise to dependence: *psychopathology* of the individual; frustrating *environment;* and *availability* of powerful, addicting, and temporarily satisfying drug.
B. According to conditioning principles, substance abuse and dependence proceed in *several phases:*
1. *Use* of sedatives-hypnotics, CNS stimulants, hallucinogens and narcotics, for relief from daily tensions and discomforts or anticipated withdrawal symptoms.
2. Habit is *reinforced* with each relief by drug use.
3. Development of *dependency*—drug has less and less efficiency in reducing tensions.
4. Dependency is further reinforced as addict *fails* to maintain adequate drug intake—increase in frequency and duration of periods of tension and discomfort.

II. Street names of common drugs and terms relating to drug use—Tables 14.3 and 14.4.

◄► III. **Assessment**
A. **Abuse**
1. **Hallucinogens:** euphoria and rapid mood swings, flight of ideas; perceptual impairment, feelings of omnipotence, "bad trip" (panic, loss of control, paranoia), flashbacks, suicide.
2. **CNS stimulants** (*amphetamines* and *cocaine* abuse): euphoria, hyperactivity, hyperalertness, irritability, persecutory delusions; insomnia, anorexia → weight loss; tachycardia; tremulousness; hypertension; hyperthermia → convulsions.
3. **Narcotics** (*opium* and its derivatives; e.g., *morphine, heroin, codeine, Demerol*): used by "snorting," "skin popping" and "mainlining."

Table 14.3   STREET NAMES OF COMMONLY ABUSED DRUGS

Type of Drug	Examples	Street Names
Uppers		
Amphetamines	*Benzedrine*	A's, Bennies, Benzies, cartwheels, hearts, peaches, roses, speed
	Dexedrine	Dexies, footballs, oranges
	Methedrine	Bonita, bambita
	Methylenedioxyamphetamine (MDA)	Ecstasy, XTC, Adam, MDM
	Methylenedioxyethamphetamine (MDEA)	Eve
	Methamphetamine hydrochloride	Ice
Cocaine		Bernice, big C, blow, burese, C, Carrie, Cecil, Charlie, cholly, coke, corine, dama blanca, dynamite, flake, gin, girl, gold dust, green gold, happy dust, happy trails, heaven dust, jet, joy powder, lady, nose candy, paradise, snort, snow, stardust, star-spangled powder, sugar, toot, white dust, white girl, zoom
	Modified cocaine	Crack (freebase cocaine), liquid lady (cocaine + alcohol), rock (freebase cocaine), speedball (cocaine + heroin)
Antiasthmatics	Aminophylline	
	Isoproterenol	
	Adrenalin	
Caffeine	Coffee, cola	Java
Downers		
Alcohol	Wine, beer, whiskey	Rose (wine), sneaky Pete (wine)
Narcotics	*Heroin*	China white, horse, Harry, smack, stuff, big H, blanco
	Morphine	Hard stuff, Miss Emma, big M, unkie
	Codeine	Fours
	Hydromorphone (*Dilaudid*)	Dillies
	Methadone	Amidone, dollies
	Opium	Auntie, black stuff, Greece
Barbiturates	Pentobarbital (*Nembutal*)	Yellow jackets, yellows, nimbies, nebbies
	Amobarbital (*Amytal*)	Blue devils, blue birds, blue heaven, blue bullets, jackup
	Seconal	Red birds, red devils, pinks, bala, M&Ms
Chloral hydrate		Mickey Finn, Mickey, Peter, chlorals, hog
Tranquilizers	*Thorazine*	
	Valium	
	Librium	Roche-tens
Marijuana and its products	Marijuana	Grass, pot, weed, joint, Acapulco gold, ace, Aunt Mary, bo-bo, broccoli, duby, gage, Mary Jane, tea, reefer
	Hashish	Black Russian, blue cheese, gram, hash, heesh, THC
Hallucinogens		
Lysergic acid diethylamide (LSD)		Acid, blue cheers, California sunshine, crackers, cubes, ghost, heavenly blue
Phencyclidine (PCP)		Elephant, PeaCee Pill
Mescaline		Cactus buttons
Peyote		Bad acid, bad seed, big chief, button, half-moon

Key: LSD = lysergic acid diethylamide; PCP = phencyclidine; THC = tetrahydrocannabinol

Source: Caroline N. *Emergency Care in the Streets* (5th ed). Boston: Little, Brown, 1995. P. 687.

Table 14.4   TERMS RELATING TO DRUG USE

Term	*Refers To*
Amped	Hyperstimulated on cocaine
Bagging	Inhaling volatile substances from a bag
Blank	Low-grade narcotics
Bodypacker	Person who smuggles cocaine by ingesting latex containers (e.g., condoms) filled with the drug
Burned	Received phony narcotics
Coasting	Under the influence of drugs
Cold turkey	Sudden cessation of drug intake
Cut	Adulterated
Dynamite	High-grade heroin
Freebasing	Breathing cocaine vapors (smoked in a pipe)
Hit	2–200 mg of cocaine
Huffing	Inhaling through a cloth soaked in a volatile substance (such as glue)
Joy pop	Inject narcotics regularly
Layout	Outfit employed by opium user
Lemonade	Poor heroin
Mainlining	Injecting drugs IV
Mule	Same as a bodypacker
On the nod	Drowsy from narcotics
Panic	Shortage of narcotics on the street
Quill	Matchbook cover for sniffing cocaine
Reader	Prescription order
Reader with tail	Forged prescription order
Run	Prolonged drug binge
Rush	Feeling of euphoric pleasure
Shooting gallery	Place where addicts inject themselves
Shooting up	Injecting narcotics IV
Skin popping	Injecting under skin (subcutaneous)
Snorting	Inhaling drugs in powdered form
Speedballing	Injecting drug combinations (especially cocaine plus alcohol)
Spoon	1 g of cocaine
Stepped on	Diluted
Track marks	Needle marks from injections
Wired	Hyperstimulated on cocaine

Source: Caroline N. *Emergency Care in the Streets* (5th ed). Boston: Little, Brown, 1995. P. 688.

May lead to abscesses and hepatitis. Decreased pain response, respiratory depression; apathy, detachment from reality; impaired judgment; loss of sexual activity; pinpoint pupils.

4. **Sedative-hypnotics** (*barbiturate* abuse): like alcohol-induced behavior; e.g., euphoria followed by depression, hostility; decreased inhibitions; impaired judgment; staggering gait; slurred speech; drowsiness; poor concentration; progressive respiratory depression.

B. Withdrawal symptoms

1. *Narcotics* (e.g., heroin): begins within 12 hr of last dose, peaks in 24–36 hr, subsides in 72 hr, and disappears in 5–6 d.
   a. Pupil *dilation*.
   b. Muscle: twitches, tremors, aches, pains.
   c. Goose flesh (piloerection).
   d. *Lacrimation, rhinorrhea, sneezing, yawning.*
   e. *Diaphoresis*, chills.
   f. Potential for fever.
   g. *Vomiting*, abdominal distress.
   h. Dehydration.
   i. Rapid weight loss.
   j. Sleep disturbance.

2. *Barbiturates:* may be gradual or abrupt ("cold turkey"); latter is dangerous or *life-threatening*; should be hospitalized.
   a. *Gradual* withdrawal reaction from barbiturates:
      (1) Postural hypotension.
      (2) Tachycardia.
      (3) Elevated temperature.
      (4) Insomnia.
      (5) Tremors.
      (6) Agitation, restlessness.
   b. *Abrupt* withdrawal from barbiturates:
      (1) Apprehension.
      (2) Muscular weakness.

(3) Tremors.

(4) Postural hypotension.

(5) Twitching.

(6) Anorexia.

(7) *Grand mal seizures.*

(8) *Psychosis-delirium.*

 3. *Amphetamines* and *cocaine:* depression, lack of energy, somnolence, agitation.

C. Signs of *overdose* or toxicity:

Drug Type	Signs of Overdose or Toxicity
Amphetamines and **cocaine**	Restlessness, *agitation*, jitters Incessant talking Insomnia, anorexia Dilated pupils Tachycardia, tachypnea, hypertension Extreme depression on *withdrawal* (dysphoric mood)
Narcotics	Constricted "pinpoint" pupils Marked respiratory depression Needle tracks (*heroin* user) Sometimes bradycardia and hypotension Drowsiness, stupor, or coma
Barbiturates	Respiratory depression Dilated pupils Hypotension
Hallucinogens	Hallucinations Panic reactions, agitation Chills, shivering Tachycardia, elevated blood pressure
PCP	Blank stare, muscular rigidity, sometimes extremely violent, self-destructive behavior

Source: Caroline N. *Emergency Care in the Streets* (5th ed). Boston: Little, Brown, 1995. P. 693.

D. *Difference* between alcohol and other abused substances (e.g., *opioid*).

1. Above drugs may need to be obtained by illegal means, making it a legal and criminal problem as well as a medical and social problem; *not* so with alcohol abuse and dependency.

2. *Opium* and its derivatives *inhibit* aggression, whereas alcohol *releases* aggression.

3. As long as she or he is on large enough doses to avoid withdrawal symptoms, abuser of *narcotics, sedatives,* or *hypnotics* is comfortable and functions well, whereas chronically intoxicated alcoholic *cannot* function normally.

4. Direct physiologic effects of long-term *opioid* abuse and dependence on above drugs are

much *less critical* than those with chronic alcohol dependence.

IV. Analysis/nursing diagnosis

A. *Risk for altered physical regulation processes* (cardiac, circulation, gastrointestinal, sleep pattern disturbance) related to use of mind-altering drugs.

B. *Altered conduct/impulse processes* related to rebellious attitudes toward authority.

C. *Altered social interaction* (manipulation, dependency) related to hostility and personal insecurity.

D. *Altered judgment* related to misinterpretation of sensory stimuli and low frustration tolerance.

E. *Altered feeling states* (denial) related to underlying self-doubt and personal insecurity.

V. Nursing care plan/implementation: generally the same as in treating antisocial personality and alcohol abuse and dependence.

A. Maintain *safety* and optimum level of *physical comfort.* Supportive physical care: vital signs, nutrition, hydration, seizure precautions.

B. *Assist with medical treatment* and offer support and *reality orientation* to reduce feelings of panic.

1. *Detoxification* (or *dechemicalization*): give medications according to detoxification schedule.

2. *Withdrawal:* may be gradual (*barbiturates, hypnotics, tranquilizers*) or abrupt ("cold turkey" for heroin). Observe for symptoms and report immediately.

3. *Methadone:* person must have been dependent on narcotics at least 2 years and have failed at other methods of withdrawal before admission to program of readdiction by methadone.

   a. *Characteristics*

   (1) Synthetic.

   (2) Appeases desire for narcotics without producing euphoria of narcotics.

   (3) Given by mouth.

   (4) Distributed under federal control (Narcotic Addict Rehabilitation Act).

   (5) Given with urinary surveillance.

   b. *Advantages*

   (1) Prevents narcotic withdrawal reaction.

   (2) Tolerance not built up.

   (3) Person remains out of prison.

   (4) Lessens perceived need for heroin or morphine.

   c. *Disadvantages:* addiction can occur and is more prolonged than for other opiates, but symptoms are less severe.

C. *Participation in group therapy—goals:* peer pressure, support, and identification.

D. *Rehabilitation phase*

1. Refer to halfway house and group living (e.g., Daytop).

2. Support *employment* as therapy (work training).

3. Expand client's *range of interests* to relieve characteristic boredom and stimulus hunger.

   a. Provide *structured* environment and planned routine.

    b. Provide educational therapy (academic and vocational).

    c. Arrange activities to include current events discussion groups, lectures, drama, music, and art appreciation.

  E. Achieve role of *stabilizer* and *supportive* authoritative figure; this can be achieved through frequent, regular contacts with the same client.

  F. *Health teaching:* how to cope with pain, fatigue, and anxiety without drugs.

VI. Evaluation/outcome criteria: replaces addictive lifestyle with self-reliant behavior.

Study and Memory Aids

Alcohol detoxification: care

Drugs: anticonvulsants to prevent seizures; sedatives to ↓ insomnia, agitation, tremors

Diet: Protein; ↑ CHO, vitamins B and C

Alcoholism: goals for long-term rehabilitation—"COPING"

Community resources (AA, Alanon)
Other coping means, rather than denial
Personal responsibility for not drinking
↓**I**solation: encourage activity without alcohol
Nutrition: high CHO, vitamins B and C
Group treatment

Alcohol-dependent behaviors—"Five D's"

Denial (disown, block out thoughts of being an alcoholic)
Dependent (and resentful); co-dependent relationships
Demanding (↓ frustration tolerance)
Destructive (self)
Domineering (controlling behaviors, to hide low self-esteem)

Alcohol withdrawal: need to treat "HI²TS⁴"

Hallucinations
Insomnia; **I**ncreased vital signs
Tremens: delirium tremens (can be lethal)
S⁴: **S**hakes, **S**weats, **S**eizures, **S**tomach pain

Source: Adapted from Rogers PT. *The Medical Student's Guide to Top Board Scores.* Boston: Little, Brown, 1996. P. 46.

Antabuse (disulfiram)

AVOID Alcohol-based products, including:
  Mouthwashes
  OTC cold medicines and cough syrups
  Food sauces made with wine
  Flavor extracts (e.g., vanilla)
  Vinegar
  Aftershave lotions
  Skin products and rubbing lotions

Summary of Key Points*

Substance Abuse

1. *Self-destructive* pattern of substance use continues despite negative consequences (e.g., physical danger or harm; recurrent academic, occupational or legal problems; impaired functioning at home or in social environment).
2. *Nursing implication:* safety concerns.

Substance Dependence

1. Development of *tolerance* and/or withdrawal; may use the substance to avoid or reduce withdrawal symptoms.
2. *Compulsive* use, including use of substance in greater amounts than intended, with excessive time spent getting or using the substance; ↓ other activities in favor of substance use.

3. *Nursing implication:* deal with denial and rationalization; encourage use of groups like Alcoholics Anonymous.

Substance Withdrawal

1. Sudden stoppage of a substance (e.g., alcohol, barbiturates) that has been used for a long time results in symptoms that cause severe distress and can be life-threatening.
2. *Nursing implication:* early awareness of signs and symptoms of withdrawal and immediate *medical* attention are crucial.

*Adapted from: Breaden R, et al., *Rx Prescription for the Boards, USMLE Step 2, a Student-to-Student Guide.* Boston: Little, Brown, 1996.

Wernicke-Korsakoff syndrome is an alcohol-related neurologic disorder caused by thiamine deficiency.

- **Wernicke's encephalopathy** is the *acute* phase.
- **Korsakoff's psychosis** is the *chronic* phase.

Wernicke-Korsakoff syndrome: assessment—"COAT RACK"

Wernicke's encephalopathy (acute phase):
   Confusion
   Ophthalmoplegia
   Ataxia
   Thiamine deficiency

Korsakoff's psychosis (chronic phase):
   Retrograde amnesia (↓ memory for *old* information)
   Anterograde amnesia (↓ memory for *new* information)
   Confabulation
   Korsakoff's psychosis

Source: Rogers PT. *The Medical Student's Guide to Top Board Scores.* Boston: Little, Brown, 1996. P. 44.

Glossary

abuse   Misuse of a chemical substance with mind-altering properties, which may lead to disturbed social and family relationships, loss of job and health, and legal problems.

addiction   A group of cognitive, physical, and behavioral symptoms in an individual who is using a drug or drugs, which give evidence to the individual's lack of control of the substance(s). It is characterized by physical dependence, tolerance, and psychological dependence on the drug(s). (Also known as *chemical dependence*.)

alcohol withdrawal delirium   A serious reaction to discontinuing drinking; characterized by anxiety, tremors, disorientation, and hallucinations. (Formerly called *delirium tremens*.)

co-dependency   Relationship in which an individual becomes involved with, relies on, and takes care of a substance-abusing person as a way to meet own needs for survival, security, and/or control. Can result in perpetuation of the affected individual's impairment.

dependence   Misuse of a substance that leads to significant health problems, with development of *tolerance, psychological dependence,* and *physical dependence*.

psychological **dependence**   A craving for the effect of a substance.

physical **dependence**   the body's need for a substance; can result in withdrawal reaction when substance is discontinued.

detoxification   Steps taken to medically remove a toxic substance from the body.

dysarthria   Impaired speech (e.g., stuttering) caused by emotional or physical disorders.

dyskinesia   Impaired voluntary movement.

dystonia   Impaired muscle tone.

euphoria   An exaggerated mood of well-being.

fetal alcohol syndrome   Condition affecting babies born to alcoholic mothers that includes signs of alcohol dependence, physical abnormalities, and intellectual impairment.

hallucinogens   A classification of abused drugs that produce a psychotic-like experience.

narcotics   A classification of drugs that produce analgesia and euphoria.

substance   A general term for a drug that can be used to alter perception and mood, including alcohol, over-the-counter medications, illegal drugs, and prescription drugs.

tolerance   The increasing need for more frequent and larger doses of a drug in order to get the effect previously experienced.

Questions

1. The nurse should look for which complication related to sudden alcohol withdrawal?
   1. Seizures and hallucinations.
   2. Low blood pressure and anorexia.
   3. Headaches and diarrhea.
   4. Agnosia and aphasia.

2. Which environmental factor is it most important to avoid for a patient with impending alcohol withdrawal delirium (DTs)?
   1. Unfamiliar staff.
   2. Strong odors.
   3. Shadows on the wall.
   4. Single-bedded room.

3. When doing an admission assessment of a patient with a history of alcoholism, the most important factor to assess is:
   1. The presence of track marks.
   2. When the patient last had a drink.
   3. Previous coping skills.
   4. Whether the patient has had previous treatment.

4. When would it be important for the nurse to recognize impending signs and symptoms of alcohol withdrawal delirium (DTs) in a hospitalized patient who is alcohol-dependent?
   1. During the first few hours after admission.
   2. 8–12 hours after admission.
   3. 24–48 hours after admission.
   4. 3–5 days after admission.

5. The best environment for a patient experiencing alcohol withdrawal would be a:
   1. Brightly lit room.
   2. Dim night-light on the floor.
   3. Soft, filtered, indirect light.
   4. Room as dark as possible.

6. In order for nursing interventions to be most effective, for which common and significant coping mechanism should the nurse watch when beginning to work with a patient who is alcohol-dependent?
   1. Rationalization.

2. Denial.
3. Displacement.
4. Ambivalence.

7. The nurse should anticipate that the medical management of a patient admitted with a long-term history of alcohol abuse will include:
   1. Restraints and sedation.
   2. Tranquilizers and a diet with increased thiamine.
   3. A fluid diet and vitamin C.
   4. Hydrotherapy and monitoring of serum lithium levels.

8. A patient who is on the alcohol detoxification unit asks the nurse's colleague what Alcoholics Anonymous (AA) is. What explanation by the nurse would indicate that the nurse needs further in-service education?
   1. AA encourages complete abstinence.
   2. AA instills hope.
   3. AA promotes a one-day-at-a-time philosophy.
   4. AA offers sympathy.

9. The nurse refers a patient to Alcoholics Anonymous because of its best aspect, which is that it:
   1. Is a substitute for the barroom.
   2. Provides a person on-call, prn.
   3. Is a support group.
   4. Reduces alienation.

10. As part of the discharge teaching for a patient going home on disulfiram (Antabuse), the nurse instructs the patient to avoid:
    1. Over-the-counter (OTC) antihistamines.
    2. Ibuprofen (Advil).
    3. Cough syrups.
    4. Toothpaste with bicarbonate.

11. The nurse should be aware that which common defense mechanisms are associated with substance dependence?
    1. Denial and projection.
    2. Rationalization and reaction formation.
    3. Displacement and denial.
    4. Repression and projection.

12. A patient has been admitted to a drug detoxification center because she appeared to act in a bizarre, suspicious manner, with extreme agitation. She tells the nurse that she was on weight-loss pills. The nurse should recognize that the patient's behavior is most likely related to the use of:
    1. Amphetamines.
    2. Barbiturates.
    3. Hallucinogens.
    4. Phencyclidine (PCP).

13. The nurse should be alert for amphetamine abuse by a patient when the most significant assessment finding is:
    1. Cardiac irregularities.
    2. Drowsiness.
    3. Constricted pupils.
    4. Increased appetite, dry mouth.

14. A 19-year-old has been admitted to the chemical dependency unit of a mental health center; the initial diagnosis is cocaine addiction. The patient's history reveals use of cocaine 3–4 times a week for the past 6 months, with a binge two days ago. The patient was brought to the center by the family, after telling them

that "people are trying to kill me." During the first day of hospitalization, the patient sleeps continuously and only gets out of bed for medications and to go to the bathroom. The most appropriate plan for this patient at this time is to:
    1. Allow the patient to sleep and rest the first few days of treatment.
    2. Set firm limits and restrict sleeping to nighttime hours.
    3. Allow short naps, but require the patient to attend all group sessions.
    4. Verbally confront the patient about motivation and commitment to change.

15. The nurse understands that cocaine acts on the body as a:
    1. Central nervous system depressant.
    2. Vasodilator, which lowers blood pressure.
    3. Physical stimulant and euphoriant.
    4. Synthetic pain reliever.

16. In orienting a new staff member to the drug unit, the nurse needs to stress that the most lethal method of cocaine consumption is:
    1. Intravenous injection.
    2. Snorting up the nasal canals.
    3. Freebasing.
    4. Smoking.

17. The nurse should assess for which of the following behaviors related to withdrawal from cocaine?
    1. Dysphoric mood, fatigue, and agitation.
    2. Headache, nausea, and vomiting.
    3. Hyperactivity, tachycardia, and diaphoresis.
    4. Heightened self-esteem, agitation, and elevated blood pressure.

18. After prolonged use of cocaine, the brain's pleasure center is no longer capable of responding to natural pleasures. How long can the nurse expect it will take for the chemical balance of a cocaine abuser's brain to return to normal, without medication?
    1. Several days to months.
    2. One year.
    3. Several years.
    4. Indefinitely.

19. A person who is a cocaine abuser says to the nurse, "I hate myself for being this way. Don't waste your time talking to me; I'm dead meat." The nurse's best response would be:
    1. "Go on, tell me more."
    2. "Have you considered killing yourself?"
    3. "I'm concerned about you, and I don't think you are a waste of my time."
    4. "What do you mean when you say 'dead meat'?"

Answers/Rationale

1. **(1)** The danger from sudden withdrawal from alcohol is the possibility of death related to seizures. These are signs of *actual*, not impending alcohol withdrawal delirium (DTs). *Hypertension* is associated with sudden alcohol withdrawal, *not* hypotension (**No. 2**). While headaches and diarrhea (**No. 3**) are early signs of *im-*

pending DTs, they are *not* as critical as signs and symptoms of *actual* DTs (seizures and hallucinations). Agnosia and aphasia (**No. 4**) are *not* related to sudden withdrawal from alcohol. **AS,2,PhI**

2. (**3**) Visual hallucinations are common when visual cues (such as shadows) are misinterpreted. Common visual hallucinations such as seeing crawling insects can be frightening. Excitation (in the form of fear) definitely needs to be avoided in order to reduce the chance of DTs. Unfamiliar staff (**No. 1**) is *not* a special concern for a patient with impending DTs. Strong odors (**No. 2**) might be best avoided, since most external environmental stimuli (visual, auditory, *and* olfactory) should be reduced, but olfactory overstimulation is not the *main* concern in avoiding DTs. A single-bedded room (**No. 4**) *should* be assigned, rather than avoided, to reduce environmental stimuli. **IMP, 2, SECE**

3. (**2**) The nurse needs to be concerned about the *onset of* alcohol withdrawal symptoms, which is usually within 8 hours of the last drink. This can be a life-threatening condition and needs immediate medical intervention. Alcohol is *not* usually injected; therefore checking for track marks (**No. 1**) is irrelevant. The focus needs to be on the present, *not previous* coping skills (**No. 3**), nor *previous* treatment (**No. 4**). **AS, 2, PhI**

💡 *Test-taking tip:* The *key words* are "most important factor"; in this case, a factor related to a possible problem affecting physiologic integrity (impending DTs).

4. (**2**) The impending signs are likely to be observed within 8–12 hours following withdrawal from alcohol. At this time the condition can be detected, treated, and controlled before it is a clinical emergency, when convulsions and death can occur if not treated. **No. 1** is usually too soon to observe DTs (the body's response to abrupt withdrawal from alcohol); **No. 3** is when the *onset* and *serious* signs of alcohol withdrawl delirium are detected; **No. 4** is referred to as *continuing* delirium with severe psychomotor activity, sleeplessness, hallucinations, and uncontrolled tachycardia. **EV, 2, PhI**

5. (**1**) The more light, the less likely the patient is to distort shadows, decreasing the opportunity for "seeing things" (visual hallucinations). Dim light (**No. 2**), soft, filtered, indirect light (**No. 3**), and darkness (**No. 4**) are all opposites of "brightly lit." **PL, 1, SECE**

💡 *Test-taking tip:* Three options are similar (dim, indirect light, dark), and one is different (brightly lit). When you

have to make an "educated guess," focus on the one option that is different.

6. (**2**) Denial of a problem with alcohol is the *underlying* coping mechanism. Rationalization (**No. 1**) and displacement (**No. 3**) *stem from the underlying* denial. For example, early in the nurse-patient relationship, the patient with alcohol dependency may make this typical statement to the nurse: "I'm not an alcoholic" (denial); "I only drink a few beers on the way home" (rationalization); "when the boss gives me a bad time at work" (displacement). Rather than ambivalence (**No. 4**), *resistance* is more common as a coping mechanism. Patients with alcohol abuse/dependency use *denial* to *resist* identifying alcoholism as a problem. **AS, 7, PsI**

💡 *Test-taking tip:* When two or three options appear correct (in this case, **Nos. 1, 2, and 3**), choose the one that encompasses them all like an *umbrella.*

7. (**2**) A thiamine deficiency is commonly present and needs to be corrected to decrease symptoms of peripheral neuropathy. Tranquilizers are used in detoxification to prevent alcohol withdrawal delirium. Restraints (**No. 1**) would not be necessary unless there were signs of impending alcohol withdrawal delirium, with agitation and the possibility of self-inflicted injuries. Nutritional therapy would not necessarily call for a fluid diet (**No. 3**) unless the patient was not able to eat solids. Vitamin C, although important for a regular diet, is not as essential as sources of thiamine in alcohol abuse. Monitoring serum lithium levels (**No. 4**) is not appropriate; it would be indicated in bipolar disorders. **PL, 4, PhI**

8. (**4**) On the contrary, AA encourages and reinforces self-control (with support by the AA group, as needed), rather than feeling sorry for the alcoholic. Self-pity, denial, and excuses for problems related to alcoholic dependency are not supported. **Nos. 1, 2, and 3** *are* all aspects of AA's approach. **EV, 7, PsI**

9. (**3**) Although all options are true, a support group encompasses the other three. A support group is a substitute for the barroom (**No. 1**); it provides help with an on-call buddy system to help the person avoid drinking (**No. 2**); and it reduces alienation and isolation (**No. 4**). **PL, 7, PsI**

💡 *Test-taking tip:* This is an example of an "umbrella" answer, which covers all the other options. When all (or most) options are good, choose the one that is most comprehensive and under which the other options fall.

10. (**3**) Alcohol is a common ingredient in cough syrups; it can cause a severe nausea and vomiting reaction when used with *Antabuse.* None of the products in **Nos. 1, 2, and 4** contain alcohol. **IMP, 1, PhI**

11. (**1**) The most common defense mechanisms used by people who have problems with substance dependence include denial, projection, and rationalization. Reaction formation (**No. 2**), displacement (**No. 3**), and repression (**No. 4**) are not common defense mechanisms used in substance dependence. **AS, 7, PsI**

12. (**1**) *Dexedrine*, an amphetamine, has been used for weight loss; its side effects also include hyperactivity,

---

Key to Codes

Nursing process: AS = Assessment; **AN** = Analysis; **PL** = Planning; **IMP** = Implementation; **EV** = Evaluation. (See Appendix E for explanation of nursing process steps.)

Category of human function: 1 = Protective; **2** = Sensory-Perceptual; **3** = Comfort, Rest, Activity, and Mobility; **4** = Nutrition; **5** = Growth and Development; **6** = Fluid-Gas Transport; **7** = Psychosocial-Cultural; **8** = Elimination.

Client need: SECE = Safe, Effective Care Environment; **PhI** = Physiologic Integrity; **PsI** = Psychosocial Integrity; **HPM** = Health Promotion/Maintenance.

delusions, and hallucinations similar to paranoid schizophrenia. Barbiturates (**No. 2**) are *not* used for weight loss. Side effects include: behavioral inhibitions, unsteady gait, verbosity, slurred speech. Although the side effects of hallucinogens (**No. 3**) may include delusions and unpredictable behaviors (in addition to hallucinations), hallucinogens are *not* used for weight loss. PCP (**No. 4**) is *not* used for weight loss. Additionally, dependence on PCP is characterized by *extremely violent* behavior followed by unresponsiveness; individuals on PCP show unpredictable behavior and are considered dangerous to self and others. Other side effects are: agitation, poor judgment, ataxia, and decreased pain response. **AN, 7, PsI**

13. (**1**) The nurse should suspect amphetamine abuse if assessment reveals an increased or decreased cardiac rate, with arrhythmias and chest pain. Drowsiness (**No. 2**) is a sign of abuse of *opiates*, along with slurred speech and memory and attention deficits. *Hyperalertness* would be most characteristic of amphetamine abuse. *Dilated* pupils, rather than constricted (**No. 3**), are characteristic of amphetamine abuse. Increased appetite and dry mouth (**No. 4**) are more characteristic of *cannabis* abuse. *Anorexia* and weight loss is seen in amphetamine abuse. **AS, 6, PhI**

14. (**1**) After a cocaine binge, the patient may "crash" due to exhaustion and may need to sleep. The patient may report bizarre dreams and nightmares. **Nos. 2 and 4** could lead to a power struggle, and would not be supportive to the patient. **No. 3** is not a good choice because the patient will have difficulty concentrating, and is not ready for group therapy. **PL, 3, PsI**

15. (**3**) Cocaine is abused because it acts as a stimulant and gives the user a euphoric feeling. **Nos. 1, 2, and 4** are the actions of other drugs, *not* cocaine. **AN, 3, PhI**

16. (**3**) Freebasers are most likely to die, due to the speed of absorption from the vapors, not the size of the dose. Intravenous injection (**No. 1**) is the second most lethal method, followed by snorting (**No. 2**) and smoking (**No. 4**). **IMP, 1, SECE**

17. (**1**) This option describes the classic picture of cocaine withdrawal. **Nos. 2 and 3** list symptoms of withdrawal from *depressants*. The effects listed in **No. 4** would occur with stimulant *intoxication*. **AS, 7, PsI**

18. (**1**) It may take several days to months to restore the brain's balance. Research shows that cocaine acts just like catecholamines produced by the brain; with cocaine abuse, the brain "believes" that it has too much catecholamine and, depending on the individual, may stop producing natural catecholamines. **Nos. 2, 3, and 4** are incorrect because the time periods are too long. **EV, 1, PhI**

19. (**2**) A direct suicide assessment technique is most crucial to the person's safety at this time. **No. 1** is incorrect because it only encourages conversation; it may not reveal suicide plans. **No. 3** is not the best choice because, although it may help the person's self-esteem, this comment should be made *later* in therapy. **No. 4** is not a good choice because, although it helps to clarify, it may not reveal suicide ideations. **IMP, 7, PsI**

Personality Disorders

Chapter Outline

Personality disorders are various maladaptive patterns of thinking, feeling, and relating to others that are repetitive and inflexible, and may impair relationships and functioning. Inner difficulties are revealed through general behaviors and by a pattern of living that seeks *immediate gratification of impulses* and instinctual needs without regard to society's laws, mores, and customs and *without censorship* of personal conscience. *Types:* antisocial, borderline, histrionic, narcissistic, avoidant, dependent. There are many subtypes within and among these categories.

Antisocial Personality Disorder

I. Concepts and principles

A. One defense against severe anxiety is *"acting-out,"* or dealing with distressful feelings or issues through action.

B. Faulty or arrested emotional development in preoedipal period has interfered with development of adequate social control or superego.

C. Since there is a malfunctioning or *weakened superego,* there is little internal demand and therefore no tension between ego and superego to evoke guilt feelings.

D. The defect is *not* intellectual; person shows *lack of moral responsibility, inability to control emotions* and impulses, and *deficiency in normal feeling* responses.

E. *"Pleasure principle"* is dominant.

F. *Initial* stage of treatment is most crucial; treatment situation is very threatening because it mobilizes client's anxiety, and client ends treatment abruptly.

G. Key underlying emotion: *fear of closeness,* with threat of exploitation, control, and abandonment.

◄ II. Assessment

A. Usually behaviors and traits are observed *before* age 15.

B. History of behavior that *conflicts with society:* truancy, expulsion, or suspension from school for misconduct; delinquency, thefts, vandalism; running away from home; persistent lying; repeated substance abuse; initiating fights; chronic violation of rules at home or school; school grades below IQ level.

C. Inability to sustain consistent *work* behavior (e.g., frequent job changes or absenteeism).

D. Lack of ability to function as *responsible* parent (e.g., evidence of child's malnutrition or illness due to lack of minimal hygiene standards; failure to obtain medical care for seriously ill child; failure to arrange for caretaker when parent is away from home).

E. Failure to accept *social norms* with respect to *lawful* behavior (e.g., thefts, multiple arrests).

F. Inability to maintain enduring *intimate* relationship (e.g., multiple relations, desertion, multiple divorces); lack of respect or loyalty.

G. *Irritability* and *aggressiveness* (spouse, child abuse; repeated physical fights).

H. Failure to honor *financial* obligations.

I. Failure to *plan ahead.*

J. *Disregard for truth* (e.g., lying, "conning" others for personal gain).

175

K. *Recklessness* (e.g., driving while intoxicated, recurrent speeding).

L. *Violating* rights of others.

M. Does not appear to profit from experience; *repeats* same punishable or antisocial behavior; usually does not feel guilt or depression.

N. Exhibits *poor judgment;* may have intellectual, but not emotional, insight to guide judgments. Inadequate problem solving and reality testing.

O. Uses *manipulative behavior patterns* in treatment setting (see Chap. 7, pp. 95–96).

  1. Demands and controls.

  2. Pressures and coerces; threatens.

  3. Violates rules, routines, procedures.

  4. Requests special privileges.

  5. Betrays confidences; lies.

  6. Ingratiates.

  7. Monopolizes conversation.

III. Analysis/nursing diagnosis

A. *Ineffective individual coping* related to:

  1. Inability to tolerate frustration (altered conduct/impulse processes).

  2. Verbal, nonverbal manipulation (*lying*).

  3. Destructive behavior toward self or others.

  4. Overuse of: denial, projection, rationalization, intellectualization.

  5. Inability to learn from experience.

B. *Personal identity disturbance* related to:

  1. Chronic low *self-esteem* as evidenced by grandiosity, depression.

  2. Lack of responsibility, accountability, commitment.

  3. Distancing relationships.

C. *Social intrusiveness* related to fear of real or potential loss.

D. *Noncompliance* related to excess need for independence.

IV. Nursing care plan/implementation

A. **Long-term goal:** help person accept responsibility and consequences of own actions.

B. **Short-term goal:** minimize manipulation and acting-out.

C. Set *fair, firm, consistent limits* and *follow through on consequences* of behavior; let client know what she or he can expect from staff and what the unit's regulations are, as well as the consequences of violations. Be explicit.

D. *Avoid* letting staff be played against one another by a particular client; staff should present a unified approach.

E. Nurses should *control* their *own* feelings of anger and defensiveness aroused by any person's manipulative behavior.

F. Change focus when client persists in raising inappropriate subjects (such as personal life of a nurse).

G. Encourage expression of *feelings* as an alternative to acting-out.

H. Aid client in realizing and accepting responsibility for own actions and *social responsibility* to others.

I. Use group therapy as a means of *peer control* and multiple feedback about behavior.

J. *Health teaching:* teach family how to use behavior-modification techniques to reward client's acceptable behavior (i.e., when he or she accepts responsibility for own behavior, is responsive to rights of others, adheres to social and legal norms).

V. Evaluation/outcome criteria: less use of lying, blaming others for own behavior; more evidence of following rules; less impulsive, explosive behavior.

Borderline Personality Disorder

Borderline personality disorder is characterized by wide fluctuations of mood; unstable: relationships, self-image, affect, and impulse control.

I. Assessment

A. *Behavior:* reckless, impulsive (e.g., sex, substance abuse, driving, binge eating, shoplifting, spending); self destructive (recurrent threats, gestures, behaviors); controlling; manipulative.

B. *Mood:* intense; extreme emotional lability (lasting for short periods), inappropriate anger.

C. *Relationships:* unstable, conflictual, intense.

D. *Feelings:* chronic boredom, isolation, and emptiness related to real or perceived abandonment.

II. Analysis/nursing diagnosis

A. *Ineffective individual coping* related to ineffective problem solving; restricted affect and humor; boredom and splitting; lying; blaming/projecting.

B. *High risk for injury* related to assaultive, destructive behaviors.

C. *Self-esteem disturbance* related to abandonment fears, maladaptive denial, rigid and perfectionistic behavior.

D. *High risk for violence* related to poor impulse control, anger, aggression.

E. *Defensive coping* related to passive aggressive reactions; narcissistic behaviors; mistrust/suspicion; lack of insight; personal identity disturbance; role relationship disturbance.

III. Nursing care plan/implementation

A. Be aware of manipulative behavior (e.g., flattery, hostility, seductiveness).

B. Approach: consistent, matter-of-fact.

C. Confront and give feedback regarding inappropriate behavior.

D. *Avoid* rejecting or rescuing.

E. Set limits on disregard for rights of others and manipulation.

F. Handle manipulation on-the-spot. (See **Manipulation,** pp. 95–96).

G. Give positive reinforcement for appropriate responses and behaviors, and especially for constructive ways of expressing anger.

✖ **IV. Evaluation/outcome criteria:** Little overall improvement or change in behavior, i.e., some reduction in intensity of acting-out; some reduction in aggression toward self and others; some increase in impulse control; some increase in following rules.

Histrionic Personality Disorder

Histrionic personality disorder is characterized by self-focused and dramatic attention-seeking patterns; always "on."

✖ **I. Assessment**
   A. *Behavior:* tantrums; inappropriate sexual seductiveness in behavior and appearance; flamboyance; very impressionable and suggestible.
   B. *Relationships:* dependence on authority figures, lack of commitment in relationships, delusional belief that relationships are more intimate than actually so.
   C. *Feelings:* exaggerated and labile emotions.

✖ **II. Analysis/nursing diagnosis, Nursing care plan/implementation, Evaluation/outcome criteria:** see borderline personality disorder (p. 176).

Narcissistic Personality Disorder

Narcissistic personality disorder is characterized by a rigid pattern of grandiosity (belief that one should associate only with other superior individuals); imbalance in self-esteem and expression of it (may have low or high self-esteem); and a strong sense of being entitled to special treatment and privileges.

✖ **I. Assessment**
   A. *Behavior:* attention-seeking, success- and power-driven; need for admiration; preoccupation with thoughts of beauty and intelligence; rationalizes failures.
   B. *Relationships:* difficulty in maintaining; evidence of sexual confusion and promiscuity; exploitation of others.
   C. *Feelings:* exaggerated sense of self-importance, grandiosity, lack of empathy.

✖ **II. Analysis/nursing diagnosis, Nursing care plan/implementation, Evaluation/outcome criteria:** see borderline personality disorder (p. 176).

Avoidant Personality Disorder

Avoidant personality disorder is characterized by a pervasive pattern of social inhibition, feelings of inadequacy, fearfulness, hypersensitivity to possible rejection and criticism, and avoidance of intimacy, along with fear of being alone.

✖ **I. Assessment**
   A. *Behavior:* unwilling to take risks in new activities; avoidance of occupations that involve contact with people.
   B. *Relationships:* desires affection, but withdraws from others due to fear of not being liked.
   C. *Feelings:* serious, blunted affect; very sensitive to criticism and reactions of others; fears of: failure, rejection, and being alone; self-devaluation of abilities and achievements (believes self to be inferior to others, inept, and unappealing).

✖ **II. Analysis/nursing diagnosis**
   A. *Ineffective individual coping* related to knowledge deficit regarding effective social skills.
   B. *Self-esteem disturbance* related to lifestyle of avoidance and dependency; powerlessness; developmental conflicts.
   C. *Social isolation* related to abandonment fears.

✖ **III. Nursing care plan/implementation**
   A. Establish consistent nurse-patient relationship (NPR) with clear expectations for behavior, responsibility, and achievement.
   B. Encourage expression of feelings: fear, anger, rejection, inferiority.
   C. Encourage goal attainment and task completion.
   D. Give feedback about nonproductive, unsatisfying behaviors.
   E. *Avoid* arguments.
   F. **Teach:** assertiveness, decision-making skills.

✖ **IV. Evaluation/outcome criteria**
   A. Some degree of awareness of effect of own behavior on others.
   B. Some improvement in behavior patterns.

Dependent Personality Disorder

Dependent personality disorder is characterized by the pervasive and excessive need to be taken care of; passive acceptance of control by dominant people; and submissiveness.

✖ **I. Assessment**
   A. *Behavior:* submissive, indecisive about everyday decisions; needs excessive advice and for others to take over responsibilities.
   B. *Relationships:* dependent, overly reliant, clinging.
   C. *Feelings:* devaluation of own abilities and achievements, lack of self-confidence, low self-esteem; feels helpless when alone; preoccupation with fear of separation and of being left alone to care for self.

✖ **II. Analysis/nursing diagnosis, Nursing care plan/implementation, Evaluation/outcome criteria:** see avoidant personality disorder (p. 177).

🗝 Summary of Key Points

Personality Disorders

Personality disorders are syndromes (with many subtypes) in which an individual's inner difficulties are revealed through general behavior and through a pattern of living that seeks *immediate gratification of impulses* and instinctual needs without regard to society's laws, mores, and customs and *without censorship*.

Care of a Patient with Antisocial Personality Disorder

1. Direct nursing approach is needed; i.e., set *limits*, be *consistent*, use a *team* approach to avoid manipulation.
2. Reinforce *responsible* behavior.

Care of a Patient with Borderline, Narcissistic, and Histrionic Personality Disorder

1. Make a *contract* with the patient for desired changes in behavior.
2. A consistent approach is needed: limit-setting, enforcement of rules with consequences for unacceptable behavior.
3. Watch for manipulative behavior.

Care of a Patient with Avoidant and Dependent Personality Disorder

1. Encourage expression of feelings of: inferiority, fear of rejection, and anger.
2. Assist with goal setting and attainment.
3. Teach assertiveness.

💡 Study and Memory Aids

Antisocial personality disorder—prognosis

Because the patient typically lacks insight into own behavior, prognosis is poor; it is unlikely that long-term behavioral changes will occur.

Treatment mode for borderline personality disorder:

Use behavior modification techniques.

Histrionic personality disorder—most typical characteristic:

Exaggerated affect and behavior

Avoidant personality disorder—characteristic behaviors:

Withdrawn, fearful

Dependent personality disorder—characteristic behaviors

The characteristic behaviors of dependent personality disorder—submissiveness, indecisiveness, and separation anxiety—stem from low self-esteem.

Glossary

antisocial personality disorder   A disorder of behavior in which feelings and behavior are asocial, with impaired judgment and inability to learn from experience; the intellect remains intact. There is a pattern of manipulation and disregard for rules, laws, and rights of others; characterized by irresponsibility, impulsiveness, and deceitfulness with lack of remorse. (Also known as *sociopathic* disorder.)

avoidant personality disorder   A pattern of avoiding activities involving others (social inhibition), preoccupation with fears of rejection, and hypersensitivity to criticism.

borderline personality disorder   Behavioral pattern characterized by: *unstable* mood, relationships, and identity (self-image); *poor* impulse control (in sex, substance use, spending money, stealing, etc.); intense anger; and self-mutilating actions.

conduct disorder   Behavior patterns in which rules are violated, especially rules related to the rights of others and age-appropriate expectations.

dependent personality disorder   A pattern of behavior based on fear of being left alone, with an excessive need to get others to take care of basic decisions and responsibilities; submissive to control by others.

histrionic personality disorder A pattern of excessive attention-seeking behaviors; emotional lability with exaggerated emotional expressions; and dramatic, egocentric behaviors.

narcissistic personality disorder A pattern of arrogance and preoccupation with self-importance and superiority, lack of empathy, and need for excessive admiration. Exaggerated self-love, with all attention focused on own comfort, pleasure, abilities, appearance, etc.

obsessive-compulsive personality disorder A personality disorder *subtype* where there is a pattern of rigidity and preoccupation with perfection (rules, lists, details, and schedules) to the exclusion of flexibility, openness, and leisure activities; fear of loss of control over people, situations, and objects.

paranoid personality disorder A personality disorder *subtype* with the main characteristic being a persistent and unwarranted suspiciousness about others being deceptive, threatening, and/or exploitive.

personality disorders Broad category of nonpsychotic illness characterized by various persistent, maladaptive traits or patterns of perceiving and thinking about oneself and the environment in ways that interfere with relationships and functioning. Inner difficulties are revealed by *antisocial* behavior (e.g., *acts*), not by specific symptoms. The person uses inflexible behavior patterns to fulfill own needs and get self-satisfaction, often at the expense of others and society in general.

pleasure principle According to psychoanalytic theory, the tendency for the *id* to seek pleasure and avoid pain. Demands of the pleasure principle become modified by the reality principle, and this develops a capacity to delay immediate gratification needs.

psychopath *Older*, inexact term for one of a variety of *personality* disorders in which an individual has poor impulse control, releasing tension through immediate action, without social or moral conscience.

schizoid personality disorder A behavioral pattern of aloofness in social relationships, withdrawal, shyness, and introversion, with preference to be alone; limited expression of emotion; unusual ideas and peculiar behaviors.

Questions

1. A patient with antisocial disorder gets along very well with a nursing student, who asks the staff why they are so hard on the patient. The supervising nurse's response would be:
   1. "This antisocial behavior is very complicated and difficult to understand."
   2. "You are too inexperienced."
   3. "This is exactly what the patient is trying to accomplish."
   4. "Yes, we should be more sympathetic."

2. In planning the care of an antisocial patient with a broken leg, the nurse needs to consider the need for:
   1. Kindness and reassurance.
   2. Multiple staff to encourage socialization.
   3. Intellectual activities to develop problem-solving skills.

   4. Direct, consistent statements about behavior and consequences.

3. A patient diagnosed with an antisocial personality disorder will have:
   1. The ability to tolerate frustration well.
   2. A poor academic and employment history, due to less-than-average intelligence.
   3. Good relationships, due to the ability to flatter others.
   4. A relative absence of anxiety or guilt feelings.

4. Prognosis for a patient with an antisocial personality disorder is:
   1. Good, because the patient is free of emotional pain.
   2. Fair, because the disorder develops in early childhood.
   3. Poor, because the patient is unable to learn from experience.
   4. Undeterminable, because there are many types of personality disorders.

5. For what common characteristic of borderline personality would the nurse assess the patient?
   1. Violent outbursts.
   2. Hypercriticism.
   3. Passivity.
   4. Negative thinking.

6. A patient with borderline personality disorder is seen by the nurse after a suicide attempt. The patient tells the nurse that she envies the nurse and wishes to be like the nurse. What characteristic symptom of borderline personality disorder is this patient exhibiting?
   1. Denial.
   2. Unstable self-image.
   3. Depersonalization.
   4. Dependency.

7. A colleague reports at the unit meeting that one of the patients seems insecure and continually asks other patients and staff whether what she is doing in occupational therapy is right or not. The primary care nurse recognizes that the patient's behavior is indicative of:
   1. Conduct disorder.
   2. Compensation.
   3. Dependency.
   4. Avoidant disorder.

8. A woman with a dependent personality disorder has relied on her husband for all aspects of their daily lives for many years, and has allowed his wishes and directions to prevail over hers. Following his death, the nurse should expect this woman's response to be one of:
   1. Newly gained independence, after the initial grief.
   2. Blaming him for wanting to leave her alone and helpless.
   3. Increased dependency needs.
   4. Fearfulness about forming other relationships.

9. Which finding on assessment of a patient's behavior would be characteristic of histrionic personality disorder?
   1. Disregard for social rules.
   2. Attention seeking through dramatic behaviors.
   3. Exaggerated attention to details, with fear of loss of control of situations, objects, and people.

4. Unstable relationships, with wide mood swings.
10. A 17-year-old is preoccupied with talk about her family's status and wealth. She treats others in a servile way, believing that she is entitled to special privileges. Which type of personality disorder most likely applies to this patient?
    1. Borderline personality disorder.
    2. Histrionic disorder.
    ✓3. Narcissistic disorder.
    4. Antisocial disorder.
11. Which behavior, when observed by the nurse in a patient with a narcissistic personality disorder, would indicate a nursing diagnosis of impaired social interaction?
    ✓1. Exploitation of others.
    2. Social inhibition.
    3. Submissiveness.
    4. Lack of feelings of remorse.

Answers/Rationale

1. (3) The point of theory to recall is the patient's manipulative behavior, playing on the nursing student's sympathy, as well as playing one staff against another. While **No. 1** is true, and certainly applies to the underlying concept of manipulation, it is a "put-off." **No. 2** sounds like a "put-down" of the nursing student. **No. 4** is definitely a *non*therapeutic response; sympathy (as opposed to empathy) is almost always contraindicated as a nursing response or attitude. **IMP, 7, PsI**

💡 *Test-taking tip:* Sound out the options, to eliminate responses that sound like a "put-off" or "put-down" (**Nos. 1 and 2**) as well as responses that are trite (**No. 4**).

2. (4) The goal is to reduce manipulative behaviors through statement of consistent, clear, enforceable rules, and sanctions for violations. Kindness and reassurance (**No. 1**) are the *opposite* of the correct response (a direct, confronting approach). **No. 2** is incorrect because the *opposite* is necessary: the *fewer* staff, the better, to reduce opportunities to split the staff and play one staff member against another. Consistency, rather than diversity, is key. **No. 3** is irrelevant because the least-affected aspect is the intellect. Problem-solving is *not* the concern; exploitation and demanding behaviors *are*. **PL, 7, PsI**

3. (4) According to theory, a person diagnosed with antisocial personality usually does *not* feel guilty or anxious,

but will primarily exhibit anxiety *when* manipulative behaviors are *thwarted.* The patient with antisocial behavior does *not* tolerate frustration well (**No. 1**). The id is very strong ("I want what I want when I want it") and impulse control is poor. The patient with antisocial behavior tends to have *higher* than average intelligence (*not* less than average, **No. 2**), and uses this ability to manipulate the situation and others. The patient with antisocial behavior generally tends to have *poor* relationships (not good relationships, **No. 3**), because others do not like flattery, nor being manipulated. **AS, 7, PsI**

4. (3) It is well-documented that it is difficult to do therapy with a patient with antisocial personality disorder because the patient repeats antisocial acts over and over again. The excitement comes from the challenge of "getting away" with antisocial acts. "It's all right to steal, as long as you don't get caught" may well be the motto. *Feeling* emotional pain (*rather than* a *lack* of pain, **No. 1**) may improve chances for learning to occur; feeling pain may serve as a deterrent to other antisocial acts. **No. 2** is incorrect because it has not been established that this disorder develops in *early* childhood. Even if in fact it does develop in *early* childhood, the behavior would most likely be more entrenched, and the prognosis would *not* be "fair." **No. 4** is incorrect because prognosis is still poor regardless of the subtypes under personality disorders. **EV, 7, PsI**

5. (1) A common sequence in borderline personality behavior is a sudden outburst of uncontrollable rage, followed by remorse with apology for the behavior. Hypercriticism (**No. 2**) is more typical of a person with paranoid disorder. Passive behavior (**No. 3**) is more characteristic of an avoidant personality disorder. Negative thinking (**No. 4**) is commonly related to depression. **AS, 7, PsI**

6. (2) Patients with borderline personality disorder have a persistent identity disturbance, in which others are seen as idols or as undesirable people. Denial (**No. 1**) is manifested by refusal to acknowledge one's own feelings. Depersonalization (**No. 3**) is manifested by a feeling of *loss of self,* of what is normal (e.g., a person feels like a robot, rather than a human). Dependency (**No. 4**) is characterized by *indecisiveness*, with clingy and submissive behaviors. **AN, 7, PsI**

7. (3) This behavior is part of a dependent personality disorder, in which there is an excessive need to be taken care of, with difficulty in doing things on one's own. Depending on others for approval stems from low self-esteem. Conduct disorder (**No. 1**) is a consistent pattern of behavior that goes against social rules and infringes on the rights of others. Compensation (**No. 2**) means making up for perceived failure in one quality or trait by emphasizing another. By definition, this option does not fit the behavior described. Avoidant disorder (**No. 4**) is a personality disorder that is characterized by procrastination and not doing something when the person doesn't want to. **AN, 7, PsI**

8. (3) With increased stress (such as the death of a spouse), symptoms of a disorder tend to increase; in a dependent personality, dependency needs will increase. **No. 1** is the *opposite* of the correct answer; this option

---

Key to Codes

Nursing process: AS = Assessment; **AN** = Analysis; **PL** = Planning; **IMP** = Implementation; **EV** = Evaluation. (See Appendix E for explanation of nursing process steps.)

Category of human function: 1 = Protective; **2** = Sensory-Perceptual; **3** = Comfort, Rest, Activity, and Mobility; **4** = Nutrition; **5** = Growth and Development; **6** = Fluid-Gas Transport; **7** = Psychosocial-Cultural; **8** = Elimination.

Client need: SECE = Safe, Effective Care Environment; **PhI** = Physiologic Integrity; **PsI** = Psychosocial Integrity; **HPM** = Health Promotion/Maintenance.

describes a *change* in, rather than persistence of, a personality pattern. **No. 2** describes *paranoid* personality disorder. **No. 4** relates to *avoidant* personality disorder. **AS, 7, PsI**

9. **(2)** Constant acting, role playing, and being "on stage" is characteristic of histrionic personality disorder. **No. 1** describes antisocial personality (sociopathic) disorder. **No. 3** describes obsessive-compulsive personality disorder. **No. 4** describes borderline personality disorder. **AS, 7, PsI**

10. **(3)** The description of self-importance supports narcissistic disorder. These behaviors do *not* describe borderline (**No. 1**), histrionic (**No. 2**), or antisocial (**No. 4**) disorders. **AN, 7, PsI**

11. **(1)** A strong sense of being superior to others and a belief that special treatment is deserved lead to a lack of empathy and exploitation of others. Social inhibition (**No. 2**) is more characteristic of *avoidant* personality disorder. Submissiveness (**No. 3**) is more characteristic of *dependent* personality disorder. A lack of feelings of remorse (**No. 4**) is characteristic of an *antisocial* personality disorder. **AS, 7, PsI**

Special Populations and Concerns

Chapter Outline

Mental and Emotional Disorders in Children

Children have certain developmental tasks to master in the various stages of development (e.g., learning to trust, control primary instincts, and resolve basic social roles; see Chapter 1).

Concepts and Principles Related to Mental and Emotional Disorders in Children

I. Most emotional disorders of children are related to family dynamics and the place the child occupies in the family group.

II. Children must be understood and treated within the context of their *families*.

III. Many disorders are related to the *phases of development* through which the children are passing. (Erik Erikson's developmental tasks for children are: trust, autonomy, initiative, industry, identity, and intimacy.)

IV. Table 16.1 summarizes key age-related disturbances, lists main *symptoms* and *analyses of causes,* and highlights medical interventions and *nursing plan/implementation.*

V. Children are *not* miniature adults; they have special needs.

VI. *Play* and *food* are important media to make contact with children and help them release emotions in socially acceptable forms, prepare them for traumatic events, and develop skills.

VII. Children who are physically or emotionally ill regress, giving up previously useful habits.

VIII. Strong feelings may be evoked in nurses working with children; these feelings should be expressed, and each nurse should be supported by team members.

⋈ Assessment of Selected Disorders

Autistic Disorders

I. Autistic disorders (previously called *childhood schizophrenia* with unknown etiology):
    A. Disturbance in how *perceptual* information is processed; normal abilities present.

TABLE 16.1   EMOTIONAL DISTURBANCES IN CHILDREN

Stage	Disturbance	◢ *Assessment: Symptoms or Characteristics*	◢ *Analysis: Altered Growth and Development Related to*	◢ *Plan/Implementation*
Oral (Birth–1 yr)	**Feeding and eating disorder**	Refusal of food	Rigid feeding schedule *Psychological* stress Incompatible formula *Physiologic:* pyloric stenosis	Pediatric evaluation, especially if infant is not gaining weight or is losing weight Rule out physiologic etiology or incompatible formula Evaluate *feeding style* of caretaker. Is baby on demand feeding? Is caregiver sensitive to infant's needs or communications about holding, hunger, or satiation?
		Colic. Crying is usually confined to one part of day and starts after a feeding; commonly lasts from first to third mo.	Periodic tension in infant's immature nervous system, causing gas and sharp intestinal pains	Reassure parents and teach about condition and how to relieve it with *hot water bottle, rocking, rubbing back, pacifier,* which may soothe infant
	Sleeping disturbances	Infant resists being put down for sleep or going to sleep	Need for parental attention A pattern formed during period of colic or other illness Emotional disturbance related to *anxiety*	If it is attention-getting behavior, suggest parental lack of response for few nights to break pattern If emotional disturbance is suspected, evaluate *infant-caregiver interaction* and refer for psychotherapeutic intervention
	Failure to thrive	Infant does not grow or develop over a period of time	*Physiologic:* heart, kidneys, central nervous system (CNS) malfunction. *Psychological:* inadequate caretaking	*Hospitalization* is essential. Assist in evaluation of physiologic functioning, especially heart, kidneys, and CNS *Nurturing plan* for infant, using specifically assigned personnel and the caregiver parent. If the infant grows and develops with nurturing, thus confirming problems of parenting as causative factor, *psychotherapeutic* and *child protective* interventions are necessary

continues

TABLE 16.1   EMOTIONAL DISTURBANCES IN CHILDREN (CONTINUED)

Stage	Disturbance	✕ Assessment: Symptoms or Characteristics	✕ Analysis: Altered Growth and Development Related to	✕ Plan/Implementation
Oral (Birth–1 yr) *continued*	**Severe disturbances**	**Autistic disorder:** very early onset; lack of response to others; bizarre, repetitive behavior; normal to above normal intelligence; failure to develop language or use communicative speech Autism is one of the most severe and debilitating psychiatric disturbances	Uncertain etiology; *regression* or *fixation* at earlier developmental stage, before child differentiates "me" from "not me" A *"nature vs. nurture"* controversy exists over the causative factors: *Environment only:* infant is tabula rasa and all disturbance is directly attributable to the environment (primarily the parenting) *Heredity only:* For genetic, biochemical, or other predetermined reasons, some infants will be psychotic regardless of the environment *Combination* of environment and heredity *plus* the interaction between them: A *susceptible* infant, *less* than optimal parenting, and *negative* interaction between parent and infant combine to produce disturbance	The severely disturbed child requires intensive psychotherapy and often milieu therapy available in residential or daycare programs. Therapy is usually indicated for parents also. Nurses can work on a *primary level of prevention* by assessing parenting skills of prospective parents and *teaching* them these skills. On a *secondary level of prevention*, nurses can be knowledgeable about and *teach* others the early signs of childhood psychosis, making appropriate referrals. The earlier the intervention, the better the prognosis. On a *tertiary level of prevention*, nurses work with severely disturbed children and their families in child guidance clinics and residential and daycare settings. *Health teaching* would include: play activities that foster support, acceptance, and a nonthreatening mode of communication and interaction with a significant other. *continues*

1. Behave *as though they cannot* hear, see, etc.
2. *Do not react to external* stimulus.
3. Mute or echolalic.
B. Lack of self-awareness as a unified whole; may not relate bodily needs or parts as extension of themselves.
C. Severe difficulty in communicating with others; may be *mute* and isolated.
D. *Bizarre* postures and gestures (head-banging, rocking back and forth).
E. Disturbances in *learning*.

TABLE 16.1   EMOTIONAL DISTURBANCES IN CHILDREN (CONTINUED)

Stage	Disturbance	✄ Assessment: Symptoms or Characteristics	✄ Analysis: Altered Growth and Development Related to	✄ Plan/Implementation
Oral (Birth–1 yr) *continued*	**Severe disturbances** *continued*	**Symbiotic psychosis:** Identified later than autistic type, usually between 2 and 5 yr; Seem to be unable to function independently of the caregiving parent; A *situational stress*, such as hospitalization of parent or child or entry into school, may precipitate a psychotic break in the child.	The same *"nature versus nurture"* controversy with respect to the origin of symbiotic psychosis; Child's progression beyond the self-absorbed autistic stage to form an object relationship with another (usually the mother). Having progressed to this stage, the child then *fails to differentiate his or her own identity* from that of the mother.	
Anal (1–3 yr)	**Disturbances related to toilet training**	Constipation	*Diet* Child withholding due to history of one or two painful, *hard bowel movements*; *Psychological* causation: child withholds from parents to *express anger, opposition*, or passage through a very *independent* development stage	Evaluate *diet* and consistency of stools; ☞ Fecal softener may be prescribed if necessary; In all cases, *help parent avoid* making an issue of constipation with the child; Enemas are *contraindicated*; If child is withholding, *work with parents* around *not* forcing rigid toilet training on child; Most children are more cooperative about *toilet training* at 18–24 mo.
		Encopresis (soiling)	Child's expression of anger or hostility: it is usually directed toward the parent with whom the child is experiencing conflict and is *rarely* physiologic	Medical evaluation, then assessment and intervention in the child-parent relationship; Therapy for child (and possibly for parent) may be indicated

continues

TABLE 16.1 EMOTIONAL DISTURBANCES IN CHILDREN (CONTINUED)

Stage	Disturbance	⋈ *Assessment: Symptoms or Characteristics*	⋈ *Analysis: Altered Growth and Development Related to*	⋈ *Plan/Implementation*
Anal (1–3 yr) *continued*	**Disturbances related to toilet training** *continued*	**Enuresis.** Ordinarily refers to wetting while asleep (nocturnal enuresis), though some enuretic children wet themselves during the day also Enuresis is a *symptom*, not a diagnosis or disease entity.	*Faulty toilet training* (especially if child wets during the day also) or *Psychological* stress *Physiologic* etiology, such as genitourinary (GU) tract infections or CNS disease, is rare (The child under 4 yr is usually not considered enuretic but is included in this section because bladder training is part of toilet training) Uncertain etiology.	Many approaches have been tried with varying degrees of success. These include ⊂ *Tofranil, fluid restriction, behavioral intervention* (in which a buzzer wakes the child when the child starts to wet), and psychotherapy *Educating parents in bladder training* techniques and attitudes can help solve the problem on a *primary* level It is important when working with enuretic children or their parents to *suggest* ways to help the child *overcome feelings of shame and guilt.* These feelings are often exacerbated by well-meaning but misguided parents.
	Excessive rebelliousness	Frequent temper tantrums, fighting, destruction of toys and other objects, consistent oppositional behavior	Fear caused by inconsistency in handling the child, the setting of rigid limits, or the parents' refusal or inability to set limits, which can all create *insecurity and fear* in the child Excessive rebelliousness usually indicating a *frightened* child, should *not* be confused with expression of negativism normal at around age 2, which is a necessary (though trying) developmental stage	The nurse should offer parent counseling if necessary When working with the child, the nurse needs to be receptive and empathetic while establishing and maintaining firm limits

continues

TABLE 16.1   EMOTIONAL DISTURBANCES IN CHILDREN (CONTINUED)

Stage	Disturbance	▶ Assessment: Symptoms or Characteristics	▶ Analysis: Altered Growth and Development Related to	▶ Plan/Implementation
Anal (1–3 yr) *continued*	**Excessive conformity**	Lack of spontaneity, anxious desire always to please all adult authority figures, timidity, refusal to assert own needs, passivity	Very rigid control established in an attempt to handle fears Harsh *toilet training*, resulting in an over-compliant child. These children need help as much as over-rebellious children, but they get it less frequently because their behavior is not a "problem"—i.e., it is not difficult for parents to tolerate	Excessive conformity can lead to compulsive, ritualistic, or obsessive behavior later The nurse needs to be able to identify such a child, then work with the child and parents to encourage *self-expression* in the child Referral for psychotherapy may be necessary to help the child deal with *repressed anger*
Oedipal (3–6 yr)	**Excessive fears**	Child is frightened even in nonthreatening situations *Nightmares* and other *sleep disturbances* occur Usually, child will be very "clingy" with parents in an attempt to gain reassurance	*Anxiety* as the causative factor. Anxiety that is induced by: Parental *failure to set appropriate limits* *Physical or psychological abuse* *Illness* Fear of *mutilation* *Imaginary worries* that are common at this age, e.g., a 4-year-old who is suddenly afraid of the dark, or dogs, or fire engines is not necessarily suffering from excessive fears	If possible, identify and deal with the factors that are producing the anxiety Offer child calm reassurance *Night-light* and *open doors* can help allay night fears, but *counsel parents* that it is unwise to allow the child to sleep with the parents, which may make the child feel that the Oedipal retaliation has succeeded With the hospitalized child, the nurse needs to be aware of and work with the *mutilation fears* common at this age Fears around certain procedures (like injections) can often be resolved by helping the child *play out fears*

continues

F. Prognosis depends on severity of symptoms and age of onset.

Developmental Disorders

I. Developmental disorders (*brain injury*) characteristics:

A. Hyperactivity.
B. Explosive outbursts.
C. Distractibility.
D. Impulsiveness.
E. Perceptual difficulties (*visual* distortions, such as figure-ground distortion and mirror-reading;

TABLE 16.1   EMOTIONAL DISTURBANCES IN CHILDREN (CONTINUED)

Stage	Disturbance	⋈ Assessment: Symptoms or Characteristics	⋈ Analysis: Altered Growth and Development Related to	⋈ Plan/Implementation
Oedipal (3–6 yr) *continued*	**Excessive masturbation**	Touching and fondling of genitals excessively, sometimes in a preoccupied or absentminded manner	*Insecurity* If exploration and stimulation of the genital area (*normal* and common in this age group) is compulsive, the behavior is a signal that the child is *insecure* A *specific fear* (e.g., a boy viewing a baby sister's genitals); may have castration fears. These can be dealt with directly.	*Assess* the child's masturbating activity. When does it occur and why? Help the child develop other *strategies* for coping with anxiety *Answer questions about sexuality* in an open manner *Counsel parents* that *threats and shaming are contraindicated*, and help parents deal with *their* feelings about masturbation
	Regression	Resumption of activities (e.g., *thumb sucking, soiling* and *wetting, baby talk*) characteristic of earlier developmental levels	Child's attempt to regain a more comfortable, previous level of development in response to a *threatening* situation (such as a new baby), or A response to difficulty resolving Oedipal *conflicts*	*Counsel parents* not to make an issue of behavior Offer child emotional support and acceptance, though not approval of regressive behavior
	Stuttering	Articulation difficulty characterized by many stops and repetitions in speech pattern	Anxiety Frustration Insecurity Excitement Stuttering occurs when the affected child feels *anxious, frustrated, insecure,* or *excited* Parental concerns and attention to stuttering as focus of attention on it increases anxiety. (The origins of stuttering are not understood. It is *common* around *2–3 yr* and is not a cause for concern at that time)	*Speech therapy* is usually indicated *Psychotherapy* may also be indicated, if stuttering is an expression of anxiety and conflict, persisting *beyond age 6*

continues

TABLE 16.1   EMOTIONAL DISTURBANCES IN CHILDREN (CONTINUED)

Stage	Disturbance	⋈ *Assessment: Symptoms or Characteristics*	⋈ *Analysis: Altered Growth and Development Related to*	⋈ *Plan/Implementation*
Latency (6–12 yr)	**Attention-deficit hyperactivity disorder**	Both hyperactivity and hyperkinesis are occasionally observed in school children Characterized by: *Short attention span* Restlessness Distractibility *Impulsivity*	*Organic disturbance* of the *CNS*, of uncertain origin, as the basis of *hyperkinesis.* Because the primary symptom—difficulty with attention span—is the same as that presented by the hyperactive child, the hyperactive child is frequently and *incorrectly labeled* hyperkinetic.	For the *hyperkinetic* child, psychopharmaceutical intervention—usually ● *Ritalin*—is most often employed. Psychotherapy and special education classes may also be indicated.
			Hyperactive child—attempts to *control* anxiety through *reducement*, and *can* attend when interested or relaxed. Does not fit smoothly into environment, but problem may be with the environment rather than the child. In other words, the school situation requires a high degree of conformity. The child who does not fit the mold is *not* necessarily emotionally disturbed.	● *Ritalin* is also frequently prescribed for the *hyperactive* child—which raises the issue of whether an individual should be medicated to fit more smoothly into the environment. Therapy can help the hyperactive child *decrease anxiety* and *increase self-esteem*, thus reducing the symptoms.
	Withdrawal	Reduced body movement and verbalization Lack of close relationships *Detachment* Timidity Seclusiveness	Need to withdraw as a defensive behavior, through which the child controls anxiety by *reducing contact* with the outer world. Like the overcompliant child, the withdrawn child is frequently not identified as needing help because this behavior is not a "problem."	Offer *positive reinforcement* when child is more active Help child *assert* self and *experience success* at certain tasks The nurse needs to work with the parents who are *overprotective* Therapy may be useful to work through anxiety and provide child with a chance to form a *trusting* relationship with another

continues

TABLE 16.1   EMOTIONAL DISTURBANCES IN CHILDREN (CONTINUED)

Stage	Disturbance	⋈ *Assessment: Symptoms or Characteristics*	⋈ *Analysis: Altered Growth and Development Related to*	⋈ *Plan/Implementation*
Latency (6–12 yr) *continued*	**Psychophysiologic symptoms**	The child experiences physical symptoms (e.g., *vomiting, headaches, eczema, asthma, colitis*) with no apparent physiologic cause	*Conversion* of anxiety into physical symptoms	After medical evaluation has established lack of physiologic etiology, psychotherapy is usually indicated Family therapy may be treatment of choice since *dysfunctional interpersonal family dynamics* are common in these cases The nurse can also provide the child with a healthy interpersonal relationship Nurses are frequently in a position to talk to parents and teachers about the importance of mental health counseling for children with physical symptoms
	School "phobia"	Sudden and seemingly inexplicable fear of going to school These children often don't know what it is they fear at school Frequently occurs *after an illness* and absence from school or birth of sibling	*Acute anxiety reaction related to separation* from home—not actually a phobia.	If the child is allowed to stay home, the dread of returning to school usually increases The child and parent should have psychiatric intervention *quickly* (before the problem becomes worse) to help the child separate from the parent

continues

body-image problems; difficulty in telling left from right).

F. Receptive or expressive language problems.

Elimination Disorders

I. Elimination disorders (functional *enuresis*): related to feelings of insecurity due to unmet needs of attention and affection; important to preserve their self-esteem.

Separation Anxiety Disorders of Childhood

I. Separation anxiety disorders of childhood (*school phobias*): anxiety about school is accompanied by

physical distress. Usually observed with fear of leaving home, rejection by mother, fear of loss of mother, or history of separation from mother in early years.

Conduct Disorders

I. Conduct disorders include lying, stealing, running away, truancy, substance abuse, sexual delinquency, vandalism, and fire-setting; chief motivating force is either overt or covert *hostility*; history of *disturbed parent-child relations*.

⋈ **II. Analysis/nursing diagnosis**

    A. *Altered feeling states:* anxiety, fear, hostility related

TABLE 16.1   EMOTIONAL DISTURBANCES IN CHILDREN (CONTINUED)

Stage	Disturbance	◄ *Assessment: Symptoms or Characteristics*	◄ *Analysis: Altered Growth and Development Related to*	◄ *Plan/Implementation*
Latency (6–12 yr) *continued*	**Learning disorder**	Failure or difficulty in learning at school	Emotional disorders that can cause school failure Feelings of *inferiority, discouragement,* and loss of confidence from school failure Learning disabilities that may be caused by many factors or combinations of factors, including *anxiety, poor sensory or sensorimotor integration, dyslexia, receptive aphasia*	A comprehensive evaluation is essential. Ideally, this would include assessments by a pediatric neurologist, a mental health worker such as a psychiatric nurse or psychiatrist, a learning disabilities teacher specialist, and possibly an occupational therapist trained to work with sensory integration Treatment is then based on the specific problem or problems.
	Behavior problems	Behavior that is nonproductive; that is repeated in spite of threats, punishments, or rational argument; and that usually leads to punishment Persistent *stealing* and *truancy* are examples	*Conflicts* that are expressed and communicated through behavior rather than verbally Child knowing what he or she is doing but is unaware of the underlying motivations for the problem behavior	Counseling or therapy for the child by a child psychiatric nurse or other mental health worker can allow the child to resolve the basic conflict, thus making the problem behavior unnecessary

Source: Adapted from Wilson HS, Kneisl CR, *Psychiatric Nursing* (3rd ed) Addison-Wesley: Redwood City, CA, 1983.

to personal vulnerability and poorly developed or inappropriate use of defense mechanisms.

B. *Altered interpersonal processes*

    1. *Impaired verbal communication* related to cerebral deficits and psychological barriers.

    2. *Altered conduct/impulse processes:* aggressive, violent behaviors toward self, others, environment related to feelings of distrust and altered judgment.

    3. *Dysfunctional behaviors:* age-inappropriate behaviors, bizarre behaviors; disorganized and unpredictable behaviors related to inability to discharge emotions verbally.

    4. *Impaired social interaction:* social isolation/withdrawal related to feelings of suspicion and mistrust.

    5. *Altered values:* inability to internalize values associated with refusing limits, related to unresolved emotions and altered judgment.

C. *Altered parenting* related to ambivalent family relationships and failure of child to meet role expectations.

D. *Sensory-perceptual alterations:* altered attention related to disturbed mental activities.

E. *Altered cognition process:* altered decision making, judgment, knowledge and learning processes; altered thought content and processes related to perceptual or cognitive impairment and emotional dysfunctioning.

◄ **III. Nursing care plan/implementation** in mental and emotional disorders in children:

    A. *General goals:* corrective behavior—*behavior modification.*

    B. Help children gain self-awareness.

    C. Provide *structured* environment to orient children to reality.

D. Impose *limits* on destructive behavior toward themselves or others without rejecting the children.
   1. *Prevent* destructive behavior.
   2. *Stop* destructive behavior.
   3. *Redirect* nongrowth behavior into constructive channels.
E. Be *consistent*.
F. Meet *developmental* and *dependency* needs.
G. Recognize and encourage each child's strengths, growth behavior, and reverse regression.
H. Help these children reach the next step in social growth and development scale.
I. Use *play* and *projective media* to aid working out feelings and conflicts and in making contact.
J. Offer support to parents and strengthen the parent-child relationship.
K. *Health teaching:* teach parents methods of behavior modification.

✖ **IV. Evaluation/outcome criteria**
   A. Destructive behavior is inhibited.
   B. Demonstrates age-appropriate behavior on developmental scale.

Adolescent Behaviors: Normal, Problematic, and Emotional Disorders

I. Definition: The early adolescent period usually begins at 12–13, and late adolescent period extends through the teenage years, until 20–21 years of age.
✖ **II. Assessment**
   A. Growth and development milestones—achievement of developmental tasks:
   1. Evolution of *identity* (*self, gender,* in relation to family and society).
   2. Individuation (*self-realization*).
   3. *Value-clarification* and *prioritization* of beliefs and interests.
   4. Establishment of meaningful relationships with same and opposite sex.
   5. Achievement of *intimacy*.
   6. Building competence and sharpening *skills*.
   7. Thinking of career goals, life-style.
   B. Physical factors associated with adolescent disorders
   1. *Hormonal* changes, affecting body image, mood, drives.
   2. Changes in *genital* development, affecting psychosexuality and body image.
   C. Normal behavior seen in adolescents—common age-related areas of *conflict:*
   1. Body image.
   2. Identity: process of individuation.
   3. Independence: moving away from parental control (*control* vs. need to *rebel; dependency* vs. *independency*).

   4. Sexuality: exploring homosexual and heterosexual relationships.
   5. Sexual behavior: fantasy, masturbation.
   6. Social role: peer group.
D. General characteristics of **problematic** adolescent behavior
   Adolescents often *act out* their underlying feelings of *insecurity, rejection, deprivation,* and *low self-esteem.*
   1. *Sexually active* adolescent: way of exploring meaning of sexual behavior, and is an acting-out behavior.
   2. *Suicidal* adolescent: expressions of self-disgust, sadness.
   3. *Runaway:* expression of family conflicts.
   4. *Violent* adolescent: aggressive and disruptive behavior.
   5. *Substance abuse:* bizarre behavior, aggressive behavior, extremely sedated behavior.
   6. *Weight problems:* e.g., anorexia nervosa, bulimia.
   7. *School phobia:* lack of relatedness with peers, reduced performance in school.
   8. *Conduct disorder:* poor impulse control.
   9. *Over*-involvement or *under*-involvement with age-related activities.
E. Environment: family history and school
   1. *Prolonged stressors:* parental marital discord and family breakup, overcrowded living conditions, low socioeconomic status, parental psychiatric condition or trouble with the law, child abuse (physical, emotional, sexual).
   2. *Lack* of guidelines.
   3. *Neglect.*
F. Family dynamics in which the adolescent patient bears the symptoms of a troubled family system:
   1. Parenting: overanxious or rigid.
   2. Communication: dysfunctional patterns, e.g., double bind.
   3. Development of own identity and separation from family: blurring of ego boundaries, with poor differentiation of individual family member identity.
G. Daily activities: assess current functioning
   1. Acceptance by peers.
   2. Acceptance of peers' norms and rules for behavior.
H. Support systems: Who are they? Where and when do they come in to play?
III. Types of adolescent disorders
   A. Conduct disorder: persistent, serious behavioral problems at home, school, and in the community. (If persists into adulthood, diagnosis is changed to *personality disorder.*) *Manifested* by violation of basic rights of others, rules, laws, and mores (norms):
   1. Verbal and physical aggression toward people, property, animals.

   2. Stealing, rape, lying, cheating, truancy from school, fire-setting.
   3. Use of drugs.
   4. Callous disregard for feelings of others.
   5. Blaming others for own behavior.
   6. Low tolerance for frustration; irritability.
   7. Lack of: empathy, remorse, guilt.
   8. Low self-esteem.

   B. **Oppositional defiant disorder:** pattern of defiance, hostility, and negativism. *Manifestations:*
   1. Loss of temper; show of anger, hostility, and vindictiveness.
   2. Argumentativeness.
   3. Defiance and refusal to follow adult rules.
   4. Deliberate annoyance of others.
   5. Swearing and obscene language.
   6. Low tolerance level.

IV. Analysis/nursing diagnosis
   A. *Ineffective individual coping* related to having a short attention span and being easily distracted.
   B. *Altered nutrition: less than body requirements* related to induced vomiting and reduced eating.
   C. *Impaired social interaction* related to inability to follow rules and need to test limits.
   D. *Social isolation* related to feelings of inadequacy or inferiority and inadequate social skills.
   E. *High risk for violence: self-directed* related to self-disgust and feelings of hopelessness.
   F. *High risk for violence: directed at others* related to feelings of anger and frustration.

V. Nursing care plan/implementation
   A. Family therapy (*always* involve family to increase support):
   1. Provide education concerning normal growth and development, with age-related realistic expectations about adolescent's ability to function at home and in community.
   2. Assess bonding issues.
   3. Establish rules of confidentiality.
   4. Do *not* take sides or assume parental role.
   B. Parental skills: assess and teach.
   C. Emotional support for all family members:
   1. Alleviate feelings of guilt and self-blame.
   2. Support strengths.
   D. Expand family's social support network: support groups, community agencies.
   E. Have a contract with adolescent to encourage self-control and sense of autonomy; *avoid* power struggles.

VI. Evaluation/outcome criteria
   A. *Demonstrates emotional control;* attends school and performs without undue frustration or inappropriate anger.
   B. *Exhibits improved interactive* skills appropriate for adolescent level of development; has meaningful interactions with staff, family, peers.
   C. *Demonstrates appropriate eating* habits and behaviors, with adequate nutritional intake.
   D. *Uses adaptive coping techniques* with decreased attempts at self-harm or violence toward others.
   E. *Uses community resources.*

Midlife Crisis: Phase-of-Life Problems

Midlife crisis is a time period that marks the passage between early maturity and middle age. Middle age is generally placed between 40–45 and 65–70 years of age.

I. Assessment
   A. Mid-life crisis commonly occurs between ages 35 and 45.
   B. Preoccupied with *visible* signs of aging, own mortality.
   C. *Feelings: urgency* that time is running out ("last chance") for career achievement and unmet goals; *boredom* with present, *ambivalence, frustration, uncertainty* about the future and *dissatisfaction* with life.
   D. Time of *reevaluation:*
   1. Reassess: meaning of time and parental role (omnipotence as a parent is challenged).
   2. Reexamine and contemplate change in career, marriage, family life.
   E. *Personality changes* may occur. *Women:* traditional definitions of femininity may be challenged as they become more assertive. *Men:* may be more introspective, sensitive to emotions, make external changes (e.g., look for younger mate, improve looks, new sports activity), mood swings.
   F. Presence of *helpful elements* necessary to turn life's obstacles into opportunities.
   1. Willingness to take risks.
   2. Strong support system.
   3. Sense of purpose.
   4. Accumulated wisdom.

II. Analysis/nursing diagnosis
   A. *Self-esteem disturbance* (*low self-esteem*) related to: loss of youth, faltering physical powers, and facing discrepancy between youthful ambitions and actual achievement (no longer a promising person with potential).
   B. *Altered role performance* (*role reversal*): related to parents who previously provided security and comfort but now need care.
   C. *Altered feeling states* (*depression*): related to disappointments and diminished optimism as life is reconsidered in light of the reality of aging and death.

III. Nursing care plan/implementation—*long-term goal:* help individual to rebuild life structure.
   A. Help client reappraise meaning of own life in terms of past, present, and future, and integrate aspects of time. Encourage introspection and reflection with questions.
   1. What have I done with my life?
   2. What do I really get from and give to my spouse, children, friends, work, community, and self?
   3. What are my strengths and liabilities?
   4. What have I done with my early dream, and do I want it now?

B. Assist client to complete *four major tasks:*

1. Terminate era of early adulthood by *reappraising* life goals identified and achieved during this era.
2. Initiate movement into middle adulthood by beginning to make *necessary changes* in *unsuccessful* aspects of the current life while trying out new choices.
3. Cope with *polarities* that divide life.
4. Directly confront *death of own parents.*

C. *Health teaching:* stress management techniques; how to do self-assessment of aptitudes, interests; how to plan for retirement, aloneness, and use of increased leisure time; dietary modification and exercise program.

IV. Evaluation/outcome criteria

A. Gives up *idealized* self of early 20s for more *realistically* attainable self.

1. Talks *less* of early *hopes of eminence* and *more* on modest goal of *competence.*
2. Shifts values from sexuality to platonic relationships: replaces romantic dreams with *satisfying* friendships and companionships.
3. Modifies early illusions about own capacities.
4. Shifts values away from physical attractiveness and strength to *intellectual* abilities.

B. Comes to accept that life is finite and reconciles what *is* with what *might have been;* appreciates everyday human experience rather than glamor or power.

C. Through self-confrontation, self-discovery, and change, experiences time of restabilization; is reinvigorated, adventuresome.

D. Develops *alternative* abilities that release new energies.

E. Tries *less* to please everyone; others' opinions less important.

F. Makes more efficient and well-seasoned decisions from well-developed sense of judgment.

Mental Health Problems of the Elderly

In general, problems affecting the elderly are *similar* to those affecting persons of *any* age. This section will highlight the *differences* from the viewpoint of etiology, frequency, and prognosis.

I. Concepts and principles related to mental health problems of the elderly.

A. The elderly *do* have capacity for growth and change.

B. Human beings, regardless of age, need sense of future and *hope* for things to come.

C. An inalienable right of all individuals should be to make or *participate* in *all decisions* concerning themselves and their possessions as long as they can.

D. Physical disability due to the aging process may enforce dependency, which may be unacceptable

to elderly patients and may evoke feelings of *anger* and *ambivalence.*

E. In an attempt to *reduce feelings of loss,* elderly patients may *cling to concrete things* that most represent, in a *symbolic* sense, all that has been significant to them.

F. As memory diminishes, *familiar objects* in environment and *familiar routines* are important in helping *to keep clients oriented* and in contact with reality.

G. *Familiarity of environment brings security;* routines bring a sense of security about what is to happen.

H. If individuals feel unwanted, they may tell *stories* about their *earlier* achievements.

I. Many of the traits in the elderly result from *cumulative* effect of *past* experiences of frustrations and *present* awareness of limitations rather than from any primary consequences of physiologic deficit.

II. Assessment

A. *Psychological characteristics of the elderly*

1. Increasingly *dependent* on others, not only for physical needs but also for emotional security; concerned with abandonment and financial exploitation.
2. Concerns focus more and more *inward,* with narrowed outside interests.
   a. Decreased emotional energy for concern with social problems unless these issues affect them.
   b. Tendency to *reminisce.*
   c. May appear selfish and unsympathetic.
3. Sources of pleasure and gratification are more childlike: e.g., *food, warmth,* and *affection.*
   a. Tangible and frequent evidence of affection is important (e.g., letters, cards, and visits).
   b. May hoard articles.
4. *Attention span and memory are short;* may be forgetful and *accuse others of stealing.*
5. Deprivation of any kind is *not* tolerated:
   a. Easily frustrated.
   b. Change is poorly tolerated; e.g., need to have favorite chairs and established daily routine.
6. Main *fears* in the elderly include:
   a. *Fear of: dependency,* chronic *illness, loneliness, boredom;* of being unloved, forgotten, *deserted* by those close to them; of abuse and *neglect* by caregiver (e.g., by withholding food and drink, by omission of or over medication); of *death;* of *loss of control* of one's own life.
   b. Failing *cognition.*
   c. Loss of *purpose* and *productivity.*
7. *Nocturnal delirium (sundowner's syndrome)* may be due to problems with night vision and inability to perceive *spatial* location.

8. May have *sunriser's* syndrome of *early* morning confusion (e.g., in Alzheimer's).

B. *Psychiatric problems in aging*

1. *Loneliness:* related to *loss* of mate, diminishing circle of friends and family through death and geographic separation, *decline* in physical energy, loss of work (*retirement*), sharp loss of income, and loss of a life-long life-style.

2. *Insomnia*—pattern of sleep changes in significant ways: disappearance of *deep* sleep, frequent *awakening, daytime* sleeping.

3. *Hypochondriasis:* anxiety may shift from concern with finances, job, or social prestige to concern about own bodily function. See also hypochondriasis in Chap. 9.

4. *Depression:* common problem in the aging, with a *high suicide rate;* partly because of bodily changes that influence the *self-concept,* the older person may direct *hostility toward self* and therefore may be subject to feelings of depression and loneliness. See also depression in Chap. 12.

5. *Senility—four early symptoms:*
   a. Change in attention span.
   b. Memory loss for *recent* events and *names.*
   c. Altered intellectual capacity.
   d. Diminished ability to respond to others.

C. *Successful aging*

1. Being able to *perceive* signs of aging and limitations resulting from the aging process.

2. *Redefining* life in terms of effects on social and physical aspects of living.

3. Seeking *alternatives* for meeting needs and finding sources of pleasure.

4. Adopting a *different outlook* about self-worth.

5. *Reintegrating* values with goals of life.

D. *Causative factors* of mental disorder in the elderly related to:

1. *Nutritional* problems and *physical ill health* related to neglect and *acute and chronic illness:*
   a. Cardiovascular disease (e.g., heart failure, stroke, hypertension).
   b. Respiratory infection.
   c. Cancer.
   d. Alcohol dependence and abuse.
   e. Dentition problems.

2. *Faulty adaptation* related to *physical* changes of aging; e.g., depression, hypochondriasis.

3. Problems related to *loss, grief,* and *bereavement.*

4. *Retirement* shock related to loss of status and financial security.

5. Social isolation and loneliness related to *inadequate sensory stimulation.*

6. *Environmental change* (e.g., relocation within a community or from home to institution): loss of family and privacy.

7. *Hopelessness, helplessness* related to condition and circumstances and neglect.

8. *Altered body image* (i.e., negative) related to aging process.

9. Depression related to *helplessness, inability to express anger.*

▶ III. Analysis/nursing diagnosis

A. *Self-esteem disturbance* related to body image disturbance and altered family role.

B. *Impaired social interaction* related to social isolation and environmental changes.

C. *Dysfunctional grieving* related to loss and bereavement.

D. *Altered feeling states and spiritual distress* related to hopelessness, anxiety, fear, powerlessness.

E. *Altered physical regulation processes* related to physical ill health, neglect, poor hygiene.

F. *Sleep pattern disturbance* related to insomnia and altered sleep/arousal patterns.

▶ IV. Nursing care plan/implementation

A. Long-term goal: to help reduce hopelessness and helplessness.

B. Short-term goal: to keep free from injury; to focus on ego assets.

C. Help elderly *preserve* what facet of life they can and *regain* that which has already been lost.

1. Help *minimize regression* as much as possible.

2. Help retain their *adult* status.

3. Help preserve their *self-image* as useful individuals.

4. Identify and preserve their *abilities* to perform, emphasizing what they *can* do.

5. Report elder abuse.

D. Attempt to *prevent* loss of dignity and loss of worth; address them by titles (e.g., "Mr.," "Dr."), not "Gramps."

E. *Reduce* feelings of *alienation* and loneliness. Provide *sensory* experiences for those with visual problems:

1. Let them *touch* objects of various textures and consistencies.

2. Encourage heightened *use of remaining senses* to make up for those that are diminished or lost.

F. *Reduce* depression and feelings of isolation.

1. Allow time to *reminisce.*

2. *Avoid changes* in surroundings or routine.

G. *Protect* from rush and excitement.

1. Use simple, unhurried conversation.

2. Allow *extra* time to organize thoughts.

H. Be sensitive to *concrete* things they may want to *keep.*

I. *Health teaching*

1. How to keep track of time (e.g., by marking off days on a calendar), to promote orientation.

2. How to keep track of medications.

3. Exercises to promote blood flow.

4. *Retirement counseling*
   a. Obtaining satisfaction from leisure time.
   b. Nurturing relationships with younger generations.

      c. Adjusting to changes: physical health, retirement, loss of loved ones.

      d. Developing connections with own age group.

      e. Taking on new social roles.

      f. Maintaining a satisfactory and appropriate living situation.

      g. Coping with dependence on others, especially one's children.

✕ **V. Evaluation/outcome criteria**

    A. Less confusion and fewer mood swings.

    B. Increased interest in activities of daily living and interaction with others.

    C. Lessened preoccupation with death, dying, physical symptoms, feelings of sadness.

    D. Reduced insomnia and anorexia.

    E. Expresses feelings of belonging and being needed.

Victims of Violence and Abuse

Battered Woman

I. Characteristics

    A. *Victims:* feel helpless, powerless to prevent assault; blame themselves; ambivalent about leaving the relationship.

    B. *Abusers:* often blame the victims; have poor impulse control; use power (physical strength or weapon) to threaten and subject victims to their assault.

    C. *Cycle* of stages, with increase in severity of the battering:

      1. *Buildup of tension* (through verbal abuse): abuser is often drinking or taking other drugs; victim blames self.

      2. *Battering:* abuser does not remember brutal beating; victim is in shock and detached.

      3. *Calm:* abuser "makes up," apologizes, and promises "never again"; victim believes and forgives the abuser, and feels loved.

II. Risk factors

    A. *Learned responses:* abuser and victim have had past experience with violence in family; victim has "learned helplessness."

    B. *Pregnant* women and those with one or more *preschool children,* who see no alternative to staying in the battering relationship.

    C. Women who *fear* punishment from the abuser.

✕ **III. Assessment**

    A. Injury to parts of body, especially face, head, genitals (e.g., welts, bruises, fracture of nose).

    B. Presents in the emergency department with report of "accidental injury."

    C. Severe anxiety.

    D. Depression.

✕ **IV. Analysis/nursing diagnosis**

    A. *Risk for injury* related to physical harm.

    B. *Posttraumatic response* related to assault.

    C. *Fear* related to threat of death or change in health status.

    D. *Pain* related to physical and psychological harm.

    E. *Powerlessness* related to interpersonal interaction.

    F. *Ineffective individual coping* related to situational crisis.

    G. *Spiritual distress* related to intense suffering and challenged value system.

✕ **V. Nursing care plan/implementation**

    A. Provide safe environment; refer to community resources for shelter.

    B. Treat physical injuries.

    C. Document injuries.

    D. Supportive, nonjudgmental approach: identify woman's strengths; help her to accept that she cannot control the abuser; encourage description of home situation; help her to see choices.

    E. Encourage individual and family therapy for victim and abuser.

✕ **VI. Evaluation/outcome criteria**

    A. Physical symptoms have been treated.

    B. Discusses plans for safety (for self and any children) to protect against further injury.

Rape-Trauma Syndrome

I. Definition: forcible perpetration of an act of sexual intercourse on the body of an unwilling person.

✕ **II. Assessment**

    A. **Physical trauma**

      1. *Signs:* physical findings of entry.

      2. *Symptoms:* verbatim statements regarding type of sexual attack.

    B. **Emotional trauma**

      1. *Signs:*

        a. Shame, embarrassment, and guilt; self-blame.

        b. Extreme anxiety: tears, hyperventilating.

        c. Withdrawal.

        d. Sleeping and eating disturbances.

        e. Anger; desire for revenge.

        f. Fears.

      2. *Symptoms:* statements regarding method of force used and threats made.

✕ **III. Analysis/nursing diagnosis**—*Rape-trauma syndrome* related to phases of response to rape:

    A. *Acute response:* volatility, disorganization, disbelief, shock, incoherence, agitated motor activity, nightmares, guilt (should have been able to protect self), phobias (crowds, being alone, sex).

    B. *Outward coping:* denial and suppression of anxiety and fear (silent rape syndrome), feelings appear controlled.

    C. *Integration and resolution:* confronts anger with attacker; realistic perspective.

✕ **IV. Nursing care plan/implementation** in counseling rape victims. Figure 16.1 is a summary of self-care decisions a victim faces during the acute phase following a sexual assault.

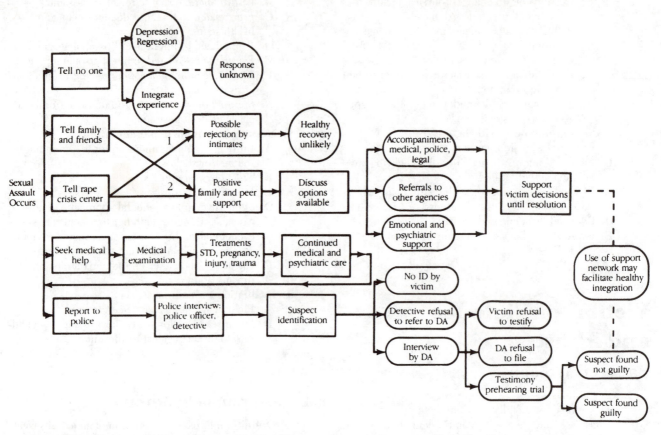

FIGURE 16.1   **VICTIM DECISIONS FOLLOWING A SEXUAL ASSAULT**
(From the Rape Crisis Services of the YWCA. Greater Harrisburg, PA.)

A. *Overall goals*—help victim to:
  1. Acknowledge feelings.
  2. Face feelings.
  3. Resolve feelings.
  4. Maintain and restore *self-respect, dignity, integrity,* and *self-determination.*
B. *Work through issues*
  1. Handle *legal* matters and police contacts.
  2. Clarify *facts.*
  3. Get *medical* attention if needed.
  4. Notify *family and friends.*
  5. Understand emotional reaction.
  6. Attend to *practical* concerns.
  7. Evaluate need for psychiatric consultations.
C. *Acute phase*
  1. Decrease victim's stress, anxiety, fear.
  2. Seek medical care.
  3. Increase self-confidence and self-esteem.
  4. Identify and accept feelings and needs (to be in control, cared about, to achieve).
  5. Reorient perceptions, feelings, and statements about self.
  6. Help resume normal life-style.
D. *Outward coping phase*
  1. Remain available and supportive.
  2. Reflect words, feelings, and thoughts.

  3. Explore real problems.
  4. Explore alternatives regarding contraception, legal issues.
  5. Evaluate response of family and friends to victim and rape.
E. *Integration* and *resolution* phase
  1. Assist exploration of feelings (anger) regarding attacker.
  2. Explore feelings (guilt and shame) regarding self.
  3. Assist in making own decisions regarding health care.
F. Maintain *confidentiality* and *neutrality;* facilitate person's own decision.
G. Search for alternatives to advice-giving.
H. *Health teaching*
  1. Explain procedures and services to victim.
  2. Counsel to avoid isolated areas and being helpful to strangers.
  3. Counsel where and how to resist attack (scream, run unless assailant has weapon), refer to self-defense courses.
  4. Offer options about what to do if pregnancy or STD are outcome.
V. **Evaluation/outcome criteria:** little or no evidence of possible long-term effects of rape (guilt, shame, phobias, denial).

Battered Child

✉ **I. Assessment**—clues to the identification of a battered child°

    A. Clues in the *history*

        1. Significant *delay* in seeking medical care.

        2. Major *discrepancies* in the history:

            a. Discrepancy between different people's versions of the story.

            b. Discrepancy between the history and the observed injuries.

            c. Discrepancy between the history and the child's developmental capabilities.

        3. History of multiple emergency department visits for various injuries.

        4. A story that is *vague* and *contradictory*

    B. Clues in the *physical examination*

        1. Child who seems withdrawn, apathetic and *does not cry* despite his injuries.

        2. Child who *does not turn to parents for comfort;* or unusual desire to please parent; unusual fear of parent(s).

        3. *Child who is poorly nourished* and *poorly cared for.*

        4. The presence of *bruises: multiple bruises,* welts, and abrasions, especially around the trunk and buttocks; *old bruises in addition to fresh ones* (Table 16.2).

        5. The presence of *suspicious burns:*

            a. Cigarette burns.

            b. Scalds without splash marks or involving the buttocks, hands, or feet but sparing skin folds.

            c. Rope marks

        6. Clues in parent behavior—exaggerate care and concern.

✉ **II. Analysis/nursing diagnosis**

    A. Same as for battered woman, see p. 197.

    B. Altered parenting.

    C. Low self-esteem.

✉ **III. Nursing care plan/implementation**

    A. Same as for battered woman, see p. 197, V. A., B., C.

    B. Report suspected child abuse to appropriate source.

    C. Conduct assessment interview in private, with child and parent separated.

    D. Be supportive and nonjudgmental.

✉ **IV. Evaluation/outcome criteria**

    A. Same as battered woman, see p. 197, VI. A.

    B. Child safety has been ensured.

    C. Parent(s) or caregivers have agreed to seek help.

°Adapted from Caroline N. *Emergency Care in the Streets* (5th ed). Boston: Little, Brown, 1995. P. 761.

Table 16.2	GAUGING THE AGE OF A SOFT TISSUE INJURY
Time Since Injury	**Color of the Bruise**
0–2 hr	No discoloration (may be swollen and tender)
1–5 d	Reddish blue
5–7 d	Greenish
7–10 d	Yellow
10–14 d	Brown

Source: Caroline N. *Emergency Care in the Streets* (5th ed). Boston: Little, Brown, 1995. P. 761.

Sexually Abused Child

✉ **I. Assessment**—characteristic behaviors:

    A. *Relationship* of abuser to victim: many filling paternal role (uncle, grandfather, cousin) with repeated, unquestioned access to the child.

    B. Methods of *pressuring* victim into sexual activity: offering material goods, misrepresenting moral standards ("it's OK"), exploiting need for human contact and warmth.

    C. Method of pressuring victim to *secrecy* (in order to conceal the act) is inducing fear of: punishment, not being believed, rejection, being blamed for the activity, abandonment.

    D. *Disclosure* of sexual activity via:

        1. Direct visual or verbal confrontation and *observation* by others.

        2. *Verbalization* of act by victim.

        3. *Visible clues:* excess money and candy, new clothes, pictures, notes.

        4. *Signs and symptoms:* trauma to genitalia, STD, bed-wetting, excessive bathing, tears, avoiding school, somatic complaints (*GI* and *urinary* tract pains).

        5. Overly solicitous parental attitude toward child.

✉ **II. Analysis/nursing diagnosis**

    A. *Altered protection* related to inflicted pain.

    B. *Risk for injury* related to neglect, abuse.

    C. *Personal identity disturbance* related to abuse as child and feeling guilty and responsible for being a victim.

    D. *Ineffective individual coping* related to high stress level.

    E. *Sleep pattern disturbance* related to traumatic sexual experiences.

    F. *Ineffective family coping.*

    G. *Altered family processes* related to use of violence.

    H. *Altered parenting* related to violence.

    I. *Powerlessness* related to feelings of being dependent on abuser.

    J. *Social isolation/withdrawal* related to shame about family violence.

K. *Risk for altered abuse response patterns.*

☝ **III. Nursing care plan/implementation**

    A. Establish *safe* environment and the *termination* of trauma.

    B. Encourage child to verbalize feelings about incident to dispel tension built up by secrecy.

    C. Ask child to draw a picture or use dolls and toys to show what happened.

    D. Observe for symptoms over a period of time.

        1. *Phobic* reactions when seeing or hearing abuser's name.

        2. *Sleep pattern* changes, recurrent dreams, nightmares.

    E. Look for *silent reaction* to being an accessory to sex (i.e., child keeping burden of the secret activity within self); help deal with unresolved issues.

    F. Establish therapeutic alliance with abusive parent.

    G. *Health teaching*

        1. Teach child that his or her body is private and to inform a responsible adult when someone violates privacy without consent.

        2. Teach adults in family to respond to victim with sensitivity, support, and concern.

☝ **IV. Evaluation/outcome criteria**

    A. Child's needs for affection, attention, personal recognition, or love met without sexual exploitation.

    B. Perpetrator accepts therapy.

    C. Conspiracy of silence is broken.

Patients with Hearing Impairment

   I. Definition: Hearing impairment is the inability to hear adequately as a result of the aging process (*presbycusis*) or other physical or psychological condition. Each type of loss imposes life-style changes that require compensation for the impairment.

☝ **II. Assessment**

    A. Auditory distortions.

    B. Change in usual response to stimuli.

    C. Related factors: accumulated cerumen; nerve damage from toxic drugs; chronic ear infections; anxiety with narrowed perception.

☝ **III. Analysis/nursing diagnosis:** *altered sensory perception (auditory).*

☝ **IV. Nursing care plan/implementation**

    A. Assess auditory perception: abilities, limitations in activities of daily living (ADL) imposed by hearing loss.

    B. Assess need for and provide referral for supplementary aids (hearing aids).

    C. *Communication skills* that are meaningful for the patient with auditory deficit:

        1. Face the patient.

        2. Speak slowly, clearly.

        3. *Avoid* shouting.

        4. Use a *low*-pitched tone.

        5. *Avoid* covering mouth or chewing gum when speaking.

        6. Use repetition if patient responds inappropriately.

        7. Make sure hearing aid, if used, is turned on; encourage use of hearing aid if not used. Encourage use of assistive devices such as amplifiers for phone instruments.

        8. Refer to community services that assist hearing impaired individuals (see Appendix C).

☝ **V. Evaluation/outcome criteria:** optimal hearing perception as evidenced by patient's awareness; incorporation of life-style changes to compensate for auditory loss.

Patients with Visual Impairment

   I. Definition: Visual impairment is the inability to see adequately as a result of the aging process (*presbyopia*) or other physical or psychological condition. Life-style changes are imposed that require intervention to compensate for impairment.

☝ **II. Assessment**

    A. Visual distortions.

    B. Change in usual response to stimuli.

    C. Related factors: chronic illness, neurologic deficit or disease, hypoxia, alteration in sense organ (eyes), psychological stress, anxiety with narrowed perceptual fields.

☝ **III. Analysis/nursing diagnosis:** *altered sensory perception (visual).*

☝ **IV. Nursing care plan/implementation**

    A. Assess visual perception, limitations in ADL imposed by sensory loss and need for supplementary aids.

    ☞ **1.** Assist in ambulation by placing patient's hand on nurse's elbow and have the patient follow the nurse.

    B. Use as many sensory modes as possible, as is comfortable (e.g., use touch and verbalization, music, tape recording).

    C. Interact in well-lit room, free from outside distractions.

    D. *Communication skills* that are meaningful for the patient with a particular visual deficit:

        1. Allow time to process and respond to communication.

        2. Announce arrival and departure.

        3. Announce touch before doing so.

        4. Speak in a moderate, not loud, tone.

        5. Speak *to* the patient, not about the patient.

        6. Sit directly in front of the patient (for lip reading).

        7. Make sure patient is using glasses or contact lenses, if prescribed.

        8. Encourage use of assistive devices (e.g., reading material in large print or Braille, big numbers on phone dials).

9. Refer to community services that assist visually impaired individuals and their families (see Appendix C).

✉ V. **Evaluation/outcome criteria**
  A. *Short-term: adequate* visual perception as evidenced by awareness of need for life-style change to compensate for visual loss.
  B. *Long-term: optimal* visual perception, related to adoption of life-style changes into daily living.

💡 Study and Memory Aids

Assessment of adolescents

Make age-appropriate assessment based on age-typical development stage.

Rule out abnormal—not age-related—changes in elderly

1. With elderly patients, the nurse needs to differentiate age-related changes (e.g., impaired short-term memory, slower response times) from abnormal changes (e.g., dementia).
2. With elderly patients, it is especially important to distinguish *depression* from *dementia*. See Summary of Key Points, p. 202.

Counseling rape victims—nursing role

Mainly supportive, as a source of referral; collect and document physical evidence

Glossary

adjustment disorder   Common in adolescents; characterized by maladaptive response to an identifiable psychosocial stressor (e.g., birth of a sibling, death of a parent). Reaction occurs within 3 months of the stressor event and is manifested by impaired social or occupational functioning that is more intense than the "normal" expected response.

adolescence   A stage of growth and development; a transitional period from beginning of puberty to maturity, with major physiologic, cognitive, and behavioral changes taking place. Development of the many different functions may be reached at different times. Time period: 12–21 for girls; 13–23 for boys.

authority figure   Person seen as exerting influence over another because of role, status, and superiority in attributes such as knowledge, strength, etc.

autonomy   Independence; self-determination.

identification   Merging or submerging of one's own values with another's.

life review   The process of recalling and going over past experiences.

mental retardation   Mental deficiency or defect in normal development of intelligence that makes intellectual abilities lower than normal for chronologic age. May result from a condition at birth, from injury during or after birth, or from disease after birth.

midlife crisis   A period of disequilibrium between the ages of 35 and 45, during which individuals note various signs of aging and experience feelings of dissatisfaction with life and uncertainty about the future.

peer   An "equal" with whom one associates; e.g., for an adolescent, another adolescent the same age, in the same grade in school, or in the same sports group.

preadolescence   An arbitrary period generally considered to be the 2 years prior to puberty (i.e., ages 10–12 years).

puberty   The period during which secondary sex characteristics develop and reproductive organs become capable of functioning. In girls, menstruation marks the onset; in boys, a sign is pigmentation in axillary hair.

reality orientation   A therapeutic process used to keep an individual alert to here-and-now events.

sundowner's syndrome   *Late* evening confusion in elderly individuals who have cognitive impairment.

sunriser's syndrome   *Early* morning confusion in elderly individuals who have cognitive impairment.

tic disorder   Occurs in children; characterized by eye blinking, squatting, grimacing, grunting, or barking.

Questions

1. What should the nurse do if a child with autism crawls under a bench while the nurse is with him?
   √1. Sit on the ground near him.
   2. Pull him out.
   3. Entice him with a cookie.
   4. Watch him from a distance.
2. A 6-year-old recently hospitalized develops enuresis. What should be the primary nurse's chief goal?
   1. Preventing regressive behavior.
   √2. Protecting self-esteem.
   3. Providing opportunity for discussion of possible causes.
   4. Ignoring the enuresis.
3. An adolescent boy with acting-out behavior is introduced to the other adolescents in group therapy. The most significant factor that the nurse should consider in initiating group therapy is that:
   1. Confrontation could lead to elopement.
   2. He may refuse to verbalize.
   3. Group members may ignore him.
   4. He may act out during group therapy.
4. The nurse determines that a 45-year-old single woman is not exhibiting an age-typical maturational crisis when she seems agitated and repetitively expresses serious concerns about:
   1. Her economic security.

🔑 Summary of Key Points

Care of Children with Autism

1. Build trust.
2. Accept nonverbal communication.
3. *Avoid* touch.
4. Speak simply; use concrete terms and be direct ("Please sit in this chair").

Adolescents: Special Difficulties for Nursing Interventions Due to Age-Typical Behaviors:

1. Silence.
2. Need for confidentiality.
3. Negativism.
4. Resistance.
5. Need for limit-setting.
6. Attention-seeking.

Middle-Age: Phase-of-Life Crisis

Nursing implications:
1. Help with *reappraisal* of values and capabilities.
2. Encourage modifications and shifts in values that are made necessary by age and stage of development.
3. Encourage *self-discovery* of alternative abilities through willingness to *make changes* and take risks.

Care of the Elderly Needs to Include Comparison of Dementia and Depression

	Dementia	Depression
Affect	Labile	Remains depressed
Mood	Anxiety	Apathy
Onset	Gradual	More readily identifiable (i.e., able to "pinpoint")
Response to memory loss	Loss is covered up	No attempt to cover up

Care of a Patient with Rape-Trauma Syndrome

1. *Initial care:* Provide privacy and stay with patient. Encourage her to talk about the event. Assist with physical exam; help her to bathe and change clothes.
2. Help notify family and friends.
3. Refer to rape crisis center.
4. Help victim with legal decisions.
5. Reassure/reinforce that she is not at fault.

Care of Battered Children and Adults

1. Assess for physical evidence of abuse.
2. Listen for conflicting stories or placing blame on the victim.
3. Suspected abuse must be reported to the appropriate authorities.
4. *Battered woman:* work with her ambivalence and anger; help her to see and act on choices; identify strengths and areas in which she *is* in control; help her with plan to "escape" from home if she decides to go back; provide list of safe places to stay; refer to community resources. Help her to accept that she cannot control the abuser.

Care of Sexually Abused Child

1. Report suspected abuse.
2. Ensure safety of the child.
3. Refer parent(s) or caregiver(s) for assistance and therapy.

Care of a Patient with Hearing or Vision Problems

Nursing implications—priorities:
1. Promote *safety*.
2. *Minimize* deficits.
3. Provide *compensatory* activities and aids.

---

  2. Dying with dignity.
  3. Her social isolation.
  4. Her body image.

5. What parental behavior during the admission procedure for a child should cause the nurse to suspect child abuse?
  1. Acting overly solicitous toward the child.
  2. Ignoring the child.
  3. Expressions of guilt.
  4. Flat affect.

6. Which assessment findings for a child would *most* suggest sexual abuse?
  1. Trauma to genitalia and sexually transmitted disease.
  2. Nightmares and depression.
  3. Somatic complaints and enuresis.
  4. Sexual jokes and nudity.

7. Which emotional response is the admitting nurse in the emergency department most likely to see as predominant in a woman who is a victim of rape?
  1. Rage.
  2. Guilt.
  3. Phobia.
  4. Anxiety.

8. A woman comes in with bruises on her face, neck, wrists, and legs. The nurse suspects abuse by the spouse, although the woman offers a different story. What should the nurse say to this woman?
  1. "Here's the name of a home for women who need a safe place to go."
  2. "Here's the day and time of a support group for your husband."
  3. "It is all right to admit that you have been abused."

4. *"You should discuss this with the doctor."*
9. While assessing an elderly patient who is suspected of being abused, for which sign of the most common type of abuse in the elderly should the nurse assess?
   1. Bruising from beatings.
   2. Dehydration and malnutrition.
   3. Skin lesions from tight restraints.
   4. Confusion from overmedication.
10. An elderly woman comes in with bruises and says she fell; the nurse suspects she has been abused. How would the nurse question this elderly patient?
    1. With no one else present.
    2. With a relative present.
    3. With another nurse present.
    4. With a doctor present.
11. An elderly client says, "I can't hear you." How should the nurse speak?
    1. Louder.
    2. Slowly, with exaggerated mouthing.
    3. In a higher-pitched tone.
    4. In a lower-pitched tone.
12. The nurse demonstrates the best way of helping a patient who is blind to walk down the hallway by:
    1. Holding the patient by the hand and leading the patient.
    2. Holding the patient by the elbow and steering the patient around obstacles.
    3. Placing both of the patient's hands on the nurse's shoulders and walking slowly.
    4. Placing the patient's hand on the nurse's elbow and having the patient follow the nurse.

Answers/Rationale

1. **(1)** This response conveys *acceptance*, an especially important concept in the therapeutic use of self when working with autistic children. Force (**No. 2**) is *not* therapeutic. **No. 3** is not a good choice *unless* the question clearly calls for using behavior modification (which this question does not); *then* maybe the use of a "cookie" as a reward for inducing desired behavior may be acceptable. Watching the child from a distance (**No. 4**) would *not* readily convey acceptance. Picture the nonverbal interaction: sitting from afar and watching the child. What feeling tones are conveyed by this posture? "Big Nurse is watching you." **PL, 7, PsI**

Key to Codes

Nursing process: AS = Assessment; **AN** = Analysis; **PL** = Planning; **IMP** = Implementation; **EV** = Evaluation. (See Appendix E for explanation of nursing process steps.)

Category of human function: 1 = Protective; **2** = Sensory-Perceptual; **3** = Comfort, Rest, Activity, and Mobility; **4** = Nutrition; **5** = Growth and Development; **6** = Fluid-Gas Transport; **7** = Psychosocial-Cultural; **8** = Elimination.

Client need: SECE = Safe, Effective Care Environment; **PhI** = Physiologic Integrity; **PsI** = Psychosocial Integrity; **HPM** = Health Promotion/Maintenance.

💡 *Test-taking tip:* Look for two contradictory options. Force (**No. 2**) is the opposite of acceptance (**No. 1**); one of these (in this case, force) must be incorrect.

2. **(2)** This *general* concept (self-esteem) meets the condition of the question stem ("chief goal" is a *general* term). Preventing regressive behavior (**No. 1**) is one *particular* way to help protect self-esteem, which is the chief *general* goal. **No. 3** focuses on *talking* about an embarrassing situation, which doesn't help with self-esteem. The nurse *does need* to look into possible causes and protect self-esteem, and so must *not* ignore the bed-wetting (**No. 4**). **PL, 8, PsI**

💡 *Test-taking tip:* A *general* question usually calls for a *general* answer.

3. **(1)** If a confrontation develops *too soon*, the adolescent may feel threatened and run away from the group. Although the other options are all accurate, they have *less significant consequences*. The adolescent's refusal to verbalize (**No. 2**) is expected only *initially*, because he probably will not trust the group members at first. The other group members may also feel threatened by a new member and may not trust him at *first* (**No. 3**). Acting-out (**No. 4**) is a coping mechanism that is used to mask fear of a new situation or the sense of feeling threatened. If the patient is at least *present* in the group (even though acting-out), it provides an opportunity for observation and corrective interventions. **AN, 7, PsI**

4. **(2)** Dying with dignity is a more typical concern of an *elderly* individual, not a middle-aged person. The other options *are* age-typical in the middle years: financial concerns (**No. 1**) with approaching retirement ("Is that all there is . . . all that there is going to be . . . in my bank account?"); concern about being alone (**No. 3**), with the advent of age-related illnesses; and awareness of physiologic changes (**No. 4**) as well as psychological changes. **AS, 5, HPM**

5. **(1)** There is a pattern of parental behaviors that includes covering up the abuse by going to the other extreme of exaggerated care and concern. (Remember Shakespeare: "Methinks the [parent] doth protest too much.") Lack of attention (**No. 2**) and absence of emotion (**No. 4**) are the *opposite* of the correct response, which involves an exaggerated display of emotion. It is *not* expressions of *guilt* (**No. 3**), but of inordinate care and concern that are often seen. **EV, 7, PsI**

6. **(1)** These are the most typical *objective* findings, occurring in most cases. The findings in **Nos. 2 and 3** may *also* be present, but they are *subjective* findings, and do not necessarily occur in most cases. *Shame* and *withdrawal* are more likely than overt behaviors, such as sexual jokes and nudity (**No. 4**). **AS, 7, PsI**

💡 *Test-taking tip:* Look at the pattern: Which option is not like the others? *Two options list subjective findings:* **No. 2** nightmares and depression and **No. 3** somatic *complaints*; but one option lists *objective* findings, **No. 1**, trauma to genitalia and STD. When you need to guess, choose the option that is different (**No. 1**).

7. **(2)** *Shame* and *guilt* are the main feelings expressed by rape victims on admission. They feel violated, and many feel (or are induced to feel) that in some way they were partly responsible for what happened. Anger and rage **(No. 1)** is a *later* reaction in response to being a victim of rape. Phobias **(No. 3)** occur *later,* if at all (e.g., a morbid fear of strangers, of darkness, of being alone), whereas reality-based *fears* are common initially (e.g., fear of pregnancy, fear of having contracted a sexually transmitted disease). Anxiety **(No. 4),** while likely to be present, is an *underlying* state, not a *predominant* feeling like guilt. **EV, 7, PsI**

8. **(1)** The goal is to provide safety; this is the only option that provides it. (Note the word "safe" in the option.) The focus should *not* be on the husband **(No. 2);** the nurse must stay *client*-centered, focusing on safety for the woman. **Nos. 3 and 4** do *not* focus on safety. Moreover, the woman does *not* need to discuss this matter with the doctor **(No. 4);** discussions with the *nurse* are *not* contraindicated. **IMP, 1, SECE**

💡 *Test-taking tip:* Patient-centered and safety-oriented concerns are good answers.

9. **(2)** Neglect is the least obvious, but most common form of abuse of the elderly, e.g., by not providing adequate food or withholding food and drink. The signs of abuse are further obscured, and assessment therefore more complicated, because the elderly normally have a diminished appetite. Beatings **(No. 1)** and tight restraints **(No. 3)** are, fortunately, not as common. It would be difficult for the nurse to determine the cause of confusion **(No. 4)** that is not part of age-typical development. **AS, 4, PsI**

10. **(1)** The nurse needs to do crisis counseling (listening with concern) and *ease* the way for the person to talk-

out the experience, to express shame and guilt related to lack of family support system. Because there is fear (related to an environmental stressor), a threat to personal values and beliefs, and a diminished sense of control over self and own environment, this is best accomplished with no one else present. If someone else is present **(Nos. 2, 3, and 4),** the inherent fear and guilt will probably prevent the person from "talking-out" the experience. **PL, 7, PsI**

💡 *Test-taking tip:* When you need to guess, look at the option that is not like the others: in this case, three options have others present, but one **(No. 1)** has "no one" present.

11. **(4)** When talking to someone who is hard of hearing, the nurse should *lower* the pitch of the voice, because hearing loss in most elderly people primarily involves high-pitched sounds. **No. 3** is incorrect because this is the range likely to be most affected by the hearing loss. Similarly, speaking *loudly* **(No. 1)** may be counterproductive, since the *pitch* usually rises along with the volume. **No. 2** would not help, unless perhaps the nurse knows that the person reads lips. **IMP, 2, PsI**

💡 *Test-taking tip:* Focus on two options that contradict each other (here, **No. 3** is "higher" and **No. 4** is "lower"); then rely on knowledge about hearing loss.

12. **(4)** This gives the patient a feeling of control and guidance. Holding the patient's hand **(No. 1)** or elbow **(No. 2)** gives the patient *neither* control nor the chance to develop self-confidence. Placing both of the patient's hands on the nurse's shoulder **(No. 3)** poses a safety *hazard* (tripping). In addition, being *led* again does not allow the patient to have control nor to develop self-confidence. **IMP, 3, SECE**

Special Issues

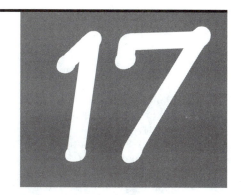

Nursing Ethics

Nursing ethics are rules and principles to guide right conduct in terms of moral duties and obligations to protect the rights of human beings. In nursing, ethical codes provide professional standards and formal guidelines for nursing activities to protect both the nurse and the client.

I. Code of ethics—serves as a frame of reference when judging priorities or possible courses of action. *Purposes:*
  A. To provide a basis for regulating relationships between nurse, client, coworkers, society, and profession.
  B. To provide a standard for excluding unscrupulous nursing practitioners and for defending nurses unjustly accused.
  C. To serve as a basis for nursing curricula.
  D. To orient new nurses and the public to ethical professional conduct.

ANA Code for Nurses*

1. The nurse provides services with respect for human dignity and the uniqueness of the client unrestricted by considerations of social or economic status, personal attributes, or the nature of health problems.
2. The nurse safeguards the client's right to privacy by judiciously protecting information of a confidential nature.
3. The nurse acts to safeguard the client and the public when health care and safety are affected by the incompetent, unethical, or illegal practice of any person.
4. The nurse assumes responsibility and account-

*American Nurses Association. *1985 Code for Nurses, with Interpretive Statements.* American Nurses Association: Kansas City, Missouri, 1985. Reprinted with permission. (Interpretive statements for each portion of the above Code for Nurses are available from ANA.)

ability for individual nursing judgments and actions.

5. The nurse maintains competence in nursing.
6. The nurse exercises informed judgment and uses individual competence and qualifications as criteria in seeking consultation, accepting responsibilities, and delegating nursing activities to others.
7. The nurse participates in activities that contribute to the ongoing development of the profession's body of knowledge.
8. The nurse participates in the profession's efforts to implement and improve standards of nursing.
9. The nurse participates in the profession's efforts to establish and maintain conditions of employment conducive to high-quality nursing care.
10. The nurse participates in the profession's effort to protect the public from misinformation and misrepresentation and to maintain the integrity of nursing.
11. The nurse collaborates with members of the health professions and other citizens in promoting community and national efforts to meet the health needs of the public.

II. The **ANA Standards of Clinical Nursing Practice** address the following standards of care and standards of professional performance[a]
   A. Use of *nursing process:* assessment, nursing diagnosis, outcome identification, planning, implementation, evaluation.
   B. Quality of care.
   C. Performance appraisal review.
   D. Continuing education.
   E. Collegiality; peer review.
   F. Ethics.
   G. Interdisciplinary collaboration.
   H. Research.
   I. Resource utilization: utilization of community health systems.
III. **Bioethics:** a philosophical field that applies ethical reasoning process for achieving clear and convincing reasons to issues and dilemmas (conflicts between two obligations) in health care.[b]
   A. Purpose of applying ethical reflection to nursing concerns:
      1. Improve quality of professional nursing decisions.
      2. Increase sensitivity to others.
      3. Offer a sense of moral clarity and enlightenment.
   B. Framework for analyzing an ethical issue:
      1. Who are the relevant participants in the situation?
      2. What is the required action?
      3. What are the probable and possible consequences of the action?
      4. What is the range of alternative actions or choices?
      5. What is the intent or purpose of the action?
      6. What is the context of the action?
   C. Principles of bioethics:
      1. *Autonomy*—the right to make one's own decisions.
      2. *Nonmalfeasance*—the intention to do no wrong.
      3. *Beneficence*—the principle of attempting to do things that benefit others.
      4. *Justice*—the distribution, as fairly as possible, of benefits and burdens.
      5. *Veracity*—the intention to tell the truth.
      6. *Confidentiality*—the social contract guaranteeing another's privacy.
IV. **Patient rights**[b]
   A. Right to appropriate treatment.
   B. Right to individualized treatment plan, subject to review and reassessment.
   C. Right to active participation in treatment, with the risk, side effects, and benefits of all medication and treatment (and alternatives) to be discussed.
   D. Right to give and withhold consent (exceptions: emergencies and when under conservatorship).
   E. Right to be free of experimentation unless following recommendations of the National Commission on Protection of Human Subjects.
   F. Right to be free of restraints except in an emergency.
   G. Right to human environment.
   H. Right to confidentiality.
   I. Right of access to personal treatment record.
   J. Right to as much freedom as possible to exercise *constitutional* rights of:
      1. Association; e.g., having visitors.
      2. Expression; e.g.:
         a. Right to keep *clothing* and *personal effects* with one in the hospital.
         b. Right to *religious* freedom.
         c. Right to be *employed,* if possible.
         d. Right to execute *wills,* enter into *contractual* relationships, and make *purchases.*
         e. Right to *education.*
         f. Right to *habeas corpus.*
         g. Right to retain licenses, privileges, or permits established by law (e.g., *driver's or professional license*).
         h. Right to *marry* and *divorce.*
   K. Right to information about these rights in both written and oral form, presented in an understandable manner at outset and periodically thereafter.
   L. Right to assert grievances through a grievance mechanism that includes the power to go to court.
   M. Right to obtain *advocacy* assistance.
   N. Right to criticize or complain about conditions or services without fear of retaliatory punishment or other reprisals.
   O. Right to referral to complement the discharge plan.

---

[a]Complete description with rationale and assessment factors are in *1991 Standards of Clinical Nursing Practice.* Washington, DC: American Nurses Association, 1991.

[b]Davis AJ. Ethical Dilemmas in Nursing. Recorded at JONA and Nurse Educator's 1981 Joint Leadership Conference.

V. Conflicts and problems

A. *Personal values vs. professional duty:* nurses have the right to refuse to participate in those areas of nursing practice that are against their personal values, as long as a client's welfare is not jeopardized. *Example:* therapeutic abortions.

B. *Nurse vs. agency:* conflict may arise regarding whether to give out needed information to a client or to follow agency policy, which does not allow it. *Example:* an emotionally upset teenager asks a nurse about how to get an abortion, a discussion which is against agency policy.

C. *Nurse vs. colleagues:* conflict may arise when determining whether to ignore or report others' behavior. *Examples:* you see another nurse steal medications; you know that a peer is giving a false reason when requesting time off; or you observe an intoxicated colleague.

D. *Nurse vs. client/family:* conflict may stem from knowledge of confidential information. Should you tell? *Example:* client (or family member) relates a vital secret, such as an undesired pregnancy, to the nurse and asks not to tell the family.

E. *Conflicting responsibilities:* to whom is the nurse primarily responsible when needs of the agency and the client differ? *Example:* an MD asks a nurse not to list all supplies used for client care, as the client cannot afford to pay the bill.

F. *Ethical dilemmas:* stigma of diagnostic label (e.g., AIDS, schizophrenic, addict); involuntary psychiatric confinement; right to control individual freedom; right to suicide; right to privacy and confidentiality.

Trends in Nursing Practice

I. Overall characteristics of trends

A. Some trends are subtle and slow to emerge; others are obvious and quickly emerge.

B. Trends may conflict; some will prevail, others get modified by social forces.

II. General trends in nursing practice

A. *Broadened focus of care:* from care of ill to care of sick and healthy, from care of individual to care of family. Focus on prevention of illness, promotion of optimum level of health, holism.

B. *Increasing scientific base:* in bio-social-physical sciences, not mere reliance on intuition, experience, and observation.

C. *Increasingly complex technical skills* and use of *technologically advanced equipment,* such as monitors and computers.

D. *Increased independence* in use of judgment, such as teaching nutrition in pregnancy and providing primary prenatal care.

E. *New roles,* such as phone triage nurse, quality assurance, case management, infection control nurse, and *nurse-clinician,* require advanced skills in a particular area of practice. *Examples:* psychiatric nurse consults with staff about problems; *primary care* nurse takes medical histories and does physical assessment; one nurse coordinates 24-h care during hospital stay; *independent nurse practitioner* has own office in community where clients come for care.

F. Greater emphasis on *community nursing services* such as home health care, rather than hospital-based; needs of the healthy are served as well as those of the ill.

G. *Development of nursing standards* to reflect specific nursing functions and activities.

1. Assure *safe* standard of care to clients and families.

2. Provide criteria to measure *excellence* and *effectiveness* of care.

H. Mergers and new organizations (e.g., *Health Maintenance Organizations, Preferred Provider Organizations*) affect delivery of nursing care.

1. Supervision of more and new paraprofessionals assigned to perform patient care previously carried out by RNs.

2. Mergers have resulted in nursing layoffs.

3. Shorter hospital stays.

4. Total inpatient population more acutely ill and in need of specialized nursing care.

5. Patients discharged from hospitals still need expert care and follow-up.

III. Trends in care of childbearing family

A. *Consumerism*

1. Consumer push for humanization and individualization of health care during the childbearing cycle to reflect client's role in decision making, preferences, and cultural diversity.

2. Emphasis on family-centered care (including father, siblings, grandparents).

3. Increase in options available for conduct of birth experience and setting for birth: birthing homes, alternative birth center (ABC) in hospitals; birthing chairs; side-lying position for birth; family-centered cesarean delivery; health care provider (MD, RN, lay midwife); length of postpartum stay.

4. Increased consumer awareness of legal issues and clients' rights.

5. Major nursing role: client advocate.

B. *Social trends*

1. Alternative life-styles of families: single parenthood, communal living, surrogate motherhood, marriages without children.

2. Earlier sexual experimentation; availability of assistance to emancipated minors.

3. Increase in number of older (over 38) primiparas.

4. Legalization of abortion; availability to emancipated minors.

5. Smaller families.

6. Rising divorce rates.

C. *Technologies*

1. Development of genetic and bioengineering techniques.

2. Development of prenatal diagnostic techniques, with options for management of each pregnancy.

3. In vitro fertilization and embryo transplantation.

IV. Trends in community mental health (1960s–1990s)

A. Shift from institutional to community-based care.

B. Preventive services.

C. Consumer participation in planning and delivery of services.

D. Original 12 essential services (1975) reduced to 5(°) (1981).

　1.°24-hour in-patient care.

　2.°Outpatient care.

　3.°Partial hospitalization (day or night).

　4.°Emergency care.

　5. Consultation and education.

　6. Follow-up care.

　7. Transitional services.

　8. Services for children and adolescents.

　9. Services for elderly.

　10.°Screening services (courts).

　11. Alcohol abuse services.

　12. Drug abuse services.

E. Protecting human rights of persons in need of mental health care.

F. Developing an advocacy program for chronically mentally ill.

G. Improving delivery of services to underserved and high-risk populations (e.g., minorities, homeless).

Nursing Responsibilities

I. Four levels of nursing practice

A. *Promotion of health* to increase level of wellness. *Example:* provide dietary information to reduce risks of coronary artery diseases.

B. *Prevention of illness or injury or further injury. Example:* immunizations; report suspected child and elder abuse.

C. *Restoration of health. Example:* teach how to change dressing, care for wound; report infectious diseases.

D. *Consolation of dying. Example:* assist person to attain peaceful death.

II. Five components of nursing care

A. *Nursing care activities:* assist with basic needs, give medications and treatments; observe response and adaptation to illness and treatments; teach self-care; guide rehabilitation activities for daily living.

B. *Coordination of total client care:* all health team members should work together toward common goals.

C. *Continuity of care* when the location of care is transferred.

D. *Evaluation of care:* flexibility and responsiveness to changing needs: clients' reactions and perceptions of their needs.

E. *Delegate responsibility and direct nursing care provided by others* based on particular client/family

needs and on skills and abilities of nursing personnel; report impaired health professionals.

III. Three main nursing roles in relation to care of clients and their families. The emphasis of each role varies with the situation, with adaptation of skills and modes of care as necessary.

A. *Therapeutic role* (instrumental). *Function:* work toward "cure" in acute and subacute setting.

B. *Caring role* (expressive). *Function:* provide support through human relations, show concern, demonstrate acceptance of differences.

C. *Socializing role. Function:* offer distractions and respite from focus on illness.

Nursing Organizations

I. International Council of Nurses (ICN)

A. *Purpose:* to provide a medium through which national nursing associations can work together, share common interests. Formed in 1899.

B. *Functions*

　1. Serves as representatives of and spokespersons for nurses at international level.

　2. Promotes organization of national nurses' associations.

　3. Assists national organizations to develop and improve services for public health practice of nursing and social/economic welfare of nurses.

II. World Health Organization (WHO)—special intergovernmental agency of the UN, formed in 1948.

A. *Purpose:* to bring all people to the highest possible level of health.

B. *Functions:* provides assistance in the form of education, training, improving health standards, fighting disease, and reducing environmental pollution in member countries.

III. American Nurses Association (ANA)—national professional association in the U.S. composed of the nurses' associations of the 50 states, Guam, Virgin Islands, Puerto Rico, and Washington, D.C.

A. *Purpose:* to foster high standards of nursing practice and promote the education and welfare of nurses.

B. *Functions*

　1. Officially represents professional nurses in this country and internationally.

　2. Defines practice of nursing.

　3. Lobbies and promotes legislation affecting nurses' welfare and practice.

IV. National League for Nursing (NLN)—composed of both individuals and agencies.

A. *Purpose:* to foster the development and improvement of all nursing services and nursing education.

B. *Functions*

　1. Provides educational workshops.

　2. Assists in recruitment for nursing programs.

　3. Provides testing services for both RN and LPN (LVN) nursing programs.

　4. Performs accreditation of nursing programs.

Legal Aspects of Nursing

I. Definition of terms

A. *Common law:* accumulation of law as a result of judicial court decisions. A ruling by a court establishes precedent for all lower courts within its jurisdiction.

B. *Civil law* (private law): law that derives from legislative codes and deals with relations between private parties.

C. *Public law:* concerns relationships between an individual and the state. The thrust of public law is to attain what are deemed valid public goals, such as reporting child abuse.

D. *Criminal law:* concerns actions against the safety and welfare of the public, such as murder, robbery. It is part of the public law.

E. *Informed consent:* implies that significant benefits and risks of any procedure, as well as alternative methods of treatment, have been explained; person has had time to ask questions and have these answered; person has agreed to the treatment voluntarily and is legally competent to give consent; and communication is in a language known to the client. See also p. 213.

F. *Reasonably prudent nurse:* nurse must react as a reasonably prudent nurse trained in that specialty area would react. For example, if a nurse works with fetal monitors, she must know how to use the monitors, know how to read the strips, and know what actions to take based on the findings.

II. Nursing licensure—mandatory licensure required in order to practice nursing.

A. *Nurse Practice Act:* each state has one to protect nurses' professional capacity, to legally control nursing through licensing, and to define standards of professional nursing.

B. *American Nurses Association (1980):* "The practice of nursing means the performance for compensation of professional services requiring substantial specialized knowledge of the biological, physical, behavioral, psychological, and sociological sciences and of nursing theory as the basis for assessment, diagnosis, planning, intervention, and evaluation in the promotion and maintenance of health; the casefinding and management of illness, injury, or infirmity; the restoration of optimum function; or the achievement of a dignified death. Nursing practice includes but is not limited to administration, teaching, counseling, supervision, delegation, and evaluation of practice and execution of the medical regimen, including the administration of medications and treatments prescribed by any person authorized by state law to prescribe. Each registered nurse is directly accountable and responsible to the consumer for the quality of nursing care rendered."[1]

C. *Revoking a license:* Board of Examiners in each state in the US and each province in Canada has the power to revoke licenses for just cause, such as incompetence in nursing practice, conviction of crime, drug addiction, obtaining license through fraud, or hiding criminal history.

III. Crimes and torts

A. *Crime:* an act committed in violation of societal law and punishable by fine or imprisonment. A crime does not have to be intended (as in giving a client an accidental overdose that proves to be lethal).

　　1. *Felonies:* crimes of a serious nature (such as murder, embezzlement) punishable by imprisonment of greater than 6 mo.

　　2. *Misdemeanors:* crimes of a less serious nature (such as shoplifting), usually punishable by fines or short prison term or both.

B. *Tort:* a wrong committed by one individual against another or another's property. Fraud, negligence, invasion of privacy, and malpractice are torts (such as losing a client's hearing aid or bathing him in water that burns him).

　　1. *Fraud:* misrepresentation of fact with intentions for it to be acted upon by another person (such as falsifying college transcripts when applying for a graduate nursing program).

　　2. *Negligence:* Omission to do something that a reasonable person, guided by those *ordinary* considerations which ordinarily regulate human affairs would *do,* or doing something which a reasonable and prudent person would *not* do.[2] Types of negligent acts may relate to:

　　　　a. Sponge counts: incorrect counts or failure to count.

　　　　b. Burns: heating pads, solutions, steam vaporizers.

　　　　c. Falls: side rails left down, baby left unattended.

　　　　d. Failure to observe and take appropriate action; e.g., forgetting to take vital signs and check dressing in a newly postoperative client.

　　　　e. Wrong medicine, wrong dose and concentration, wrong route, wrong client.

　　　　f. Mistaken identity—preparing wrong client for surgery.

　　　　g. Failure to communicate—ignore, forget, fail to report complaints of client or family.

　　　　h. Loss of or damage to client's property: dentures, jewelry, money.

　　3. *Malpractice:* part of the law of negligence as applied to the *professional* person; any professional misconduct, unreasonable lack of skill, or lack of fidelity in professional duties, such as accidentally giving wrong medication,

---

[1]American Nurses Association. *The Nursing Practice Act; Suggested State Legislation,* American Nurses Association: Kansas City, Missouri, 1980. P. 6. Reprinted with permission.

[2]H. Creighton. *Law Every Nurse Should Know.* Philadelphia: Saunders, 1986.

forgetting to give correct medication, or instilling wrong strength of eyedrops into the client's eyes. Proof of intent to do harm is *not* required in acts of commission or omission.

IV. **Invasion of privacy:** compromising a person's right to withhold self and own life from public scrutiny. *Implications for nursing:*
   A. *Avoid* unnecessary discussion of client's medical condition.
   B. Client has a right to refuse to participate in clinical teaching.
   C. Obtain consent prior to teaching conference.

V. **Libel and slander:** wrongful action of communication that damages person's reputation by print, writing, or pictures (libel), or by spoken word using false words (slander). *Implications for nursing:* make comments about client only to another health team member caring for that client.

VI. **Privileged communications:** information relating to condition and treatment of client requires confidentiality and protection against invasion of privacy. This applies only to court proceedings. Selected person does not have to reveal in court a client's communication to him or her. The purpose of privileged communication is to encourage the client to communicate honestly with the treating practitioner. It is the client's privilege at any time to permit the professional to release information.

   Therefore, if the client asks the nurse to testify, the nurse must truthfully give all information. However, if the nurse is a witness against the client, without the client's permission to release information, the nurse must keep the information confidential by invoking the privileged communication rule if the state law recognizes it and if it applies to the nurse.

VII. **Assault and battery:** violating a person's right to refuse physical contact with another.
   A. *Definitions*
      1. *Assault:* the *attempt* to touch another or the threat to do so.
      2. *Battery:* physical *harm* through *willful* touching of person or clothing.
   B. *Implications for nursing:* need to obtain consent to treat, with special provisions when clients are under age, unconscious, or mentally ill.

VIII. **Good Samaritan Act:** protects health practitioners against malpractice claims resulting from assistance provided at scene of an emergency (unless there was willful wrongdoing) as long as the level of care provided is the same as any other reasonably prudent person would give under similar circumstances.

IX. **Nurses' responsibilities to the law**
   A. A nurse is liable for nursing acts, even if directed to do something by an MD.
   B. A nurse is *not* responsible for the negligence of the employer (hospital).
   C. A nurse is responsible for refusing to carry out an order for an activity believed to be *injurious* to the client.
   D. A nurse *cannot* legally diagnose illness or pre-

scribe treatment for a client. (This is the MD's responsibility.)
   E. A nurse is legally responsible when participating in a criminal act (such as assisting with criminal abortions or taking medications for own use from client's supply).
   F. A nurse should reveal client's confidential information *only* to appropriate health care team members.
   G. A nurse is responsible for explaining nursing activities but *not* for commenting on medical activities in a way that may distress the client or the MD.
   H. A nurse is responsible for recognizing and protecting the rights of clients to refuse treatment or medication, and for reporting their concerns and refusals to the MD or appropriate agency people.
   I. A nurse needs to respect the dignity of each client and family.

Questions Most Frequently Asked By Nurses About Nursing and the Law

I. **Taking orders**
   A. *Should I accept verbal phone orders from an MD?* Generally, no. Specifically, follow your hospital's bylaws, regulations, and policies regarding this. Failure to follow the hospital's rules could be considered negligence.
   B. *Should I follow an MD's orders if (a) I know it is wrong, or (b) I disagree with his judgment?*
      1. Regarding *(a)*; No, if you think a reasonable, prudent nurse would not follow it; but first inform the MD and record your decision. Report it to your supervisor.
      2. Regarding *(b)*; Yes, because the law does not allow you to substitute your nursing judgment for a doctor's medical judgment. Do record that you questioned the order and that the doctor confirmed it before you carried it out.
   C. *What can I do if the MD delegates a task to me for which I am not prepared?* Inform the MD of your lack of education and experience in performing the task. Refuse to do it. If you inform her or him and still carry out the task, *both* you and the MD could be considered negligent if the client is harmed by it. If you do not tell the MD and carry out the task, you are *solely* liable.

II. **Obtaining client's consent for medical and surgical procedures:** *Is a nurse responsible for getting a consent for medical/surgical treatment?* Obtaining consent requires explaining the procedure and risks involved, which is the MD's responsibility. A nurse may accept responsibility for *witnessing* a consent. This carries with it little legal liability other than obtaining the correct signature and describing the client's condition at time of signing.

III. **Client's records**
   A. *What should be written in the nurse's notes?* All *facts* and information regarding a person's condi-

tion, treatment, care, progress, and response to illness and treatment. *Purpose of record:* factual documentation of care given to meet legal standards; used to refute unwarranted claims of negligence or malpractice.

   B. *How should data be recorded?* Entries should:
     1. State time given.
     2. Be written and signed by caregiver or supervisor who observed action.
     3. Follow chronologic sequence.
     4. Be accurate, precise, and clear, *avoid* opinions and judgmental comments.
     5. Be legible.
     6. Use universal abbreviations.

IV. Confidential information

   A. *If called on the witness stand in court, do I have to reveal confidential information?* It depends on your state, as each state has its own laws pertaining to this. Consult a lawyer. Inform the judge and ask for specific directions before relating in court information that was given to you within a confidential, professional relationship.

   B. *Am I justified in refusing (on the basis of "invasion of privacy") to give information about the client to another health agency to which a client is being transferred?* No. You are responsible for providing *continuity of care* when the client is moved from one facility to another. Necessary and adequate information should be transferred between professional health care workers. The client's consent for this exchange of information should be obtained. Circumstances under which confidential information can be released include:
     1. By authorization and consent of the client.
     2. By order of the court.
     3. By statutory mandate, as in reporting cases of child abuse or communicable diseases.

V. Liability for mistakes—yours and others.

   A. *Is the hospital or the nurse liable for mistakes made by the nurse while following orders? Both* the hospital and the nurse can be sued for damage if a mistake made by the nurse injures the client. The nurse is responsible for her own actions. The hospital would be liable, based on the doctrine of *respondeat superior.*

   B. *Who is responsible if a nursing student or another staff nurse makes a mistake? The supervisor? The instructor?* Ordinarily the instructor and/or supervisor would not be responsible unless the court thought the instructor and/or supervisor was negligent in supervising or in assigning a task beyond the capability of the person in question. No one is responsible for another's negligence *unless* he or she contributed to or participated in that negligence. Each person is personally liable for his or her own negligent actions and failure to act as a reasonably prudent nurse.

   C. *Am I responsible for injury to a client by a staff member who was observed (but not reported) by me to be intoxicated while giving care?* Yes, you

may be responsible. You have a duty to take reasonable action to prevent a client's injury.

VI. Good Samaritan Act: *For what would I be liable if I voluntarily stopped to give care at the scene of an accident?* You would be protected under the Good Samaritan Act and required to live up to *reasonable* and *prudent* nursing standards in those specific circumstances. You would not be treated by the law as if you were performing under professional standards of properly sterile conditions, with proper technical equipment.

VII. Leaving against medical advice (AMA): *Would I or the hospital be liable if a client left "AMA," refusing to sign the appropriate hospital forms?* None of the involved parties would ordinarily be liable in this case as long as (a) the medical risks were explained, recorded, and witnessed, and (b) the client is a competent adult. The law permits clients to make decisions that may not be in their own best health interest. You *cannot* interfere with the right and exercise of the decision to accept or reject treatment.

VIII. Restraints: *Can I put restraints on a client who is combative even if there is no order for this?* Do not use unless in an emergency, for a limited *time*, for the limited *purpose* of protecting the client from injury, not for convenience of personnel. Restraints of any degree may constitute false imprisonment. Freedom from unlawful restraint is a basic human right protected by law. If you do need to use them as a last resort after other reasonable means have not been effective:

   A. Notify attending MD immediately. Consult with another staff member, obtain client's consent if possible, document facts and reasons, get coworker to witness the record.

   B. Apply restraints properly, check frequently to ensure they do not impair circulation, cause pressure sores, or other injury.

   C. Remove restraints at the first opportunity.

IX. Wills: *What do I do when a client asks me to be a witness to her or his will?* There is *no legal* obligation to participate as a witness, but there is a *moral* and *ethical* obligation to do so. You should not, however, help draw up a will as this could be considered practicing law without a license. You could witness that

   A. The client is signing the document as her or his last will and testament.

   B. At that time, to the best of your knowledge, the client (testator) was of sound mind, was lucid, and understood what she or he was doing (i.e., she or he must not be under the influence of drugs or alcohol or otherwise unable to know what she or he is doing); and

   C. The testator was under no overt coercion, as far as you could tell, but was acting freely, willingly, and under her or his own impetus.

X. Disciplinary action

   A. *For what reasons may the RN license be suspended or revoked?*
     1. Obtaining license by fraud (omission of information, false information).

2. Negligence and incompetence.
3. Substance abuse.
4. Conviction of crime (state or federal).
5. Practicing medicine without a license.
6. Practicing nursing without a license (expired, suspended).
7. Allowing unlicensed person to practice nursing or medicine.
8. Giving client care while under the influence of alcohol or other drugs.
9. Habitually using drugs.
10. Discriminatory and prejudicial practices in giving client care (pertaining to race, color, sex, age, or ethnic origin).

B. *What could happen to me if I am proven guilty of professional misconduct?*
   1. License may be revoked.
   2. License may be suspended.
   3. Behavior may be censured and reprimanded.
   4. You may be placed on probation.

C. *Who has the authority to carry out any of the above penalties?* The State Board of Registered Nursing that granted your license.

D. *I am the head nurse. One of my nurse's aides has a history of failing to appear to work and not giving notice of or reason for absence. How should I handle this?* An employee has the right to know hospital policies, what is expected of an employee, and what will happen if an employee does not meet the expectations stated in his or her job description or in hospital policies and procedures. As a head nurse, you need to document behavior factually, clearly, and concisely, as well as any discussion and decision about future course of action. The employee needs the chance to read and sign it. The head nurse then sends a copy to her or his supervisor.

XI. **Floating:** *Is a nurse hired to work in psychiatry obligated to cover in ICU when the latter is understaffed?* The issue is the *hiring contract* (implied or expressed). The contract is a composite of the mutual understanding by involved parties of rights and responsibilities, any written documents, and hospital policies. If the nurse was hired as a psychiatric nurse, he or she could legally refuse to go to the ICU. If the hospital intends to float personnel, such a policy should be clearly stated during the hiring process. Also at this time the employer should determine the employee's education, skills, and experience. On the other hand, if emergency staffing problems exist, a nurse should go to the ICU regardless of personal preference.

XII. **Dispensing medication:** *Can a nurse legally remove a drug from a pharmacy when the pharmacy is closed (during the night) if the MD insists that the nurse go to the pharmacy to get the specifically prescribed medication immediately?* Within the legal boundaries of the Pharmacy Act, a nurse may remove *one* dose of a *particular* drug from the pharmacy for a *particular* client during an *unanticipated* emergency within a *limited* time and availability of resources. However, the hospital should have a *written* policy for the nurse to follow and should authorize a specific person to use the services of the pharmacy under certain circumstances.

XIII. **Illegible orders:** *What should I do if I cannot decipher the MD's handwriting when she or he persists in leaving illegible orders?* Talk to the MD regarding the dangers of your giving the wrong amount of the wrong medication via the wrong route at the wrong time. If that does not help, follow appropriate channels. Do *not* follow an order you cannot read. You will be liable for following orders you thought were written.

XIV. **Heroic measures:** *The wife of a terminally ill client approaches me with the request that heroic measures not be used on her husband. She has not discussed this with him but knows that he feels the same way. Can I act on this request?* No. The client is the only one who can legally make the decision as long as he or she is mentally competent unless there is a living will requesting no resuscitation.

XV. **Medication:** *An MD orders pain medication prn for a client. The client asks for the medication, but when I question her she says the pain "isn't so bad." If in my judgment the client's pain is not severe, am I legally covered if I give half of the pain medication dosage ordered by the MD?* A nurse *cannot* substitute his or her judgment for the MD's. If you alter the amount of medication prescribed by the MD without a specific order to do so, you may be liable for practicing medicine without a license.

XVI. **Malfunctioning equipment:** *At the end-of-shift report the nurse going off duty tells me that the tracheal suctioning machine is malfunctioning and describes how she got it to work. Should I plan to use the machine in the evening shift and follow her suggestions about how to make it work?* Do *not* plan to use equipment that you know is not functioning properly. You could be held liable since you could reasonably foresee that proper functioning of equipment would be needed for your client. You have been put on notice that there are defects. Report this to the supervisor or person responsible for maintaining equipment in proper working order.

Ethical and Legal Considerations in Intensive Care of the Acutely Ill Neonate

I. **Responsibilities of the health agency**
   A. Provide a Newborn (Neonatal) Intensive Care Unit (NICU) or transfer to another hospital.
   B. *Personnel: adequate number trained in neonate diseases, special treatment, and equipment.*
   C. Equipment: adequate supply on hand, functioning properly (especially temperature regulator in incubator, oxygen analyzer, blood-gas machine).

II. **Dying infants**
   A. Decision regarding resuscitation in cardiac arrest, with brain damage from cerebral anoxia. It is diffi-

cult to predict the effect of anoxia in infancy on the child's later life.
  B. Decision to continue supportive measures.
  C. Issue of euthanasia, such as in severe myelomeningocele at birth.
    1. *Active* euthanasia (e.g., giving overdose).
    2. *Passive* euthanasia (e.g., not placing on respirator).
III. **Extended role of nurse in NICU:** may raise issues of nursing practice *vs.* medical practice, as when a nurse draws blood samples for blood-gas determinations without prior order. To be legally covered:
  A. The nurse must be trained to perform specialized functions.
  B. The functions must be written into the nurse's job description.
IV. **Issue of negligence**—such as cross-contamination in nursery, e.g., transmission of a communicable disease from one infant to another, not placing infant in isolation when there is a possibility of transmitting a disease.
V. **Issue of malpractice**—such as assigning care of critically ill infant on respirator to untrained student or aide.
  A. May be liable for inaccurate *bilirubin* studies for neonatal jaundice; may be legally responsible if brain damage occurs in absence of accurate laboratory tests.
  B. May be liable for brain damage in infant due to respiratory or cardiac distress. Nurse needs to make sure that there are frequent *blood-gas determinations* to ensure adequate oxygen to prevent brain damage. Nurse also needs to make sure that the infant is not receiving too high a concentration of oxygen, which may lead to retrolental fibroplasia.

Legal Aspects of Psychiatric Care

I. **Four sets of criteria to determine criminal responsibility at time of alleged offense**
  A. *M'Naghten Rule* (1832)—a person is not guilty if:
    1. Person did not know the *nature* and *quality* of the act.
    2. Person could not distinguish right from wrong; if person did not know what he or she was doing, person did not know it was wrong.
  B. *Irresistible Impulse Test* (used together with M'Naghten Rule)—person knows right from wrong, but:
    1. Driven by *impulse* to commit criminal acts regardless of consequences.
    2. Lacked premeditation in sudden violent behavior.
  C. *American Law Institute's Model Penal Code (1955) Test*
    1. Not responsible for criminal act if person lacks capacity to "appreciate" the wrongfulness of it or to "conform" conduct to requirements of law.
    2. Excludes "an abnormality manifested only by repeated criminal or antisocial conduct"—namely, psychopathology.

    3. Includes "knowledge" and "control" criteria.
  D. *Durham Test* (Product Rule—1954): accused not criminally responsible if act was a "product of mental disease." Discarded in 1972.
II. **Types of admissions**
  A. *Voluntary*
    1. Person, parent, or legal guardian applies for admission.
    2. Person agrees to receive treatment and to follow hospital rules.
    3. Civil rights are retained.
  B. *Involuntary:* process and criteria vary among states (Figure 17.1). Danger to self and others is of primary consideration.
III. **Legal and civil rights of hospitalized clients**—the right to:
  A. Wear own clothes, keep and use personal possessions and reasonable sum of money for small purchases.
  B. Have individual storage space for private use.
  C. See visitors daily.
  D. Have reasonable access to confidential phone conversations.
  E. Receive unopened correspondence and have access to stationery, stamps, and a mailbox.
  F. Refuse: shock treatments, lobotomy.
IV. **Concepts central to community mental health** (Community Mental Health Act, 1980)
  A. *Systems* perspective: scope of care moves beyond the individual to the community, with influences from biologic, psychological, and sociocultural forces.
  B. Emphasis on *prevention*
    1. *Primary* (reduce incidents by preventing harmful social conditions).
    2. *Secondary* (early identification and treatment of disorders to reduce duration).
    3. *Tertiary* (early rehabilitation to reduce impairment from disorders).
  C. *Interdisciplinary collaboration:* flexible roles based on unique areas of expertise.
  D. *Consumer participation and control.*
  E. *Comprehensive services:* outpatient care, partial hospitalization, 24-hour hospitalization, and emergency care; consultation and education; screening services.
  F. *Continuity of care.*

Legal Aspects of Preparing a Client for Surgery

I. No surgical procedure, however minor, can proceed without the *voluntary, informed,* and *written* consent of the client.
  A. Surgical permits are witnessed by the physician, nurse, or other authorized person.
  B. Surgical permits protect the client against unsanctioned surgery and also protect the surgeon and hospital staff against claims of unauthorized operations.
  C. *Informed consent* means that the operation has

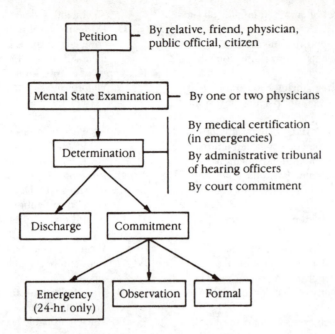

FIGURE 17.1   TYPICAL PROCEDURE FOR INVOLUNTARY COMMITMENT

been fully explained to the client, including possible complications and disfigurements, as well as whether any organ or parts of the body are to be removed.

D. Adults and emancipated minors may sign their own operative permits *if* they are mentally competent; permission for surgery of minor children and incompetent or unconscious adults must be obtained from a responsible family member or guardian.

E. The signed operative permit is placed in a prominent place on the client's chart and accompanies the client to the operating room.

F. *Legal issues in the emergency room: record keeping* plays an essential role in both the prevention and defense of malpractice suits. Detailed documentation not only provides for continuity of care but also perpetuates evidence that care was appropriately given. Records should:
  1. Be written legibly.
  2. Clearly note events and time of occurrence.
  3. Contain all lab slips and results of other tests.
  4. Describe events and clients objectively.
  5. Clearly note physician's parting instructions to the client.
  6. Be signed where appropriate, such as with doctor's orders.
  7. Contain descriptions of every event that might lead to a lawsuit, such as fights, injuries, equipment failures.

G. *Consent:* although there is no law requiring written consent before performing medical treatment, all elective procedures can only be performed if the client has been fully informed and voluntarily consents to the procedure.
  1. If informed consent cannot be obtained be-

cause of the client's condition and immediate treatment is necessary to save life or safeguard health, the *emergency rule* can be applied. This rule implies consent. However, if time allows, it is advisable to obtain either oral or written informed consent from someone who has authority to act for the client.
  2. Verbal consents should be recorded in detail, witnessed and signed by *two* individuals.
  3. Written or verbal consent can be given by alert, coherent, or otherwise competent adults, by parents, legal guardian, or person in *loco parentis* (one standing in for the parent with the parent's rights, duties, and responsibilities) of minors or incompetent adults.
  4. If the minor is *14* years or *older,* consent must be acquired from the minor as well as from the parent or legal guardian. Emancipated minors can consent for themselves.

 Study and Memory Aid

As patient advocates, it is especially important for nurses to monitor *patients' rights* to:

- Accept or refuse treatment
- Due process of the law
- Least restrictive alternatives
- Informed consent

🗝 Summary of Key Points

Nursing Ethics

Confidentiality is integral to patient care; rules of confidentiality do not apply *only if* there is potential of serious harm to the patient or others (e.g., suicidal or homicidal plans).

Client Rights

Many client rights are based on *constitutional* rights, e.g., involuntary confinement. Confinement may be enforced if client is *unable to care* for self (e.g., provide for own food, clothing, and shelter) or is thought to pose an *immediate danger to self or others.*

Trends in Nursing Practice

1. Community-based care.
2. New roles in home-health care, case management, quality assurance, phone triage.

Nursing Responsibilities

Report suspected child and elder abuse, impaired health professionals, some infectious diseases.

Nursing Organizations

Two national professional organizations (ANA and NLN) still exist, with distinct yet overlapping purposes.

Legal Aspects of Nursing

The only time that *informed consent* is not required is when the patient lacks decision-making capacity, in which case a surrogate can make decisions for the patient, or in an emergency, in which case there is a *doctrine of implied consent* (a physician can intervene in patient's best interests).

Issues of liability, confidentiality, and nursing responsibility need to be covered at time of employment.

Glossary*

confidentiality The requirement that information not be disclosed except to an *authorized* person or group.

ethics Standards of values and beliefs upon which an individual or group may base a course of action.

habeas corpus A right to be released from illegal detention.

informed consent The requirement that information *must* be given to a patient and consent obtained about proposed treatment. In order for the consent to be considered valid, the patient must be competent, understand the information, and give consent voluntarily.

insanity *Legal* term for a mental condition that is of sufficient gravity to bring an individual under special legal restrictions and immunities.

malpractice Failure of a health-care professional to give competent care, resulting in harm to a patient. Competency is measured by the standard of what *similarly* trained professionals would do in the *same* situation.

privileged communication A legal term meaning that the *recipient* of information cannot disclose it without the *speaker's* consent (i.e., the right to reveal belongs to the speaker, not the listener).

respondeat superior "Let the master answer." A legal term that states that the principal (e.g., hospital) may be responsible for the wrongful acts of its agent (e.g., a nurse).

tort A civil wrong for which a victim is entitled to compensation.

*See **Legal Aspects of Nursing**, p. 209–210, for other definitions of legal terms.

Questions

1. What criterion is used in most states for involuntary admission of a patient to a psychiatric unit?
   1. A history of chronic mental illness.
   2. The need for medication.
   3. Danger to self or others.
   4. The lack of availability of "half-way" housing.
2. A woman has AIDS. Her sister asks the nurse, "What is wrong with my sister?" What should the nurse say to her?
   1. "She has a serious illness."
   2. "What do you think is wrong?"
   3. "Tell me what information you want, and I'll ask the doctor to talk to you."
   4. "You need to ask your sister."
3. A nurse witnesses a coworker raping a semi-conscious patient. What should the nurse's first action be?
   1. Call the police.
   2. Ask to have this worker fired.
   3. Report this to the appropriate state nursing board.
   4. Tell the coworker that what the coworker is doing is wrong.
4. A patient with alcohol dependency is admitted. An LPN/LVN says: "I'll take care of him; my husband was an alcoholic and I know all about it." The primary nurse is responsible for:
   1. Assigning the patient to this LPN/LVN because of her personal experience.
   2. Assigning the patient to another nurse who has not had such a personal experience.
   3. Assessing the LPN/LVN's knowledge before assigning the patient.

4. Exploring the LPN/LVN's feelings about her spouse before assigning the patient.

5. Which legal charge would apply if the nurse placed a patient in mechanical restraints without clinical justification?
   1. Assault.
   2. False imprisonment.
   3. Malpractice.
   4. Breach of confidentiality.

6. A homeless woman was found mumbling incoherently that her heart was "lost" and that her kidneys had "turned to rubber." She refused to eat, saying she was too evil, and wanted to punish others. She is admitted for 90 days to the county patient psychiatric unit by a court-ordered involuntary commitment. On what legal basis was this person committed?
   1. The patient could not afford private care.
   2. The patient was psychotic.
   3. The patient made threatening comments.
   4. The patient was a danger to herself.

Answers/Rationale

1. **(3)** Danger to self or others is grounds for involuntary hospitalization in most states. **Nos. 1 and 2** may be considerations, but are not as critical. **No. 4** is not a reason for involuntary hospitalization. **AN, 7, PsI**

💡 *Test-taking tip:* Remember, *safety* first as the best answer.

2. **(4)** It is the patient's prerogative to make her condition known. The concept tested here is *confidentiality* in *general,* as well as *specifically* in a situation where a person

---

Key to Codes

Nursing process: AS = Assessment; **AN** = Analysis; **PL** = Planning; **IMP** = Implementation; **EV** = Evaluation. (See Appendix E for explanation of nursing process steps.)

Category of human function: 1 = Protective; **2** = Sensory-Perceptual; **3** = Comfort, Rest, Activity, and Mobility; **4** = Nutrition; **5** = Growth and Development; **6** = Fluid-Gas Transport; **7** = Psychosocial-Cultural; **8** = Elimination.

Client need: SECE = Safe, Effective Care Environment; **PhI** = Physiologic Integrity; **PsI** = Psychosocial Integrity; **HPM** = Health Promotion/Maintenance.

---

has AIDS. **Nos. 1, 2, and 3** make a statement about the patient's illness, or allow discussion about the patient and the diagnosis. **IMP, 7, SECE**

💡 *Test-taking tip:* Which option is not like the others? Three options involve *discussions* (**Nos. 1, 2, 3**), but one (**No. 4**) directs the sister *back to the patient.*

3. **(4)** An intervention is needed to *stop the act now,* to *confront* this coworker. **Nos. 1, 2, and 3** all allow the violation to go on (while the nurse leaves to call the police, to ask to have this worker fired, or to notify the state nursing board—hardly a prompt response!). **IMP, 1, SECE**

💡 *Test-taking tip:* Which option is not like the others? Three (**Nos. 1, 2, and 3**) call on *others,* involve *leaving* the scene, and are *delayed* interventions; the other *confronts* the coworker directly and "on-the-spot" (**No. 4**).

4. **(3)** Knowledge and application of knowledge about the condition (i.e., prevalent theory about dynamics of co-dependency and knowledge of the most effective strategies for interpersonal interventions) is needed to distance oneself, in order to avoid the common pitfall of becoming emotionally engulfed. Personal history (**No. 1**) and feelings (**No. 4**) interfere with needed objectivity in the emotionally charged area of personal experience with alcohol dependency. **No. 2** is incorrect because *lack* of personal experience is not the issue. The nurse needs to assess application of knowledge, and skill in use of therapeutic interventions. **PL, 1, SECE**

5. **(2)** False imprisonment is the wrongful confinement of a person so that he or she cannot escape. Assault (**No. 1**) is a threat of touching without consent. Malpractice (**No. 3**) is a civil charge that may be brought against a professional when there is failure to meet the professional standard and injury to the patient occurs. Breach of confidentiality (**No. 4**) is the release of information about the patient without the patient's consent. **IMP, 7, SECE**

6. **(4)** A legal commitment is made on the information that this person is of potential harm to self or others). Poverty (**No. 1**) is not the basis for court-ordered detention in a community facility. Psychotic behavior (**No. 2**) in itself does not necessarily mean that an individual will harm self or others. Talk of threats (**No. 3**) are *not* harmful actions. **AN, 1, SECE**

NANDA-Approved Nursing Diagnoses

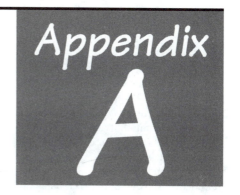

This list represents the North American Nursing Diagnosis Association (NANDA)-approved nursing diagnoses for clinical use and testing (1994).

Pattern 1: Exchanging

Altered Nutrition: More than Body Requirements
Altered Nutrition: Less than Body Requirements
Altered Nutrition: Potential for More than Body Requirements
Risk for Infection
Risk for Altered Body Temperature
Hypothermia
Hyperthermia
Ineffective Thermoregulation
Dysreflexia
Constipation
Perceived Constipation
Colonic Constipation
Diarrhea
Bowel Incontinence
Altered Urinary Elimination
Stress Incontinence
Reflex Incontinence
Urge Incontinence
Functional Incontinence
Total Incontinence
Urinary Retention
Altered (Specify Type) Tissue Perfusion (Renal, cerebral, cardiopulmonary, gastrointestinal, peripheral)
Fluid Volume Excess
Fluid Volume Deficit
Risk for Fluid Volume Deficit
Decreased Cardiac Output
Impaired Gas Exchange
Ineffective Airway Clearance
Ineffective Breathing Pattern
Inability to Sustain Spontaneous Ventilation
Dysfunctional Ventilatory Weaning Response (DVWR)
Risk for Injury
Risk for Suffocation

Risk for Poisoning
Risk for Trauma
Risk for Aspiration
Risk for Disuse Syndrome
Altered Protection
Impaired Tissue Integrity
Altered Oral Mucous Membrane
Impaired Skin Integrity
Risk for Impaired Skin Integrity
Decreased Adaptive Capacity: Intracranial
Energy Field Disturbance

Pattern 2: Communicating

Impaired Verbal Communication

Pattern 3: Relating

Impaired Social Interaction
Social Isolation
Risk for Loneliness
Altered Role Performance
Altered Parenting
Risk for Altered Parenting
Risk for Altered Parent/Infant/Child Attachment
Sexual Dysfunction
Altered Family Processes
Caregiver Role Strain
Risk for Caregiver Role Strain
Altered Family Process: Alcoholism
Parental Role Conflict
Altered Sexuality Patterns

Pattern 4: Valuing

Spiritual Distress (Distress of the Human Spirit)
Potential for Enhanced Spiritual Well-Being

Pattern 5: Choosing

Ineffective Individual Coping
Impaired Adjustment
Defensive Coping

Ineffective Denial
Ineffective Family Coping: Disabling
Ineffective Family Coping: Compromised
Family Coping: Potential for Growth
Potential for Enhanced Community Coping
Ineffective Community Coping
Ineffective Management of Therapeutic Regimen
     (Individuals)
Noncompliance (Specify)
Ineffective Management of Therapeutic Regimen: Families
Ineffective Management of Therapeutic Regimen:
     Community
Ineffective Management of Therapeutic Regimen:
     Individual
Decisional Conflict (Specify)
Health-Seeking Behaviors (Specify)

Pattern 6: Moving

Impaired Physical Mobility
Risk for Peripheral Neurovascular Dysfunction
Risk for Perioperative Positioning Injury
Activity Intolerance
Fatigue
Risk for Activity Intolerance
Sleep Pattern Disturbance
Diversional Activity Deficit
Impaired Home Maintenance Management
Altered Health Maintenance
Feeding Self-Care Deficit
Impaired Swallowing
Ineffective Breastfeeding
Interrupted Breastfeeding
Effective Breastfeeding
Ineffective Infant Feeding Pattern
Bathing/Hygiene Self-Care Deficit
Dressing/Grooming Self-Care Deficit
Toileting Self-Care Deficit
Altered Growth and Development
Relocation Stress Syndrome
Risk for Disorganized Infant Behavior

Disorganized Infant Behavior
Potential for Enhanced Organized Infant Behavior

Pattern 7: Perceiving

Body Image Disturbance
Self-Esteem Disturbance
Chronic Low Self-Esteem
Situational Low Self-Esteem
Personal Identity Disturbance
Sensory-Perceptual Alterations (Specify) (Visual, Auditory,
     Kinesthetic, Gustatory, Tactile, Olfactory)
Unilateral Neglect
Hopelessness
Powerlessness

Pattern 8: Knowing

Knowledge Deficit (Specify)
Impaired Environmental Interpretation Syndrome
Acute Confusion
Chronic Confusion
Altered Thought Processes
Impaired Memory

Pattern 9: Feeling

Pain
Chronic Pain
Dysfunctional Grieving
Anticipatory Grieving
Risk for Violence: Self-Directed or Directed at Others
Risk for Self-Mutilation
Post-Trauma Response
Rape-Trauma Syndrome
Rape-Trauma Syndrome: Compound Reaction
Rape-Trauma Syndrome: Silent Reaction
Anxiety
Fear

Psychosocial Nursing Diagnosis Related to Home Care Planning

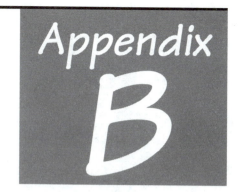

Diagnosis	Related Factors
Adjustment, impaired	Disability requiring change in life-style Inadequate support systems Impaired cognition Sensory overload Altered center of control Incomplete grieving
Anxiety	Threat to self-concept Threat of death Threat to/change in health status Threat to/change in socioeconomic status Threat to/change in roles and patterns of interaction Unmet needs
Body-image disturbance	Biomedical condition Cognitive/perceptual deficit Psychosocial problem Cultural/spiritual conflict
Caregiver role strain	Severity of illness and significant home care needs Caregiver health impairment Unpredictable cause of illness Caregiver not ready for role Family dysfunction prior to caregiving situation Poor relationship between caregiver and receiver Marginal coping patterns of caregiver
Decisional conflict	Unclear personal beliefs Perceived threat to own values Lack of relevant information Support system deficit
Defensive coping	Difficulty in reality-testing of perceptions
Denial, ineffective	Conscious or unconscious attempt to ignore meaning and impact of illness Refusal to admit fear of illness, invalidism, or death
Diversionary activity deficit	Lack of activity in environment (e.g., in long-term hospitalization)
Family coping: compromised, ineffective	Temporary family disorganization and role changes Prolonged disease or disability that exhausts supportive capacity Inadequate or incorrect information or understanding
Family coping: disabling, ineffective	Highly ambivalent family relationships Significant person with unexpressed feelings of guilt, anxiety, hostility, despair, etc.
Family coping: high risk for growth	Family member able to see *growth* impact of crisis on values, priorities, goals, relationships Family member moving toward experiences that optimize wellness

Family processes, altered	Situational transition and/or crisis Developmental transition and/or crisis
Fear	Knowledge deficit or unfamiliarity Sensory impairment Environmental stimuli Pain Separation from support system Learned response: Identification with others, modeling by others
Grieving, anticipatory	Perceived potential loss of significant other, physio-psychosocial well-being
Grieving, dysfunctional	Chronic, fatal illness Lack of resolution of previous grieving Absence of anticipatory grieving
Growth and development, altered	Environmental and stimulation deficiencies Separation from significant others Multiple caretakers Effects of disability Prescribed dependence
Hopelessness	Failing health Long-term stress Lost spiritual belief
Individual coping, ineffective	Situational crisis Maturational crisis Personal vulnerability
Self-esteem, situational low	Periodic negative feelings about self in response to a crisis, loss, or change
Self-esteem disturbance	Negative feelings about self and capabilities
Social interaction, impaired	Communication barriers Self-concept disturbance Absence of significant others or peers Limited physical mobility Environmental barriers Therapeutic isolation
Social isolation	Alterations in physical appearance/mental status Altered state of wellness Inadequate personal resources
Spiritual distress (distress of the human spirit)	Challenged belief/value system as a result of pain, suffering, moral/ethical implications of therapy
Violence, high risk for: self-directed or directed at others	Antisocial behavior Catatonic rage Manic state Panic state Rage reaction Suicidal behavior Medication reaction

Home Care Resources

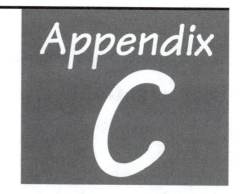

Appendix
C

Selected sources of information and services. (Every effort has been made to provide current information; however, addresses and telephone numbers do change frequently. If a number listed below is no longer in service, call Directory Assistance in the same area code for the new number.)

Health and Welfare Agencies/Associations

Alcoholics Anonymous
468 Park Ave. South
New York, NY 10016
212-686-1100

Alzheimer's Disease and Related Disorders Association
70 E. Lake St.
Chicago, IL 60601
800-621-0379

American Anorexia/Bulimia Association, Inc.
133 Cedar Ln.
Teaneck, NJ 07666
201-836-1800

American Association on Mental Deficiency
PO Box 96
Willimantic, CT 06226

American Association of Retired Persons (AARP)
1909 K St. NW
Washington, DC 20005
202-434-2277

American Cancer Society
1599 Clifton Rd. NE
Atlanta, GA 30329
404-320-3333

American Speech-Language-Hearing Association
10801 Rockville Pike
Department AP
Rockville, MD 20852
301-897-5700

Centers for Disease Control and Prevention
Department of Health and Human Services
U.S. Public Health Service
Atlanta, GA 30333
404-639-3534

Concern for Dying
250 W. 57th St.
New York, NY 10107
215-246-6962

National Safety Council
444 N. Michigan Ave.
Chicago, IL 60611
800-621-7619

Self Help for Hard of Hearing people (Shhh)
4848 Battery Ln.
Department E
Bethesda, MD 20814
301-657-2248

Sex Information and Education Council of the United States (SIECUS)
130 W. 42nd St., Suite 2500
New York, NY 10036
212-819-9770

AIDS Information and Hotlines

American Foundation for AIDS Research	212-682-7440
American Red Cross AIDS Education Office	202-737-8300
Centers for Disease Control and Prevention—Statistics:	
AIDS cases and deaths	404-330-3020
Distribution—categories	404-330-3021
Demographics	404-330-3022
Hearing Impaired AIDS Hotline	800-243-7889
National AIDS Hotline	800-342-AIDS
National AIDS Information Clearing House	800-458-5231
National AIDS Network	202-293-2437
National Gay/Lesbian Crisis Line	800-767-4297
Project Inform (Drug Information)	800-822-7422
Spanish AIDS Hotline	800-344-7432

Professional Organizations/Associations

American Academy of Nurse Practitioners
45 Foster St., Suite A
Lowell, MA 01851

The American Assembly for Men in Nursing
PO Box 31753
Independence, OH 44131

American Holistic Nurses' Association
4101 Lake Boon Tr., Suite 201
Raleigh, NC 27607

American Psychiatric Nurses' Association
6900 Grove Rd.
Thorofare, NJ 08086

Association of Nurses in AIDS Care
704 Stonyhill Rd., Suite 106
Yardley, PA 19067

Drug and Alcohol Nursing Association, Inc.
720 Light St.
Baltimore, MD 21230

Hospice Nurses Association
PO Box 8166
Van Nuys, CA 91409

National Association of Hispanic Nurses
6905 Alamo Downs Pkwy.
San Antonio, TX 78238

National Black Nurses Association, Inc.
1012 Tenth St. NW
Washington, DC 20001

National Consortium of Chemical Dependency Nurses
975 Oak St., Suite 675
Eugene, OR 97401

National Gerontological Nursing Association
3100 Homewood Pkwy.
Kensington, MD 20895

National Nurses Society on Addictions
5700 Old Orchard Rd., 1st floor
Skokie, IL 60077

North American Nursing Diagnosis Association
3525 Caroline St.
St. Louis, MO 63104

Transcultural Nursing Society
Department of Nursing
Madonna College
36600 Schoolcroft Rd.
Livonia, MI 48150

Patient Education Materials

Abbott Laboratories
Professional Services—D383
Abbott Park
N. Chicago, IL 60064

Eli Lilly and Company
Educational Resources Program
PO Box 100B
Indianapolis, IN 46206

National Clearinghouse for Alcohol and Drug Information
PO Box 2345
Rockville, MD 20852

National Council on Alcoholism
12 W. 21st St.
New York, NY 10010

National Institute on Drug Abuse (NIDA)
5600 Fishers Ln.
Rockville, MD 20857

National Mental Health Association
1021 Prince St.
Alexandria, VA 22314-2971

National Safety Council
444 N. Michigan Ave.
Chicago, IL 60611

Nutrition Education Association
PO Box 20301
Houston, TX 77225

Ross Laboratories
Creative Services and Information Department
625 Cleveland Ave.
Columbus, OH 43216

Schering Corporation
Professional Film Library
Galloping Hill Rd.
Kenilworth, NJ 07033

Common Abbreviations

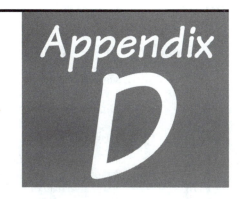

Appendix
D

Abbreviations Frequently Used in Psychosocial Aspects of Care

ADL	Activities of daily living
AODA	Alcohol and other drug abuse
CST	Convulsive shock therapy
DTs	Delirium tremens (new term: Alcohol Withdrawal Delirium)
ECT	Electroconvulsive therapy
EST	Electric shock therapy
LOC	Level of consciousness
OD	Overdose
OT	Occupational therapy

Prefixes

Aut-, Auto	Self (e.g., *aut*istic)
Dys-	Difficult (e.g., *dys*tonia, a side effect of phenothiazines)
Psych-	The mind (e.g., *psych*ology, the study of the mind)

Symbols

↑	Increased or increasing
↓	Decreased or decreasing
=	Equal to
<	Less than
≤	Less than or equal to
>	Greater than
≥	Greater than or equal to
≈	Approximately
Ø	None or no (absent)
→	Leads or leading to
×	Times

General Abbreviations*

a	Before (*ante*)
ac	Before meals (*ante cibum*)
ad lib	As much as desired (*ad libitum*)
AIDS	Acquired immunodeficiency syndrome
AK or (AKA)	Above-the-knee (amputation)
AMA	Against medical advice
A & O × 3	Alert, oriented to person, place, time
ANS	Autonomic nervous system
ASA	Acetylsalicylic acid (aspirin)
ASAP	As soon as possible
ASD	Atrial septal defect
bid	Twice daily (*bis in die*)
BK (or BKA)	Below-the-knee (amputation)
BM	Bowel movement/Bone marrow
BMR	Basal metabolic rate
BP	Blood pressure
BPH	Benign prostatic hypertrophy
bpm	Beats per minute
BUN	Blood urea nitrogen
c̄	With (*cum*)
CA	Carcinoma/Cancer
CAD	Coronary artery disease
CBC	Complete blood count
CCU	Cardiac (intensive) care unit
CF	Cystic fibrosis
CHD	Congenital heart disease
CHF	Congestive heart failure
CHO	Carbohydrate
CNS	Central nervous system
C/O	Complains of
COPD	Chronic obstructive pulmonary disease
CPK	Creatine phosphokinase
CPR	Cardiopulmonary resuscitation
CSF	Cerebrospinal fluid
CVA	Cerebrovascular accident
CVP	Central venous pressure
Δ	Change (Greek letter delta)
D/C	Discharge/Discontinue
D & C	Dilation and curettage

*Source: Adapted from Fine P. *The Wards: An Introduction to Clinical Clerkships.* Boston: Little, Brown, 1994.

DIC	Disseminated intravascular coagulation
DNR	Do not resuscitate
DOB	Date of birth
DOE	Dyspnea on exertion
DPT	Diphtheria, pertussis, and tetanus
D_5W	5% dextrose in water
Dx	Diagnosis
ECG	Electrocardiogram (also EKG)
ED	Emergency Department
EDB	Estimated date of birth
EEG	Electroencephalogram
EKG	Electrocardiogram (also ECG)
EMG	Electromyogram
EMT	Emergency medical technician
ENT	Ear, nose, and throat
EPS	Extrapyramidal symptoms
ETOH	Alcohol (ethanol)
FBS	Fasting blood sugar
FTT	Failure to thrive
FUO	Fever of unknown origin
Fx	Fracture
g	Gram
GC	Gonococcus/Gonorrhea
GI	Gastrointestinal
GTT	Glucose tolerance test
gtt(s)	Drop(s) (*guttae*)
GU	Genitourinary
GYN	Gynecologic
HCG	Human chorionic gonadotropin
Hct	Hematocrit
HDL	High-density lipoprotein
Hgb	Hemoglobin
HIV	Human immunodeficiency virus
HMO	Health maintenance organization
HOB	Head of bed
HR	Heart rate
hs	Bedtime (*hora somni*)
Hx	History
ICP	Intracranial pressure
ICU	Intensive care unit
I&D	Incision and drainage
IDDM	Insulin-dependent diabetes mellitus
IM	Intramuscular
IP	Identified patient (in family therapy)
I & O	Intake and output
IPPB	Intermittent positive pressure breathing
IUD	Intrauterine device
IV	Intravenous
IVP	Intravenous pyelogram/Intravenous push
JRA	Juvenile rheumatoid arthritis
KUB	Kidneys, ureters, bladder (flat/upright abdominal x-ray)
LLL	Left lower (lung) lobe
LLQ	Left lower quadrant
LMP	Last menstrual period
LPN	Licensed practical nurse
LSD	Lysergic acid diethylamide

LUL	Left upper (lung) lobe
LUQ	Left upper quadrant
MAOI	Monoamine-oxidase inhibitor
Med	Medication
MI	Myocardial infarction
MMR	Measles, mumps, rubella
MOM	Milk of magnesia
MR	Mental retardation
MRI	Magnetic resonance imaging
MS	Mental status/Mitral stenosis/Multiple sclerosis/Morphine sulfate
NA	Not applicable
NG	Nasogastric
NIDDM	Non–insulin-dependent diabetes mellitus
NOC	Night (nocturnal)
NPH	Neutral protamine Hagedorn (intermediate-acting insulin)
NPO	Nothing by mouth (*nil per os*)
NS	Normal saline
NSAID	Nonsteroidal anti-inflammatory drug
NTG	Nitroglycerin
NTP	Normal temperature and pressure
N/V	Nausea, vomiting
O_2	Oxygen
OB	Obstetrics
OD	Right eye (*oculus dextro*)/Overdose
OOB	Out of bed
O & P	Ova and parasites
OR	Operating room
OS	Left eye (*oculus sinistro*)
OTC	Over the counter
OU	Both eyes (*oculo utro*)
P	Para/Pulse
$\bar{p}$	Post (after)
pc	After meals (*post cibum*)
PCA	Patient-controlled analgesia (pump)
PCP	*Pneumocystis carinii* pneumonia/Phencyclidine
PDA	Patent ductus arteriosus
PERRL(A)	Pupils equally round and reactive to light (and accommodation)
PID	Pelvic inflammatory disease
PKU	Phenylketonuria
PMI	Point of maximum impulse
PMS	Premenstrual syndrome
PND	Paroxysmal nocturnal dyspnea
PO	By mouth (*per os*)
PPD	Purified protein derivative (TB skin test)
PPO	Preferred provider organization
prn	When necessary (*pro re nata*)
PSA	Prostate-specific antigen
Pt	Patient
PT	Prothrombin time/Physical therapy
PTCA	Percutaneous transluminal coronary angioplasty
PTT	Partial thromboplastin time
PUD	Peptic ulcer disease
PVC	Premature ventricular contraction

q	Each, every (*quaque*)	STD	Sexually transmitted disease
qd	Each day	Sx	Symptoms
qhs	Every night before sleep	T	Temperature
qid	Four times a day (*quater in die*)	T & A	Tonsillectomy and adenoidectomy
qod	Every other day	TB	Tuberculosis
R	Respirations	TIA	Transient ischemic attack
RBC	Red blood cell	tid	Three times a day (*ter in die*)
RHD	Rheumatic heart disease	TKO	To keep open
RLL	Right lower (lung) lobe	TLC	Total lung capacity/Tender loving care
RLQ	Right lower quadrant	TPN	Total parenteral nutrition
RML	Right middle (lung) lobe	TPR	Temperature, pulse, respirations
R/O	Rule out	TSH	Thyroid-stimulating hormone
ROM	Range of motion	TURP	Transurethral resection of prostate
RUL	Right upper (lung) lobe	Tx	Treatment
RUQ	Right upper quadrant	UA	Urinalysis
Rx	Prescription/Therapy/Treatment	UGI	Upper gastrointestinal
s̄	Without (*sine*)	UQ	Upper quadrant
SGA	Small for gestational age	URI	Upper respiratory infection
SIADH	Syndrome of inappropriate antidiuretic hormone	UTI	Urinary tract infection
SICU	Surgical intensive care unit	Vfib (VF)	Ventricular fibrillation
SLE	Systemic lupus erythematosus	VS	Vital signs
SOB	Short(ness) of breath	VSD	Ventricular septal defect
SQ	Subcutaneously	WBC	White blood count/White blood cells
S/S	Signs, symptoms	WNL	Within normal limits
Stat	Immediately (*statim*)	w/o	Without

NCLEX-RN Test Plan: Nursing Process Definitions/ Descriptions*

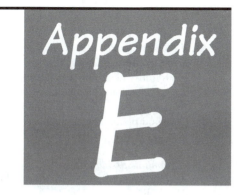

Appendix E

The phases of the nursing process include:

◢ **I. Assessment: Establishing a database**

    A. *Gather objective and subjective information relative to the client:*
- Collect information from the client, significant others, and/or health care team members; current and prior health records; and other pertinent resources.
- Utilize assessment skills appropriate to client's condition.
- Recognize *symptoms* and significant findings.
- Determine client's ability to assume care of daily health needs (self-care).
- Determine health team members' ability to provide care.
- Assess *environment* of client.
- Identify own or staff reactions to client, significant others, and/or health care team members.

    B. *Confirm data:*
- *Verify* observation or perception by obtaining additional information.
- *Question* prescriptions and decisions by other health care team members when indicated.
- *Observe* condition of client directly when indicated.
- *Validate* that an appropriate client assessment has been made.

    C. *Communicate information gained in assessment:*
- Document assessment findings thoroughly and accurately.
- Report assessment findings to relevant members of the health care team.

◢ **II. Analysis: Identifying actual or potential health care needs and/or problems based on assessment**

    A. *Interpret data:*
- Validate data.
- Organize related data.
- Determine *need for additional* data.
- Determine client's unique needs and/or problems.

    B. *Formulate client's nursing diagnoses:*
- Determine significant relationship between data and client needs and/or problems.
- Utilize *standard taxonomy* for formulating nursing diagnoses.

    C. *Communicate results of analysis:*
- *Document client's nursing diagnoses.*
- Report results of analysis to relevant members of the health care team.

◢ **III. Planning: Setting goals for meeting client's needs and designing strategies to achieve these goals**

    A. *Prioritize nursing diagnoses:*
- Involve client, significant others and/or health care team members when establishing nursing diagnoses.
- Establish *priorities* among nursing diagnoses.
- Anticipate needs and/or problems on the basis of established priorities.

    B. *Determine goals of care:*
- Involve client, significant others, and/or health care team members in setting goals.
- Establish *priorities* among goals.
- Anticipate needs and/or problems on the basis of established priorities.

    C. *Formulate outcome criteria for goals of care:*
- Involve client, significant others, and/or health care team members in formulating outcome criteria for goals of care.
- Establish *priorities* among outcome criteria for goals of care.
- Anticipate needs and/or problems on the basis of established priorities.

    D. *Develop plan of care and modify as necessary:*
- Involve the client, significant others, and/or health care team members in designing strategies.
- *Individualize* the care plan based on such information as age, gender, culture, ethnicity, and religion.
- Plan for client's safety, comfort, and maintenance of optimal functioning.
- Select nursing interventions for delivery of client's care.
- Select *appropriate teaching* approaches.

*Source: National Council of State Boards of Nursing, Inc., *NCLEX-RN Test Plan.* Chicago: National Council of State Boards of Nursing, 1994. Pp. 3–6.

E. *Collaborate with other health care team members when planning delivery of client's care:*
- Identify health or social resources available to the client and/or significant others.
- Select appropriate health care team members when planning assignments.
- Coordinate care provided by health care team members.

F. *Communicate plan of care:*
- Document plan of care thoroughly and accurately.
- Report plan of care to relevant members of the health care team.
- Review plan of care with client.

▶ **IV. Implementation: Initiating and completing actions necessary to accomplish the defined goals**

A. *Organize and manage client's care:*
- Implement a plan of care.
- Arrange for a client care conference.

B. *Counsel and teach client, significant others, and/or health care team members:*
- Assist client, significant others, and/or health care team members to recognize and manage stress.
- Facilitate client relationships with significant others and health care team members.
- *Teach* correct principles, procedures, and techniques for maintenance and promotion of health.
- Provide client with health status information.
- Refer client, significant others, and/or health care team members to appropriate *resources.*

C. *Provide care to achieve established goals of care:*
- Use *safe* and appropriate techniques when administering client care.
- Use precautionary and *preventive* interventions in providing care to client.
- *Prepare* client for surgery, delivery, or other procedures.
- Institute *interventions* to compensate for adverse responses.
- Initiate life-saving interventions for emergency situations.
- Provide an *environment* conducive to attainment of goals of care.
- Adjust care in accord with client's expressed or implied needs, problems, and/or preferences.
- Stimulate and motivate client to achieve self-care and independence.
- Encourage client to follow a treatment regime.
- Assist client to maintain optimal functioning.

D. *Supervise and coordinate the delivery of client's care provided by nursing personnel:*
- *Delegate* nursing interventions to appropriate nursing personnel.
- Monitor and follow up on delegated interventions.
- Manage health care team members' reactions to factors influencing therapeutic relationships with clients.

E. *Communicate nursing interventions:*
- Record actual client responses, nursing interventions, and other information relevant to implementation of care.
- Provide complete, accurate reports on assigned client(s) to relevant members of the health care team.

▶ **V. Evaluation: Determining the extent to which goals have been achieved and interventions have been successful.**

A. *Compare actual outcomes with expected outcomes of care:*
- Evaluate responses (*expected* and *unexpected*) in order to determine the degree of success of nursing interventions.
- Determine impact of therapeutic interventions on the client and significant others.
- Determine need for modifying the plan of care.
- Identify factors that may interfere with the client's ability to implement the plan of care.

B. *Evaluate the client's ability to implement self-care:*
- Verify that *tests or measurements are performed correctly* by the client and/or other care givers.
- Ascertain client's, and/or others' understanding of information given.

C. *Evaluate health care team members' ability to implement client care:*
- Determine impact of teaching on health care team members.
- Identify factors that might alter health care team members' response to teaching.

D. *Communicate evaluation findings:*
- Document client's response to therapy, care, and/or teaching.
- Report client's response to therapy, care, and/or teaching to relevant members of the health care team.
- Report and document others' responses to teaching.
- Document other caregivers' responses to teaching.

Notes:

1. Throughout the outline in this book, the stages of the nursing process are referred to as: assessment, analysis/nursing diagnosis, nursing care plan/implementation, evaluation/outcome criteria.

2. The practice questions in this book are coded as to the phase of the nursing process being tested; the codes are found following the answer/rationale for each question. *Key to Nursing Process Codes:*

AS	Assessment
AN	Analysis
PL	Planning
IMP	Implementation
EV	Evaluation

For an **index to questions relating to each phase of the nursing process,** see Appendix F.

Index: Questions Related to Nursing Process

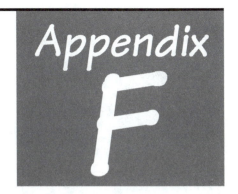

Appendix F

Use this index to locate *practice questions* throughout the book, for each of the five *phases of the nursing process.*

Unit	Assessment (AS) Question #	Analysis (AN) Question #	Planning (PL) Question #	Implementation (IMP) Question #	Evaluation (EV) Question #
1: Models of Psychosocial Nursing Care	3, 15, 16	1, 2, 5, 7, 8, 9, 10, 11, 12, 13	6, 19, 20	4, 17, 18, 22, 23, 24, 25	14, 21
2: Psychosocial Growth and Development— Selected Concepts	6	1, 2, 3	4, 8	7	5, 9
3: Assessment Tools	2, 4, 6, 7, 8	1, 3, 5			
4: Psychosocial Treatment Modes			1, 5, 6, 8, 10, 11, 12, 14, 15	2, 3, 4, 7, 13	9
5: Somatic Treatment Modes	17, 18	4, 8, 16	13, 15, 20	2, 3, 7, 9, 11, 14, 19, 21, 23, 26, 27	1, 5, 6, 10, 12, 22, 24, 25
6: Psychiatric Emergencies	3, 4, 11, 13, 14	2, 7, 8,10	9	1, 5, 12, 16	6, 15
7: Common Disruptive or Problematic Behaviors	9	8, 11, 12	1, 2, 4, 6, 7, 13, 14	5, 10, 15	3
8: Sleep Pattern Disturbances and Eating Disorders	4	1, 5, 6	2	3, 9	7, 8
9: Anxiety and Related Disorders	1, 4	2, 3, 7, 11, 12, 15, 16	5, 8, 10, 13, 14, 17	6, 18	9
10: Conditions in Which Psychological Factors Affect Medical Condition	4, 7, 8	2, 3	1, 5, 6		
11: Schizophrenia and Related Psychotic Disorders	4, 7	2, 5, 10, 12, 14, 18	3, 6, 13, 16, 20	1, 8, 9, 15, 17, 19, 21	11
12: Mood Disorders	3, 4, 6	11	2, 7, 8	9, 10, 12, 14, 15	1, 5, 13
13: Cognitive Disorders	1, 6	3, 5, 7, 8, 9, 17	10, 11, 13	2, 12, 14, 15, 16	4
14: Substance-Related Disorders	1, 3, 6, 11, 13, 17	12, 15	5, 7, 9, 14	2, 10, 16, 19	4, 8, 18
15: Personality Disorders	3, 5, 8, 9, 11	6, 7, 10	2	1	4
16: Special Populations and Concerns	4, 6, 9	3	1, 2, 10	8, 11, 12	5, 7
17: Special Issues		1, 6	4	2, 3, 5	

Index: Questions Related to Categories of Human Functions

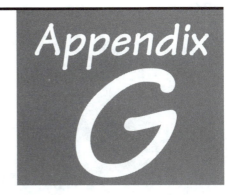

This index lists *practice questions* for you to use in reviewing *categories of human functions* (which are *detailed* examples of what is covered by the four *broad* client needs categories).

The eight categories of human functions include:

Protective Functions client's ability to maintain defenses and prevent physical and chemical trauma, injury, and threats to health status (e.g., communicable diseases, abuse, safety hazards, poisoning, skin disorders, and pre- and post-operative complications).

Sensory-Perceptual Functions client's ability to perceive, interpret, and respond to sensory and cognitive stimuli (e.g., auditory, visual, verbal impairments, brain tumors, aphasia, sensory deprivation or overload, body image, reality orientation, learning disabilities).

Comfort, Rest, Activity, and Mobility Functions client's ability to maintain mobility, desirable level of activity, adequate sleep, rest, and comfort (e.g., pain, sleep disturbances, joint impairment).

Nutrition client's ability to maintain the intake and processing of essential nutrients (e.g., obesity, gastric and metabolic disorders that primarily affect the nutritional status).

Growth and Development client's ability to maintain maturational processes throughout the life span (e.g., child bearing, child rearing, maturational crisis, changes in aging, psychosocial development).

Fluid-Gas Transport Functions client's ability to maintain fluid-gas transport (e.g., fluid volume deficit/overload, acid-base balance, CPR, anemias, cardiopulmonary diseases).

Psychosocial-Cultural Functions client's ability to function (intrapersonal/interpersonal relationships; e.g., grieving, death/dying, psychotic behaviors, self concept, therapeutic communication, ethical-legal aspects, community resources, situational crises, substance abuse).

Elimination Functions client's ability to maintain functions related to relieving the body of waste products (e.g., conditions of GI and/or GU systems).

Unit	Protective Functions (1) Question #	Sensory-Perceptual Functions (2) Question #	Comfort, Rest, Activity, and Mobility Functions (3) Question #	Nutrition (4) Question #	Growth and Development (5) Question #	Fluid-Gas Transport Functions (6) Question #	Psychosocial-Cultural Functions (7) Question #	Elimination Functions (8) Question #
1: Models of Psychosocial Nursing Care	4, 16						1, 2, 3, 5, 6, 7, 8, 9, 10, 11, 12, 13, 14, 15, 17, 18, 19, 20, 21, 22, 23, 24, 25	
2: Psychosocial Growth and Development— Selected Concepts		2			8		1, 3, 4, 5, 6, 7, 9	
3: Assessment Tools		3					1, 2, 4, 5, 6, 7, 8	
4: Psychosocial Treatment Modes		6	4				1, 2, 3, 5, 7, 8, 9, 10, 11, 12, 13, 14, 15	
5: Somatic Treatment Modes	2, 3, 7, 8, 21, 24, 26, 27	1, 13, 18	5, 6, 11, 12, 16, 22	20, 23			4, 9, 14, 17, 19, 25	10, 15
6: Psychiatric Emergencies	1, 3, 6			2		13	4, 5, 7, 8, 9, 10, 11, 12, 14, 15, 16	
7: Common Disruptive or Problematic Behaviors	6	5, 12	2				1, 3, 4, 7, 8, 9, 10, 11, 13, 14, 15	

Chapter							
8: Sleep Pattern Disturbances and Eating Disorders			9	7	2, 6	1, 3, 4, 5, 8	
9: Anxiety and Related Disorders	4, 8			6			1, 2, 3, 5, 7, 9, 10, 11, 12, 13, 14, 15, 16, 17, 18	
10: Conditions in Which Psychological Factors Affect Medical Condition	3			6			1, 2, 4, 5, 8	7
11: Schizophrenia and Related Psychotic Disorders		8		2			1, 3, 4, 5, 6, 7, 9, 10, 11, 12, 13, 14, 15, 16, 17, 18, 19, 20, 21	
12: Mood Disorders	8, 13		9, 14, 15	7, 10, 12			1, 2, 3, 4, 5, 11	6
13: Cognitive Disorders	7	14		10			1, 2, 3, 4, 5, 6, 8, 9, 11, 12, 13, 15, 16, 17	
14: Substance-Related Disorders	5, 10, 16, 18	1, 2, 3, 4	7	14, 15	13		6, 8, 9, 11, 12, 17, 19	
15: Personality Disorders							1, 2, 3, 4, 5, 6, 7, 8, 9, 10, 11	
16: Special Populations and Concerns	8	11	9	12	4		1, 3, 5, 6, 7, 10	2
17: Special Issues	3, 4, 6						1, 2, 5	

Index: Questions Related to Client Needs

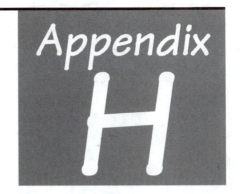

To *practice questions* in each of the four categories of *client needs* that are tested on NCLEX-RN, refer to the questions listed.

Unit	Safe, Effective Care Environment (SECE) Question #	Physiologic Integrity (PhI) Question #	Psychosocial Integrity (PsI) Question #	Health Promotion and Maintenance (HPM) Question #
1: Models of Psychosocial Nursing Care	4		1, 2, 3, 5, 6, 7, 8, 9, 10, 11, 12, 13, 14, 16, 17, 18, 19, 20, 21, 22, 23, 24, 25	15
2: Psychosocial Growth and Development—Selected Concepts			1, 3	2, 4, 5, 6, 7, 8, 9
3: Assessment Tools			1, 2, 3, 4, 5, 6, 7, 8	
4: Psychosocial Treatment Modes	1, 2, 7, 8, 10		3, 5, 6, 9, 11, 12, 13, 14, 15	4
5: Somatic Treatment Modes	4, 7, 21, 27	2, 3, 8	1, 5, 6, 9, 10, 11, 12, 13, 14, 16, 17, 18, 20, 22, 25, 26	15, 19, 23
6: Psychiatric Emergencies	6	2, 3, 13	1, 4, 5, 7, 8, 9, 10, 11, 12, 14, 15, 16	
7: Common Disruptive or Problematic Behaviors	4, 5, 6		1, 2, 3, 7, 8, 9, 10, 11, 12, 13, 14, 15	
8: Sleep Pattern Disturbances and Eating Disorders	9	6, 7	1, 2, 3, 4, 5	8
9: Anxiety and Related Disorders		4	1, 2, 3, 5, 6, 7, 8, 9, 10, 11, 12, 13, 14, 15, 16, 17, 18	
10: Conditions in Which Psychological Factors Affect Medical Condition		3, 6, 7	1, 2, 4, 5, 8	
11: Schizophrenia and Related Psychotic Disorders	4, 8	2	1, 3, 5, 6, 7, 9, 10, 11, 12, 13, 14, 15, 16, 17, 18, 19, 20, 21	
12: Mood Disorders	15	13	1, 2, 3, 4, 5, 6, 7, 8, 10, 11, 12	9, 14
13: Cognitive Disorders	7		1, 2, 3, 4, 5, 6, 8, 9, 10, 11, 12, 13, 14, 15, 16, 17	

14: Substance-Related Disorders	2, 5, 16	1, 3, 4, 7, 10, 13, 15, 18	6, 8, 9, 11, 12, 14, 17, 19	
15: Personality Disorders			1, 2, 3, 4, 5, 6, 7, 8, 9, 10, 11	
16: Special Populations and Concerns	8, 12		1, 2, 3, 5, 6, 7, 9, 10, 11	4
17: Special Issues	2, 3, 4, 5, 6		1	

The four broad categories of client needs include:

Safe, Effective Care Environment *coordinated care, environmental safety, safe* and *effective treatment* and procedures (e.g., client rights, confidentiality, principles of teaching/learning, control of infectious agents).
Physiologic Integrity *physiologic adaptation, reduction of risk potential, provision of basic care* (e.g., drug administration, emergencies, nutritional therapies).
Psychosocial Integrity *psychosocial adaptation; coping*

(e.g., behavioral norms, chemical dependency, communication skills, family systems, mental health concepts, psychodynamics of behavior, psychopathology, treatment modalities).
Health Promotion and Maintenance *normal growth and development* from birth to death, *self-care* and *support systems, prevention* and *early treatment of disease* (e.g., newborn care, normal perinatal care, family planning, human sexuality, parenting, death/dying, life-style choices, immunity).

Anxiety-Coping Mechanisms

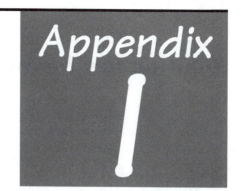

Crossword

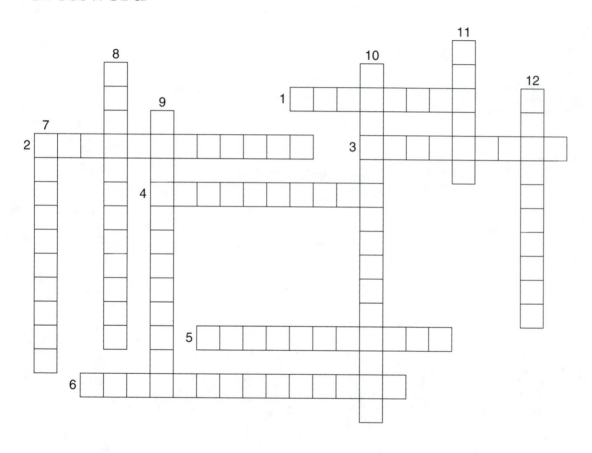

Across

1. A point in the individual's development at which certain aspects of emotional development cease to advance.
2. Anxiety from feelings of inadequacy is relieved by emphasizing a personal or social attribute.
3. A feeling is detached from an event in a person's memory.
4. Painful experiences, thoughts, impulses, and disagreeable memories are forced from consciousness.
5. Energy involved in anxiety-producing impulses is redirected into constructive and socially acceptable channels.
6. Unconsciously taking on desirable attributes found in people for whom one has admiration or affection.

Note: Solution on page 238.

Down

7. The expression of emotional conflicts through a physical symptom for which there is no demonstrable organic basis.
8. The discharge of feelings onto a person or object entirely different from the one to which they actually belong.
9. Incorporating another person to avoid the threat posed by that person or by one's own urges.
10. Attempt to make behavior appear to be a product of logical thinking rather than of unconscious desires.
11. A person truly does not recognize the existence of an event or feeling.
12. Transfers the responsibility for unacceptable ideas, impulses, wishes, and thoughts onto another person.

Solution to Crossword

Across

1. fixation
2. compensation
3. isolation
4. repression
5. sublimation
6. identification

Down

7. conversion
8. displacement
9. introjection
10. rationalization
11. denial
12. projection

Source: Taylor C, et al. *Instructor's Resource Manual and Testbank to Accompany Essentials of Psychiatric Nursing,* 14th ed. St. Louis, MO: Mosby, 1994. P44.

Bibliography

Standards

American Nurses Association. *Code for Nurses.* Washington, DC: American Nurses Publishing, 1985.

American Nurses Association. *Standards of Clinical Nursing Practice.* Washington, DC: American Nurses Publishing, 1991.

American Psychiatric Association. *Diagnostic and Statistical Manual of Mental Disorders* (DSM-IV) (4th ed). Washington, DC: American Psychiatric Association, 1994. A systematic descriptive approach to the classification of mental disorders. Provides specific diagnostic criteria. Each disorder is described in the following areas: essential features, associated features, age at onset, course, impairment, complications, predisposing factors, prevalence, and differential diagnosis.

Creighton H. *Law Every Nurse Should Know.* Philadelphia: Saunders, 1986.

International Council of Nurses. *ICN Code for Nurses: Ethical Concepts Applied to Nursing.* Geneva: International Council of Nurses, 1973.

National Commission for the Study of Nursing and Nursing Education. Summary Report and Recommendations. In J Lysaught (ed), *Action in Nursing: Progress in Professional Purpose.* New York: McGraw-Hill, 1974.

North American Nursing Diagnosis Association. *Nursing Diagnoses: Definitions and Classification for 1995–1996.* Philadelphia: NANDA, 1994.

Classic and Current Suggested Readings

Psychiatric Nursing

Antai-Otong D (ed). *Assessment and Medications for Psychiatric Nursing.* Philadelphia: Saunders, 1995.

Fortinash K, Holoday-Worret P: *Psychiatric Nursing Care Plans* (2nd ed). St. Louis: Mosby, 1995.

Taylor C, et al. *Essentials of Psychiatric Nursing* (14th ed). St. Louis: Mosby, 1994.

Varcarolis EM. *Foundations of Psychiatric Mental Health Nursing* (2nd ed). Philadelphia: Saunders, 1994. A concise yet comprehensive textbook with a variety of visual learning tools. Focuses on teaching skills to attend to psychosocial needs in a variety of settings. Discusses mental health needs regarding violence, substance abuse, and other contemporary issues.

Psychosocial Development

Duvall EM. *Marriage and Family Development.* Philadelphia: Lippincott, 1977.

Erikson E. *Childhood and Society.* New York: Norton, 1963.

Kalish R. *The Psychology of Human Behavior.* Monterey, California: Wadsworth, 1973.

Maslow A. *Motivation and Personality.* New York: Harper & Row, 1970.

Piaget J. *Origins of Intelligence in Children.* New York: Norton, 1963.

Stress and Crisis

Aguilera D. *Crisis Intervention: Theory and Methodology* (7th ed). St. Louis: Mosby, 1994.

Selye H. *Stress Without Distress.* Ontario: New American Library of Canada, 1974.

Index

The Lippincott's NurseNotes Series Disk Instructions

System Requirements
- A PC compatible computer with an Intel 386 or better processor. Windows 3.1 or later.
- 4 Megabytes RAM (minimum); but recommend 8 MB RAM on Windows 3.1.
- 8 Megabytes RAM (minimum); but recommend 12 MB RAM minimum on Windows 95.
- 3 Megabytes of available hard disk space.

Installation
Installing *NurseNotes: Psychiatric-Mental Health* for Windows
1. 'tart up Windows.
2. Insert the *Psychiatric-Mental Health* disk into the floppy disk drive.
3. From the Program Manager's File Menu, choose the Run command.
4. When the Run dialog box appears, type a:\setup (or b:\setup if you're using the B drive) in the Command Line box. Click OK or press the Enter button.
5. The installation process will begin. A dialog proposing the directory "nnpm" on the drive containing Windows will appear. If the name and location are correct, click OK. If you want to change this information, type over the existing data, then click OK.
6. When the *Psychiatric-Mental Health* setup routine is complete, a new group called "Nurse Notes" will appear on your desktop.
7. Start the *Psychiatric-Mental Health* program by double-clicking on its icon.

NurseNotes: Psychiatric-Mental Health disk program
Lippincott's *NurseNotes* Series consists of two modes: Test Mode and Study Mode.

TEST MODE
To begin a test, click the Start Over button with your mouse cursor. As a result, the first question will appear on the screen. If you decide to stop the test before you complete it, your answers will be saved. You can resume the test by selecting the Resume button from the Main Menu screen. You may clear your answers for a test at any time by clicking on the Start Over button.

NurseNotes: Psychiatric-Mental Health—Toolbar
The Toolbar contains a series of buttons that provide direct access to all test program functions. When you move the cursor over a button, an explanation of its function displays in the Status Bar which is immediately above the ToolBar.

From left to right, the Toolbar buttons are:
- Program Help
- Pause
- Mark Question
- Table of Contents
- First Question Arrow
  (go to the first question in the section)
- Prior Question Arrow
  (go to the previous question in the test)
- Next Question Arrow
  (go to the next question in the test)
- Last Question Arrow
  (go to the last question in the section)
- Stop

To get help at any time during the test, choose the Program Help button. Program Help reviews basic functions of the program. To close the Program Help window, click on the Program Help button again. Answer each question by clicking on the oval to the left of an answer selection or by selecting the appropriate letter on the keyboard (A, B, C, or D). When an answer is selected, its oval will darken. If you change your mind about an answer, simply select that choice, by mouse or keyboard, again.

To register your answer selection and proceed to the next question, click on the Next Question Arrow button or press the Enter key.

If you are unsure about an answer to a particular question, the program allows you to mark it for later review. Flag the question by clicking on the Mark Question button. To review all marked questions for a test, click on the Table of Contents button, which is immediately to the right of the Mark button. This will open the Table of Contents window.

The Table of Contents window lists every question included on the test and summarizes whether it has been answered, left unanswered, or marked for later review. Click on an item in the Table of Contents window and the program will move to that test question, or use the Arrow buttons to move to the first, previous, next, or last question. To close the Table of Contents window, click on the Table of Contents button again.

At any time during the test or when you are finished taking the test, click on the Stop button. If you wish, you may return to the session at a later time without erasing your existing answers by selecting the Resume button.

After taking the test, you may receive your score by clicking the Results Button on the Main Menu Screen. There are four different ways to review your results: Test Results, Nursing Process, Category of Human Function, and Client Need.

STUDY MODE
After taking the test and receiving your score, you may wish to enter the Study Mode. This mode supplies you with the test questions, the answers that you chose, and the rationale for correct and incorrect answers. To enter the Study Mode, click the Study Mode button with your mouse cursor. You will not be able to modify the answers you have given; however, you can select any of the answer choices for an explanation of that answer. You may also wish to use the Table of Contents button to show you which questions you marked for review. Each of these windows may be closed by clicking again on their respective buttons.

To exit the *Psychiatric-Mental Health* program, click the Exit button on the Main Menu.